Managing the Menopause

Second Edition

Managing the Menopause

Second Edition

Edited by

Nick Panay
Queen Charlotte's and Chelsea & Chelsea and Westminster Hospitals

Paula Briggs
Liverpool Women's NHS Foundation Trust

Gabor T. Kovacs
Monash University

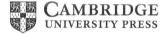

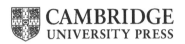

Shaftesbury Road, Cambridge CB2 8EA, United Kingdom

One Liberty Plaza, 20th Floor, New York, NY 10006, USA

477 Williamstown Road, Port Melbourne, VIC 3207, Australia

314–321, 3rd Floor, Plot 3, Splendor Forum, Jasola District Centre, New Delhi – 110025, India

103 Penang Road, #05–06/07, Visioncrest Commercial, Singapore 238467

Cambridge University Press is part of Cambridge University Press & Assessment,
a department of the University of Cambridge.

We share the University's mission to contribute to society through the pursuit of
education, learning and research at the highest international levels of excellence.

www.cambridge.org
Information on this title: www.cambridge.org/9781108798754

DOI: 10.1017/9781108869102

First edition published in 2015
© Cambridge University Press & Assessment 2020

A catalogue record for this publication is available from the British Library

Library of Congress Cataloging-in-Publication data
Names: Panay, Nick, editor. | Briggs, Paula, 1964– editor. | Kovacs, Gabor, 1947 April 6– editor.
Title: Managing the menopause / edited by Nicholas Panay, Paula Briggs, Gabor T. Kovacs.
Description: Second edition. | Cambridge, United Kingdom ; New York, NY : Cambridge University
Press, 2020. | Includes index.
Identifiers: LCCN 2019057539 (print) | LCCN 2019057540 (ebook) | ISBN 9781108798754 (paperback) |
ISBN 9781108869102 (ebook)
Subjects: MESH: Menopause | Estrogen Replacement Therapy | Female Urogenital Diseases |
Osteoporosis, Postmenopausal
Classification: LCC RG186 (print) | LCC RG186 (ebook) | NLM WP 580 | DDC 618.1/75–dc23
LC record available at https://lccn.loc.gov/2019057539
LC ebook record available at https://lccn.loc.gov/2019057540

ISBN   978-1-108-79875-4   Paperback

....

Every effort has been made in preparing this book to provide accurate and up-to-date
information which is in accord with accepted standards and practice at the time of
publication. Although case histories are drawn from actual cases, every effort has been
made to disguise the identities of the individuals involved. Nevertheless, the authors,
editors and publishers can make no warranties that the information contained herein
is totally free from error, not least because clinical standards are constantly changing
through research and regulation. The authors, editors and publishers therefore
disclaim all liability for direct or consequential damages resulting from the use of
material contained in this book. Readers are strongly advised to pay careful attention
to information provided by the manufacturer of any drugs or equipment that they plan
to use.

Contents

Contributors

Panagiotis G. Anagnostis, MD
Diabetes, Endocrinology and Metabolic Medicine, Faculty of Medicine, Imperial College London, St Mary's Campus, London, UK

Richard A. Anderson, MD, PhD, FRCO, FRCP(Ed)
Elsie Inglis Professor of Clinical Reproductive Science, MRC Centre for Reproductive Health, Queen's Medical Research Institute, University of Edinburgh, UK

Paula Briggs, MRCGP, FRCGP, FFSRH
Consultant in Sexual and Reproductive Health, Southport and Ormskirk Hospital NHS Trust, Southport, UK

Mark P. Brincat, MRCP, LRCS, FRCOG, FRCP, PhD
Obstetrician and Gynaecologist; Professor of Obstetrics and Gynaecology, St Clare's Medical Services, Ta' Xbiex, Malta

Jean Calleja-Agius, MD, FRCOG, FRCPI, MSc Clinical Emyology, PhD
Obstetrician and Gynaecologist, Associate Professor and Head of Department of Anatomy, Faculty of Medicine and Surgery, University of Malta, Malta

Marta Caretto, MD
Obstetrics and Gynaecology, Department of Clinical and Experimental Medicine, University of Pisa, Pisa, Italy

Michael C. Craig, PhD, FRCOG, FRCPsych
Female Hormone Clinic, Maudsley Hospital, London; Institute of Psychiatry, Psychology and Neuroscience, Kings College London, London, UK

Susan R. Davis, PhD FRACP
Director, Women's Health Research Program, School of Public Health and Preventive Medicine, Monash University; Consultant Endocrinologist, Cabrini Medical Centre; Head of the Women's Specialist Clinic, Alfred Hospital, Melbourne, Victoria, Australia

Nigel Denby, Registered Dietitian, BSc Hons
Nuffield Hospital, Leeds; Hormone Health, London; Lees Place Medical Centre, London, UK

Marie-Madeleine Dolmans, MD, PhD
Professor. Gynecology Department, Cliniques Universitaires St Luc, Brussels, Belgium. Universite Catholique de Louvain, Belgium

Claudine Domoney, MA, MRCOG
Consultant Obstetrician and Gynaecologist, Chelsea and Westminster Hospital, London, UK

Jacques Donnez, MD, PhD
Professor Emeritus, Universite Catholique de Louvain, Belgium

Svetlana Dragojevic-Dikic, MD, PhD
Faculty of Medicine, University of Belgrade; Gynecology-Obstetrics Clinic Narodni Front, Belgrade, Serbia

Philip J. Dutton, MBChB, MRes (Dist)
King's College School of Medicine, London, UK

John Eden, MD, FRCOG, FRANZCOG
Associate Professor of Reproductive Endocrinology, University of New South Wales; Director, Barbara Cross Research

Unit and Clinical Academic at the Royal Hospital for Women, New South Wales; Director, Women's Health and Research Institute of Australia, Sydney, Australia

Edzard Ernst, MD, PhD, FAcadMedSci, FRCP
Professor Emeritus, University of Exeter, Exeter, UK

Marco Gambacciani, MD
Obstetrics and Gynecology, Department of Clinical and Experimental Medicine, University of Pisa, Pisa, Italy

Andrea R. Genazzani, MD, PhD, HcD, FRCOG
Division of Obstetrics and Gynecology, Department of Clinical and Experimental Medicine, University of Pisa, Pisa, Italy

Andrea Giannini, MD
Obstetrics and Gynecology, Department of Clinical and Experimental Medicine, University of Pisa, Pisa, Italy

Steven R. Goldstein, MD, NCMP, CCD, FACOG, FRCOG(H)
New York University School of Medicine, New York, New York, USA

Anne Gompel, MD, PhD
University Paris Descartes, Paris, France

Sarah Gray, BSC (Hons), MBBS, MRCGP, DRCOG, DFFP, FHEA
GP Specialist in Women's Health, Nuffield Health Hospital, Plymouth, UK

Haitham Hamoda, MD, FRCOG
Consultant Gynaecologist, Kings College London, UK

Tim Hillard, FRCOG
Consultant Obstetrician and Gynaecologist, Poole Hospital NHS Foundation Trust, Poole, UK

Myra S. Hunter, PhD, Cpsychol, AFBPS
Institute of Psychiatry, Psychology and Neuroscience, King's College London, London, UK

Miomira Ivovic, MD, PhD
Faculty of Medicine, University of Belgrade, Clinic of Endocrinology, Diabetes and Diseases of Metabolism, Clinical Center of Serbia, Belgrade, Serbia

Nicola Kersey, MBchB
Southport and Ormskirk Hospital NHS Trust, SRH Mersey Deanery Trainee, Southport, UK

Gab Kovacs, MD, FRANZCOG, FRCOG
Professor of Obstetrics and Gynaecology, Monash University, Melbourne, Victoria, Australia

E. Anne MacGregor, MSc, MD, FFSRH, DIPM, MICR
Centre for Neuroscience and Trauma, Barts and the London School of Medicine and Dentistry; Centre for Reproductive Medicine, St Bartholomew's Hospital, London, UK

Ljiljana V. Marina, MD
Faculty of Medicine, University of Belgrade, Clinic of Endocrinology, Diabetes and Diseases of Metabolism, Clinical Center of Serbia, Belgrade, Serbia

Magdalena Montt Guevara, PhD
Obstetrics and Gynecology, Department of Clinical and Experimental Medicine, University of Pisa, Pisa, Italy

Rossella E. Nappi, MD, PhD, MBA
Research Center for Reproductive Medicine, Gynecological Endocrinology and Menopause, IRCCS S. Matteo Foundation, Department of Clinical, Surgical, Diagnostic and Paediatric Sciences, University of Pavia, Pavia, Italy

Nicholas Panay, BSc, FRCOG, MFSRH
Consultant Gynecologist, Specialist in
Reproductive Medicine, Queen Charlotte's
and Chelsea & Chelsea and Westminster
Hospitals; Honorary Senior Lecturer,
Imperial College London; Director,
International Centre for Hormone Health,
London, UK

Paul Posadzki, PhD, MSc
Researcher in Alcohol Synthesis, The
Centre for Public Health, Liverpool John
Moores University, Liverpool; Honorary
Research Fellow, Plymouth University
Peninsula Schools of Medicine and
Dentistry, Plymouth, UK

Eleonora Russo, PhD
Obstetrics and Gynecology, Department of
Clinical and Experimental Medicine,
University of Pisa, Pisa, Italy

Anthony J. Rutherford, FRCOG
Honorary Senior Lecturer, University of
Leeds; Consultant in Reproductive
Medicine and Gynaecological Surgery,
Leeds Teaching Hospitals NHS Trust,
Leeds, UK

**Janice M. Rymer, MD, FRCOG,
FRANZCOG, FHEA, MRCOG**
King's College School of Medicine,
London, UK

Jenifer Sassarini, MBChB
Clinical Lecturer, Obstetrics and
Gynaecology, University of Glasgow, UK

Johannes J. Sidelmann, PhD
Unit for Thrombosis Research, Institute of
Regional Health Research, Faculty of
Health Science, University of Southern
Denmark and Department of Clinical

Biochemistry, Hospital of Southwest
Denmark, Esbjerg, Denmark

Tommaso Simoncini, MD, PhD
Obstetrics and Gynecology, Department of
Clinical and Experimental Medicine,
University of Pisa, Pisa, Italy

Sven O. Skouby, MD, DMSci
Endocrinological and Reproductive
Unit, Department of Obstetrics and
Gynecology, Herlev/Gentofte Hospital,
Faculty of Health and Medical Sciences,
University of Copenhagen, Copenhagen,
Denmark

Elizabeth Stephenson, MD
Obstetrician and Gynaecologist, Poole
Hospital NHS Foundation Trust,
Poole, UK

John C. Stevenson, FRCP
Consultant Metabolic Physician and
Reader, National Heart and Lung Institute,
Imperial College London, Royal Brompton
Hospital, London, UK

Vujovic Svetlana, MD, PhD
Faculty of Medicine, University of
Belgrade; Clinic of Endocrinology,
Diabetes and Diseases of Metabolism,
Clinical Center of Serbia, Belgrade, Serbia

Milina Tančić-Gajić, MD
Faculty of Medicine, University of
Belgrade; Clinic of Endocrinology,
Diabetes and Diseases of Metabolism,
Clinical Center of Serbia, Belgrade, Serbia

Kugajeevan Vigneswaran, MRCOG
Clinical Research Fellow, King's College
Hospital NHS Foundation Trust,
London, UK

Foreword

In 1971, a general practitioner with a major interest in the management of menopausal symptoms, the late Dr Jean Hailes, approached the late Professor Bryan Hudson and me for advice as to how to introduce menopausal hormone therapy (MHT), largely unknown at the time in Australia. She had received no encouragement from senior gynaecologists. In my capacity as head of the Endocrinology Clinic at the former Prince Henry's Hospital, I organized a working space for her at the Clinic, where she saw a small number of patients each week. She then gave an interview regarding therapeutic possibilities for menopausal symptoms to one of Melbourne's daily newspapers, the *Age*, which was immediately followed by a deluge of bookings to see her. In order to be able to respond, I arranged with the Hospital authorities to establish a separate Menopause Clinic for which she was responsible and to which she invited a number of her colleagues as co-staff. At her request, I acted in an advisory role, and Jean initiated a number of research projects, including a controlled study of the efficacy of currently available MHT, and several studies of the use of testosterone in women with low libido. She was a true pioneer, and the Menopause Clinic was the third established globally, preceded only by Wulf Utian's Clinic in South Africa and the clinic established by one of his colleagues, Morris Notelowitz, after his move to the US.

In the early 1980s, our research at Prince Henry's and Monash University had successfully isolated the gonadal hormone inhibin, and we began studies of its role in the menopausal transition and menopause, in collaboration with Lorraine Dennerstein and David Robertson. A number of important research papers on the hormonal changes in women as they experienced menopause resulted, published in leading endocrine journals such as the *Journal of Clinical Endocrinology and Metabolism*.

In 1980–1, I spent a six-month sabbatical at the Human Reproduction Program at WHO in Geneva, taking on the role of Rapporteur for a Scientific Group on Research on the Menopause. Our report was published by the World Health Organization in 1981 and was a comprehensive survey of current knowledge and needs for future research. It proved to be a valuable reference source. It is noteworthy that the main controversies highlighted in the report concerned whether MHT caused breast cancer and whether it decreased cardiovascular risk, issues which are still controversial in contemporary practice.

Henry Burger, AO, MD, FRACP, FAA
Emeritus Director of the Hudson Institute of Medical Research and Past President
of the International and Australasian Menopause Societies

Chapter

1

Physiology of the Menstrual Cycle and Changes in the Perimenopause

Philip J. Dutton and Janice M. Rymer

The menopause marks the permanent cessation of menstruation and heralds the transition in a woman's life from a reproductive state to a non-reproductive one. Whilst the average age of this landmark varies slightly across the world, the menopause generally occurs in the early fifties and is only truly affected by factors such as smoking and medical and surgical induction of the menopausal state. However, clinical symptoms may precede this, and the physiological changes which occur with the menopausal transition may begin several years prior to the onset of any manifestations. The basis of the clinical and biochemical changes associated with the perimenopausal period is the depletion of ovarian follicles to a critical level.

Although the physiology of the normal menstrual cycle has been studied extensively, an understanding of the physiological changes of the menopause and their relationship to menopausal symptoms has only begun to make significant advances in the last 2 decades. The development of a validated staging system has been immensely beneficial in standardizing nomenclature surrounding the menopause as well as characterizing the changes at each stage in the transition. Despite these developments, there remain considerable gaps in the literature which require further investigation [1–11]. This chapter outlines current knowledge surrounding the staging and physiology of reproductive aging and its relationship to the troublesome symptoms experienced by the majority of women at this challenging stage of their lives. Before discussing this, however, it is important to have a firm grasp of the concepts surrounding the normal menstrual cycle.

Premenopausal Hormonal Regulation of Ovarian Function

The menstrual cycle is controlled by the hypothalamic–pituitary–ovarian axis, which, apart from its mid-cycle gonadotropin surge, acts as a negative feedback system, whereby peptide gonadotropins stimulate steroid hormone production in the ovaries, which in turn inhibits gonadotropin secretion, thus allowing cycles to occur [1–3].

The hypothalamus secretes gonadotropin-releasing hormone (GnRH). This acts on the pituitary gland in a pulsatile manner, which leads to the secretion of the gonadotropins follicle-stimulating hormone (FSH) and luteinizing hormone (LH) [1, 2]. It is the frequency and amplitude of these pulses which determine the quantity of each hormone ultimately secreted. Slower frequencies appear to precipitate FSH secretion, whereas LH secretion has a predilection for higher frequencies of GnRH stimulation [2].

At the start of the menstrual cycle, the ovary contains several antral follicles. These follicles consist of an oocyte separated from a fluid-filled sac called the antrum, both of which are surrounded by a layer of granulosa cells (cumulus cells and mural cells). These cells are surrounded by a basal membrane, around which lies another layer of theca cells. Theca cells develop LH receptors if they are part of the dominant follicle and produce androgens (progesterone or testosterone) from cholesterol. Conversely, granulosa cells have FSH receptors; androgens are absorbed by these cells and aromatized to estradiol (E2). Granulosa cells also produce the glycoprotein hormone inhibin, which includes two isoforms, A and B [1, 2].

In the late luteal phase (prior to menstruation) and the early follicular phase, levels of circulating FSH rise. This in turn stimulates follicular development and leads to selection of a dominant follicle. Whilst it is not known exactly how a dominant follicle is selected, it is thought that through varying follicular sensitivity, the most sensitive follicle goes on to mature, whilst the other follicles undergo atresia (degeneration). With its development, the dominant follicle secretes increasing levels of E2; this acts on the endometrium to stimulate proliferation. At the hypothalamus and pituitary gland, rising levels of E2 and inhibin B act to reduce FSH secretion through a negative feedback mechanism [1–3].

During the early and mid-follicular phases, E2 also exerts negative feedback on LH secretion, which ensures basal levels during this period. However, about 36 hours prior to ovulation (i.e. in the late follicular phase), E2 reaches levels in the circulation which switch this negative feedback effect to a positive feedback effect. This leads to a surge in LH (which is accompanied by a smaller surge in FSH) over a 24-hour period in the 24 hours prior to ovulation. This LH surge leads to rupture of the dominant follicular wall and release of the oocyte [2, 3].

Following ovulation, there is an abrupt fall in E2 production from the ruptured follicle. The follicle undergoes a series of changes which convert it into an endocrine structure called the corpus luteum ('yellow body'). This produces E2 and progesterone, which act on the endometrium to promote implantation. LH maintains the corpus luteum in the week following ovulation, but if pregnancy does not occur, then this begins to degenerate, leading to a gradual reduction in the production of steroid hormones. With falling E2 and progesterone levels, the loss of negative feedback leads to a subsequent rise in FSH, heralding the start of a new menstrual cycle. A summary of these processes is shown in Figure 1.1 [1, 2].

Definitions and Staging in Reproductive Aging

In order to understand the context in which the physiological changes of the menopausal transition are happening, it is necessary to consider the definitions and stages associated with reproductive aging.

The premenopause is typically defined as the phase of a woman's life from the menarche (onset of menstruation) until the beginning of the perimenopausal stage. The perimenopause comprises the time from a woman's mature reproductive state at the point when she begins to experience variability in the length of her cycle or characteristic symptoms of the menopausal transition to the year following her final menstrual period (FMP). It is only following this 12-month period of amenorrhea that a diagnosis of *menopause* can be made. The term *menopausal transition* also refers to the time when a woman's cycle changes or she experiences clinical symptoms, but ends with the FMP. The terms *menopause* and *postmenopause* are often used interchangeably to describe the phase of a woman's life from the FMP [1–11].

Menstrual cycle regulation

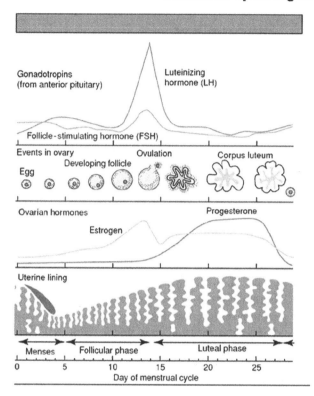

1. Hypothalamus releases GnRH, stimulating the pituitary

2. FSH secreted from pituitary stimulates follicle

3. Follicles produce estrogen-negative feedback, turning off FSH release

4. Critical level of E_2 stimulates LH peak-positive feedback ovulation

5. Corpus luteum secretes E_2 and P_4, lifespan 12–14 days

Figure 1.1 Endocrine changes during the menstrual cycle.

In 2001, the Stages of Reproductive Ageing Workshop (STRAW) met to propose criteria for defining the stages of reproductive life. They generated a staging system which provided guidance on ovarian aging in women. Prior to this, there was no generally accepted staging system. The aim of this was to improve research in women transitioning from a reproductive to a non-reproductive state by standardizing nomenclature and outlining the characteristic changes of each stage to aid consistency across studies. In a clinical context, the STRAW staging system provides health care providers and women with a guide to assessing fertility and contraceptive requirements. In 2006, the ReSTAGE collaboration assessed the validity and reliability of STRAW's criteria and made several recommendations. Ten years later, this collaboration and a greater understanding of ovarian aging have led to a revision of the STRAW staging system. The STRAW + 10 staging system is shown in Tables 1.1 and 1.2 [4].

The STRAW + 10 staging system is divided into three phases: the reproductive phase, the menopausal transition and the postmenopausal phase. The reproductive phase is subdivided into three stages (−5 to −3). The early reproductive stage (−5) refers to the period immediately following the menarche, before menstrual cycles become regular. During the peak reproductive stage (−4), menstrual cycles are regular. The late reproductive stage (−3) marks the time when fertility begins to go into decline and is

Table 1.1 The reproductive phase as outlined in the STRAW + 10 classification

Stage	−5	−4	−3b	−3a
Terminology	Reproductive phase			
	Early	Peak		Late
Duration		Variable		
Menstrual cycle	Variable to regular	Regular	Regular	Subtle changes in cycle length/flow
FSH			Normal	Variable[a]
AMH			Low	Low
Inhibin B			Low	Low
AFC (2–10 mm)			Low	Low

Note. FSH = follicle-stimulating hormone; AMH = anti-Müllerian hormone; AFC = antral follicle count.
[a] Based on blood samples taken at days 2–5 of cycle.

subdivided into two stages. During stage −3b, menstrual cycles are regular, but anti-Müllerian hormone (AMH) levels continue to fall (a process which starts from the menarche) as a result of a gradual depletion in the antral follicle count (AFC) [1, 4, 6]. Stage −3a is characterized by subtle changes in menstrual cycle length and flow. Cycles tend to become shorter and periods heavier [1, 3, 7]. FSH levels rise with increasing variability, whilst AFC, AMH and inhibin B are low [4].

From the onset of the early menopausal transition, also known as the perimenopause (−2), cycle variability increases with a persistent difference of 7 days or more in the length of consecutive cycles. Anatomical and biochemical changes are similar to those of stage −3a, but with increasing variability in FSH levels. The late menopausal transition (−1) is characterized by an interval of amenorrhea lasting at least 60 days [4]. There is an increased prevalence of anovulation and further variability in cycle length and hormonal levels [4, 7, 8]. Indeed, during this stage, FSH levels are typically defined as being greater than 25 IU/L and are often associated with high E2 levels. However, E2 does start to fall [3, 4, 6, 8]. This stage is expected to last between 1 and 3 years, and it is during this time that menopausal symptoms, and in particular vasomotor symptoms (VMS), usually arise [4].

The late menopausal transition concludes with the final menstrual period (FMP) (0) and gives way to the postmenopausal phase (+1 to +2). Stage +1 is defined as the early postmenopausal stage and is subdivided into three stages. Stage +1a lasts 1 year following the FMP, and the end of this stage is defined as the menopause (a period of amenorrhea lasting 12 months). The end of this stage marks the end of the perimenopause, and 1 year into the postmenopausal phase, although this diagnosis can only be made retrospectively [4]. During stages +1a and +1b (which also lasts 1 year), FSH levels continue to rise, whilst E2 levels continue to fall [3, 4, 6, 8]. Thereafter, stabilization of these hormones occurs. Menopausal symptoms, and particularly VMS, are most likely to occur during these stages. Stage +1c marks a period of stabilization in levels of FSH and E2 which lasts between 3 and 6 years. The late postmenopausal stage (+2) lasts for the remaining

Table 1.2 The menopausal transition and postmenopausal phase as outlined in the STRAW + 10 classification

Stage	-2	-1	0	+1a	+1b	+1c	+2
Terminology	**Menopausal transition**		**FMP**	**Postmenopausal phase**			
	Early	Late			Early		Late
		Perimenopause					
Duration	Variable	1–3 years		2 years (1+1)		3–6 years	Remainder of life
Menstrual cycle	Persistent ≥7 day difference in length of consecutive cycles	Interval of amenorrhea of ≥60 days					
FSH	↑ variable[1]	↑>25 IU/L[b]		↑ variable[a]		Stabilizes	
AMH	Low	Low		Low		Very low	
Inhibin B	Low	Low		Low		Very low	
AFC	Low	Low		Very low		Very low	
Symptoms		Vasomotor symptoms likely		Vasomotor symptoms most likely			Increasing urogenital symptoms

Note. FSH = follicle-stimulating hormone; AMH = anti-Müllerian hormone; AFC = antral follicle count; ↑ = elevated.
a Based on blood samples taken at days 2–5 of cycle.
b Based on assays using current international pituitary standard.

lifespan of a woman, during which FSH levels tend to fall gradually. Generalized somatic aging processes rather than reproductive aging characterize this period. The prevalence of urogenital symptoms increases at this time [4].

Whilst the STRAW + 10 system is regarded as the gold standard of reproductive aging given its broad applicability to women regardless of age, ethnicity, BMI and smoking status, there remain three key areas where the model cannot be applied. The first is women who are either using hormonal contraception, have had endometrial ablation or have had a hysterectomy. In these instances we must rely on hormonal and clinical criteria alone. The second is women with polycystic ovarian syndrome (PCOS), who have oligomenorrhea as well as a higher AFC and AMH. The final example is those with chronic illness, such as those undergoing chemotherapy for cancer or those living with HIV [4, 10].

Physiological Changes in the Menopausal Transition

At the root of the physiological changes taking place in the menopausal transition is a gradual reduction in the number and quality of ovarian follicles to critical levels [1–11]. During fetal development, oocyte production occurs until approximately 20 weeks of gestation, at which levels reach between 6 million and 7 million [1, 2]. Thereafter, there is no further oocyte production, and levels begin to decline through a combination of follicular atresia and oocyte release. Fewer than 100 follicles remain in each ovary at the onset of the perimenopause [1, 2, 7, 8, 11]. In addition, the oocyte and its surrounding layer of granulosa cells are thought to become increasingly incompetent with age [2, 3].

With the declining antral follicle count in the late reproductive stage and early menopausal transition, there is a reduced amount of inhibin B production by the granulosa cells. As discussed earlier, inhibin B normally acts on the pituitary gland in a negative feedback mechanism to reduce rising levels of FSH. Lower levels of inhibin B fail to keep this mechanism in check, which leads to higher levels of FSH during the early follicular phase [3, 7–9].

This in turn leads to increased activity of a single dominant follicle, or the recruitment of multiple dominant follicles, and thus higher levels of E2 production [1, 7]. As E2 levels rise to a critical level at an earlier stage, the LH surge occurs earlier and the follicular phase is shortened, which in turn reduces the overall cycle length [1, 3]. It should be noted that the luteal phase does not change in duration until later in the transition [1]. This shortened menstrual cycle length does not occur in all women entering the perimenopause.

As women move into the late menopausal transition, menstrual cycles become progressively longer in duration. The proportion of cycles which are anovulatory also increases. This may be due to a variety of reasons. Concerning the hypothalamic–pituitary–ovarian axis, there appears to be progressive deregulation of positive and negative feedback mechanisms. Indeed, high levels of E2, which would normally elicit an LH surge during the middle of the cycle, have been found to fail in this, whilst a fall in E2 in the luteal phase has failed to lower levels of circulating LH. Thus there may be an element of hypothalamic or pituitary insensitivity. In the ovary, response to FSH may be reduced. In about one-third of women in the menopausal transition, there is higher luteal phase E2, leading to a very early second ovulation. This is called a luteal-out-of-phase (LOOP) event. Whilst data are sparse, progesterone levels appear to fall steadily throughout the menopausal transition. This may be in part due to reduced progesterone production by the corpus luteum as well as an increase in the frequency of anovulatory cycles [3, 5, 7, 8].

Levels of E2 only appear to fall in the 2 years preceding the FMP (this has been noted in prolonged ovulatory cycles), whilst levels of FSH continue to rise [3, 6, 8]. Only following the 12-month period of amenorrhea which is defined as the menopause are E2 levels persistently low [1, 7]. In postmenopausal women, it is estrone (E1) which predominates in the circulation. This is generated through the aromatization of androgens (secreted by the adrenal glands and postmenopausal ovaries) predominantly in the adipose tissue, but also the ovaries and other extragonadal sites [1].

In the early years after the FMP, levels of FSH are 15-fold higher, and levels of LH are 10-fold higher. This is in part due to low levels of inhibitory ovarian hormone production but also to a longer half-life of FSH and LH following alterations in isoform composition in the absence of E2. However, following the menopause, these levels fall slowly due to reduced GnRH pulse frequency and age-related changes in the pituitary reducing GnRH response [11].

Whilst there is little change in circulating testosterone concentrations across the transition, levels of sex hormone binding globulin fall, leading to an increased proportion of free testosterone. Yet following the menopause, testosterone production decreases by 25 per cent [3, 9].

Anti-Müllerian hormone is a glycoprotein produced by primary, preantral and antral follicles which differs from the other hormones of the menstrual cycle, as it does not appear to be directly involved in feedback mechanisms (gonadotropin independent). Interestingly, the number of antral follicles appears to reflect the size of the primordial pool [2, 7]. Thus, its levels are high at the menarche and decline thereafter [1, 7]. It is for this reason that AMH is of interest as a potential biomarker of reproductive aging and fecundity [2, 6–8]. However, in order to be used in this context, it would require further validation, as well as the development of more sensitive assays, as it is almost undetectable in the 5 years preceding the menopause [6]. This is discussed in more detail in Chapter 3.

Menopausal Symptoms

The menopausal transition and postmenopausal period are characterized by a broad range of physical and psychological symptoms, which can prove extremely debilitating to women undergoing the physiological changes of this period. Physical symptoms comprise vasomotor symptoms, urogenital symptoms, headaches, palpitations, breast tenderness, menorrhagia, musculoskeletal pain, restless leg syndrome, sleep disturbance and fatigue. Psychological symptoms include depression, irritability, poor concentration and memory loss. Sexual dysfunction appears to have somatic and psychogenic origins. Of these symptoms, vasomotor and urogenital symptoms appear to have the most profound effect on quality of life, and it is for these symptoms that women generally seek medical assistance [1, 5, 7, 9].

Physical Symptoms

Vasomotor Symptoms

Vasomotor symptoms are the most common manifestation of the menopausal transition and postmenopausal period, occurring in approximately three-quarters of women, and present as either hot flashes or night sweats. According to the STRAW + 10 staging system, VMS generally arise in the late menopausal transition and are worst in the early postmenopausal period, and whilst symptoms generally last up to 5 years after the FMP, they can last as long as 15 years [1, 4, 9].

The exact physiology of VMS is not fully understood, but it is thought that the central thermoregulatory zone (where a person can maintain their body temperature without vasodilatation or sweating) becomes narrowed towards the end of the menopausal transition, so that vasodilatation and sweating are triggered at a lower temperature. This is supported by findings of VMS in those with pituitary insufficiency and following hypophysectomy (removal of the pituitary gland). There appears to be an association with low E2. Indeed, the increased prevalence of symptoms in the late menopausal transition and early postmenopausal period when E2 levels are falling, and the improvement of these symptoms with estrogen therapy, provides support to this notion. Supplementary progestogens have also been shown to have a beneficial effect on VMS [1, 5, 9].

A hot flash or night sweat is typically characterized by vasodilatation and sweating of the head, neck and chest. Other cardiovascular changes include an increase in heart rate and baseline electrocardiographic changes. Whilst the skin temperature rises by several degrees Celsius, the core body temperature appears to fall. They can be triggered by high temperatures, stress and hot food and drink. Symptoms generally last up to 5 min but can last up to an hour, and several episodes occur each day [1, 9]. There also appears to be a predilection for night-time symptoms, which in turn leads to insomnia and psychological symptoms including depression, irritability, poor concentration and memory loss [1, 5, 7, 9].

Several factors affect the frequency and severity of VMS. African American women experience VMS more frequently than their white counterparts. Women who have undergone a sudden-onset medically or surgically induced menopause experience significantly worse symptoms than those who have undergone a natural menopause [1, 9]. VMS symptoms are also discussed in Chapter 2.

Urogenital Symptoms

Whilst VMS occur in the late menopausal transition and early postmenopausal period, as outlined in the STRAW + 10 staging system, urogenital symptoms appear to be a predominating issue in the late postmenopause and worsen in severity over time. Approximately 50 per cent of women are affected. These symptoms are now collectively referred to as genitourinary syndrome of the menopause (GSM). At the root of this are estrogen and progesterone receptors which line the urogenital tract. With deficiencies in E2 and progesterone, a number of physiological changes take place [1, 4, 5].

In the vaginal tract, a loss of elasticity leads to shortening and narrowing. There is a reduction in epithelial cover, lubrication, musculature and vascularity. The vaginal rugae are lost. The vulva and vagina become paler, and there is a reduction in pubic hair as well as an increase in adiposity. Symptoms that arise from these changes include dryness, irritation, dyspareunia and traumatic bleeding. Moreover, fewer acid-producing bacilli in the vaginal tract make the pH more alkaline (>5) in postmenopausal women, and this can lead to a heightened susceptibility to infections. In the urological tract, the onset of the postmenopausal period can lead to urinary frequency, urgency, nocturia and incontinence. Women are also at an increased risk of urinary tract infections [1, 5]. Pelvic organ prolapse is also a predominating feature of the postmenopausal period. These symptoms are discussed in more detail in Chapters 4, 6 and 7.

Other Physical Symptoms

Little is known about the physiological mechanisms which give rise to other physical symptoms characteristic of the menopausal transition. Concerning headaches, migraines can be a problematic feature of the perimenopause; this may be due to fluctuating E2 levels. Palpitations are a common occurrence in perimenopausal women, and are thought to be related to increased sympathetic activity. During the early menopausal transition, women commonly report breast tenderness, although symptom frequency and severity falls with advancing age. High levels of exogenous estrogen or progestogen have both been found to induce breast tenderness [1]. With progressive ovarian follicular depletion and an increase in anovulatory cycles, women often report menorrhagia. This is thought to result from high E2 levels, although progesterone deficiency may also play a contributing factor [1, 7]. Back pain and joint stiffness are common debilitating features of the perimenopausal period [1]. Many women also report sleep disturbance. This can be attributed to physical symptoms including VMS and restless leg syndrome, but it may also be the result of psychological symptoms and external factors. Disturbed sleep patterns can lead to weakness and tiredness [1, 9].

Psychological Symptoms

Psychological symptoms are a common feature of the menopausal transition and include depression, irritability, poor concentration and memory loss. Estrogen, progesterone and testosterone receptors have all been located in several brain centres, whilst estrogen has been shown to have an effect on several neurotransmitters, so it is possible that changes in these hormones may influence psychological symptoms [1]. To date, there is limited evidence that the endocrine changes of the perimenopausal period are responsible for these symptoms, and external factors may play a significant role [1, 9]. Despite this, hormone replacement therapy (HRT) does appear to improve symptoms of depression in the menopausal transition [1]. This is discussed in more detail in Chapters 8 and 9.

Sexuality

Ascertaining the cause of changes in sexuality during the menopausal transition and postmenopause is extremely challenging due to the complex interplay of physical and psychological factors. Many women report a loss of libido, as well as changes in sensitivity during this period. This may be directly due to hormone deficiency. Complications associated with aging may play a role; with advancing age, people are increasingly prone to chronic disease processes which may impede their ability to have sexual intercourse, and they may be on medications which may adversely affect their libido. Women can also experience a change in self-image at the time of the menopausal transition; the loss of reproductive capacity, age-related changes and surgical processes such as mastectomies may affect a woman's confidence. Most likely, a combination of these factors attributes to an increased prevalence of diminished sexual activity in the menopausal transition and postmenopausal phase [1]. Further information on this can be found in Chapter 10.

Other Physiological Consequences of the Menopausal Transition

Metabolic Syndrome and Cardiovascular Disease

Presently, the effect of the menopausal transition on a woman's risk of subsequent metabolic syndrome and cardiovascular disease (CVD) is not fully understood. Postmenopausal women have a significantly increased risk of metabolic syndrome, which is defined as a group of clinical disorders including hypertension, insulin resistance, glucose intolerance, dyslipidemia and obesity. Premenopausal women rarely have CVD, but its incidence is equal across the sexes by the eighth decade [7, 9].

It is known that estrogen can impact on blood pressure, lipid metabolism and insulin action. Concerning blood pressure, estrogen is a potent vasodilator which downregulates the renin angiotensin system and prevents angiotensin II formation (a potent vasoconstrictor), and activates endothelial nitric oxide synthase. With falling estrogen levels following the menopausal transition, these protective mechanisms are lost [7, 9]. Further information can be found in Chapter 15.

Weight gain is a common feature of the menopause. Estrogen deficiency appears to be associated with weight gain, whilst treatment with estrogen therapy can reduce the degree of weight gain or lead to weight loss. With the menopausal transition, the distribution of fat also appears to change. This can in part be explained by estrogen, which has a predilection to promote gluteofemoral adipose tissue accumulation. With the loss of estrogen at the time of the menopause, women start to store their fat abdominally, and this can lead to increased insulin resistance [7, 9].

Loss of Bone Mineral Density

Although osteoporosis and increased fracture risk are common features in postmenopausal women, it appears that rapid bone loss occurs during the menopausal transition through uncoupling of bone remodelling which leads to excess bone resorption. This in turn appears to result from a downward swing in estrogen levels [7]. Indeed, estrogen therapy leads to an improvement in bone mass and a reduction in the risk of vertebral and hip fractures, whilst its cessation causes a reversal of these changes [9]. Falling progesterone levels appear to reduce the rate of bone formation [7]. This is discussed in more detail in Chapter 14.

Breast and Endometrial Cancer

The menopausal transition has been identified as a time of increased risk for the development of both breast and endometrial cancer. Indeed, perimenopausal women (in their forties) are more likely to develop breast cancer than their menopausal counterparts (in their fifties). In this period, higher levels of endogenous E2 and lower levels of progesterone are a common finding [7].

Conclusion

In this chapter, we have provided grounding in the physiology of the normal menstrual cycle, and its dynamic changes through the late reproductive stage, menopausal transition and the postmenopausal period. The STRAW + 10 staging system provides an excellent means of defining and characterizing these changes, and with more research, these stages can be delineated further. Whilst the nature of menopausal symptoms and complications is well understood, the processes which give rise to these changes still require extensive study.

References

1. Bruce D, Rymer J. Symptoms of the menopause. *Best Pract Res Clin Obstet Gynaecol* 2009;23:25–32.

2. Devoto L, Palomino A, Céspedes P, Kohen P. Neuroendocrinology and ovarian aging. *Gynecol Endocrinol* 2012;28 Suppl 1:14–17.

3. Butler L, Santoro N. The reproductive endocrinology of the menopausal transition. *Steroids* 2011;76:627–35.

4. Harlow SD, Gass M, Hall JE, et al. Executive summary of the Stages of Reproductive Aging Workshop + 10: addressing the unfinished agenda of staging reproductive aging. *J Clin Endocrinol Metab* 2012;97:1159–68.

5. Takahashi TA, Johnson KM. Menopause. *Med Clin North Am* 2015;99:521–34.

6. Su HI, Freeman EW. Hormonal changes associated with the menopausal transition. *Minerva Ginecol* 2009;61:483–9.

7. Prior JC, Hitchcock CL. The endocrinology of perimenopause: need for a paradigm shift. *Front Biosci (Schol Ed)* 2011;3:474–86.

8. Burger HG, Hale GE, Robertson DM, Dennerstein L. A review of hormonal changes during the menopausal transition: focus on findings from the Melbourne Women's Midlife Health Project. *Hum Reprod Update* 2007;13:559–65.

9. Edwards BJ, Li J. Endocrinology of menopause. *Peridontol 2000* 2013;61:177–94.

10. Harlow SD. Menstrual cycle changes as women approach the final menses: what matters? *Obstet Gynecol Clin North Am* 2018;45:599–611.

11. Hall JE. Endocrinology of the menopause. *Endocrinol Metab Clin North Am* 2015;44:485–96.

Chapter 2

Clinical Features of the Menopause/Postmenopause

Gab Kovacs

Before considering the various symptoms potentially attributable to the 'menopause', let us define the terminology.

Whilst 'menopause' means the 'end of menstruation', 'menopausal symptoms' refer to a number of different symptoms associated with the climacteric, the transition from mature reproductive function, through the perimenopause to no ovarian follicular function. The hormonal changes leading up to this stage commence several years earlier, and this period is called the 'perimenopause' or 'menopausal transition'.

Postmenopause is the period a woman enters once she has not menstruated for at least 12 months. The symptoms, which then persist for life, are due to the ovary not producing estrogen any longer, and thus reflect a permanent hormone deficiency syndrome, that of hypoestrogenism.

The physiological basis of these changes relates to the changes in a woman's ability to regularly ovulate (Chapter 1). Normal ovulation is the culmination of a complex interaction between the various elements of the hypothalamo–pituitary–ovarian axis. Loss of regulation of these complex hormonal changes results in the loss of a predictable cycle at this time and is associated with widely fluctuating levels of estrogen and the development of menopausal symptoms.

Before the menopausal transition, estrogen and progesterone circulate throughout the body, and have many different effects on various systems, some of which we do not necessarily understand as yet. The development of the Graafian follicles with maturation of the oocyte, ovulation and then subsequent formation of the corpus luteum is a complex process. Should any component of the menstrual cycle not function properly, there will be changing levels of circulating hormones, which can have deleterious effects.

A woman has about 400 000 potential oocytes in the ovary at menarche, and she loses these at a rate of about 1000 per month. This is not influenced by taking the combined oral contraceptive pill, which, although it inhibits ovulation, does not spare oocytes. It is well recognized that with aging, there are less and less potential oocytes, and less effective ovulation. Therefore, frequently ovulatory cycles have a deficient corpus luteum function, with lower levels and/or a shortened period of progesterone secretion, and many cycles are anovulatory with no progesterone secreted at all. The consequent imbalance in estrogen and progesterone is thought to be responsible for some of the symptoms during the perimenopause, especially those associated with menstrual problems. Once a woman becomes postmenopausal, ovarian function ceases completely, and the symptoms of the postmenopause relate to an estrogen deficiency syndrome. This chapter focuses on the menopausal transition, also known as the climacteric.

As these symptoms and signs are usually reported as a continuum, we usually consider them together, and classify them into several types:

1. Vasomotor: these include 'hot flushes', palpitations, night sweats and altered sleep pattern and fatigue.
2. Neuromuscular: these include headaches and joint and muscle pain. Other degenerative changes may occur such as hair and skin changes, which can include a crawling sensation (formication) and itchy skin.
3. Psychogenic: these include poor concentration, forgetfulness, depression, anxiety, claustrophobia, agoraphobia, irritability, difficulty coping and tearfulness and lack of drive including sex drive.
4. Urogenital: symptoms of vaginal dryness, utero-vaginal prolapse and urinary symptoms of urge incontinence/overactive bladder. Although stress incontinence is more common in postmenopausal women, the aetiology of this is probably not due to estrogen deficiency but disruption of the pelvic diaphragm so that the proximal urethra becomes extra abdominal, and a pressure gradient develops when there is raised intra-abdominal pressure.
5. Indirect symptoms of menopausal osteoporosis: which may result in repeated fractures, especially the wrist and hip.

There is huge variation in the frequency and severity of menopausal symptoms between different women. About 20 per cent of women have no significant symptoms, 60 per cent have mild to moderate symptoms and 20 per cent have very severe symptoms.

Women who have a sudden menopause induced by surgery (oophorectomy) or chemo/radiotherapy usually have more severe symptoms.

Vasomotor Symptoms

These are the classic symptoms heralding the onset of the menopause. About 75 per cent of women in the US report experiencing troublesome flushes – or flashes as they are called in the US [1]. Hot flushes adversely affect the quality of life and the day-to-day functioning of many women during the 'perimenopause'. Data on the duration of these symptoms are available from the Melbourne Women's Midlife Health Project [2]. The researchers found that out of 205 women who never used hormone replacement therapy (HRT) and were followed up for 13 years the mean duration of troublesome symptoms was 5.2 years (median 4 years and standard deviation of 3.8 years). Interestingly, even in women who used HRT (total sample 438 women) the duration did not change, with a mean of 5.5 years (median of 4 years, standard deviation of 4.0 years).

Thus it appears that vasomotor symptoms in a cross section of women on average persist for about 5 years.

The Mechanism of Hot Flushes

The basic physiological mechanism for hot flushes is an activation of the heat dissipation response most likely due to a hypothalamic mechanism triggered by decreasing estrogen levels [1]. It is thought that estrogen deprivation results in a loss of negative feedback for hypothalamic noradrenaline synthesis [3].

Peripheral changes that result in altered vascular activity, and a narrowed thermo-neutral zone, have also been implicated [4]. Consequently, fluctuations in temperature that would not normally trigger vasodilatation and sweating (cooling-down mechanisms) result in inappropriate flushing due to narrowing of the thermoneutral zone. Women suffering from hot flushes lose the ability to respond to an ice stimulus with vasoconstriction. It is thought likely that the α-adrenergic system, specifically noradrenaline, is the chemical trigger.

Flushes can be aggravated by stress and anxiety, and even by diet, lifestyle and medications.

The intensity of hot flushes can be measured by the increase in finger blood flow, respiratory exchange ratio, core body temperature and skin temperature changes. In laboratory studies, sternal skin conductance is usually measured with good reproducibility [1].

Although night sweats can keep women awake at night, insomnia associated with the menopause is likely to be due to a separate mechanism (loss of neuronal modulation of energy metabolism), and one can occur without the other [5].

Neuromuscular Symptoms

Joint pain is a common complaint in perimenopausal women and was reported by 77 per cent of participants in the WHI study at baseline. When estrogen-only MHT use was compared to placebo, pain was reported less commonly in the estrogen group than the placebo group (76.3 per cent vs 79.2 per cent, $P = 0.0001$) at 1 year and, 72.5 per cent of women in the estrogen group reported joint pain compared to 81.7 per cent of those in the placebo group ($P = 0.006$) reported joint pain after 3 years. Estrogen is thought to attenuate inflammation and promote cartilage turnover [6].

Headache and migraine are also common symptoms in the perimenopause, although the exact nature of the association between estrogen levels and headache are unknown and in some women treated with estrogen, symptoms remit, whilst in others there is a deterioration in symptom control [7]. In women with migraine, continuous hormone replacement therapy should be considered, preferably using a non-oral route and the lowest effective dose. For women who have contraindications to estrogen therapy or do not wish to use it, preparations that inhibit serotonin reuptake, such as venlafaxine, fluoxetine and paroxetine, have all shown efficacy [8]. In addition to the above treatment options, lifestyle changes, alone or combined with isoflavones, may be considered for the prevention of migraine associated with the menopause transition, although evidence of efficacy is limited. Gabapentin is an additional non-hormonal option to reduce frequency and severity of migraine. Although clonidine is licensed in several countries for migraine prophylaxis and treatment of vasomotor symptoms, any benefit from treatment is often offset by adverse events [8].

Psychogenic Symptoms

Emotions are the result of the interaction of many environmental factors. During the perimenopausal period, there are many life factors operating, such as fear of ageing (and wrinkles!), changing body shape, financial pressures, relationship issues, a changing role with children becoming independent and of course estrogen imbalance may aggravate any/all of these. Women who have a past history of depression, or have a history of premenstrual syndrome are more likely to experience psychogenic changes during the perimenopause.

Providing MHT will alleviate estrogen deficiency, but cannot compensate for many of the factors which may be responsible for low mood. However, certain types of depression which are due to estrogen deficiency are best treated by MHT [9].

Urogenital Symptoms

Pelvic organ prolapse (POP) and urinary incontinence are described in full in Chapter 12.

Vaginal symptoms are common and usually under-reported. Vaginal dryness as a result of estrogen deficiency can cause sexual problems as a result of lack of lubrication and loss of tissue elasticity. Loss of normal vaginal secretions can also be associated with an overgrowth of vaginal commensal organisms, resulting in vaginal discharge. In addition to the vagina, the urogenital tract is also affected by lack of estrogen and this may present as urgency or urge incontinence. Urogenital problems respond best to local estrogen therapy. This may require to be used in conjunction with systemic therapy for vasomotor symptoms. There are several options available for local estrogen therapy including creams, tablets and vaginal rings. Only intravaginal Vagifem in the lower dose of 10 micrograms, twice a week is licensed to be used without additional progestogen in women with an intact uterus.

Osteoporosis

Whilst osteoporosis is not a symptom, it is a very important part of female aging, especially after ovarian failure. We know women lose 1 per cent of their bone mass each year after ovarian failure, and that estrogen replacement can inhibit this. This important aspect of the postmenopausal estrogen deficiency is covered in Chapter 14. The reader is directed to this chapters for discussion of bone density, its investigation and available therapeutic measures.

To document the severity of symptoms, a quantitative score sheet has been developed. This enables women to self score symptoms on a scale of 0 to 3, and for the total score to be calculated. Not only does this allow the severity of symptoms to be more accurately assessed, but it also allows semi-quantitative assessment of any change/improvement as a result of therapy. An example of a score sheet used by the authors is attached as Table 2.1.

Differential Diagnosis

Before we ascribe a woman's symptoms as being due to the climacteric, we need to be sure that we are not missing a medical problem. The three commonest problems which can be confused with menopausal symptoms are hypothyroidism, anaemia and depression. Depression is particularly difficult, as this is far more common in women during the perimenopause.

Conclusion

When consulting a woman with problems relating to the peri/postmenopause the following should be followed:

Table 2.1 Menopausal symptomatology scoring sheet

SYMPTOM	SCORE: 0 = nil, 1 = mild, 2 = moderate, 3 = severe
VASOMOTOR SYMPTOMS	
Hot flushes	
Night sweats	
Crawling feelings under the skin (formication)	
Dry skin	
NEUROMUSCULAR SYMPTOMS	
Muscle pains	
Backache	
Headaches	
Joint pains	
PSYCHOLOGICAL SYMPTOMS	
Depression	
Irritability	
Mood swings	
Anxiety	
Inability to sleep	
Tiredness	
Loss of sex drive	
Unloved feelings	
Tearfulness	
UROGENITAL SYMPTOMS	
Dry vagina	
Painful sex	
Urinary frequency/urgency	

A total score is then obtained by adding together all the scores. The maximum possible score is $20 \times 3 = 60$.

At baseline, take a medical history and establish a baseline BP and BMI. BP ideally should be within normal limits or controlled prior to commencing menopausal hormone therapy (MHT).

Measuring gonadotrophin levels will be of very little help in her management, as values often vary widely during the menopause transition.

Fortunately, like many endocrine deficiency disorders (e.g. underactive thyroid), estrogen deficiency in the menopause transition can be managed with estrogen replacement therapy. For healthy women below the age of 60, provision of hormone replacement therapy carries no increase in risk, but results in control of symptoms and has other potential benefits such as maintenance of bone health.

It is also important to know whether the woman has an intact uterus.

If the answer to this question is no, she can be provided with estrogen alone. There are a number of delivery route options including oral, transdermal – gels or patches – and subcutaneous (implants).

Non-oral delivery does not increase the risk of VTE over and above the individual's inherent risk, based upon their individual risk factors (Chapter 22), but if there are no underlying risk factors then the choice of delivery rests with the patient and this will influence compliance and symptom control.

If she has an intact uterus, then using supplementary progestogen to prevent endometrial hyperplasia/neoplasia is essential. For women during their perimenopausal years a sequential progestogen therapy is recommended to minimize the risk of abnormal vaginal bleeding. Whilst estrogen can be administered every day progestogen is used for 10–14 days/month, which then results in a withdrawal bleed. Women who are postmenopausal are usually prescribed a 'combined continuous' regimen with estrogen and progestogen being taken each day.

Does she require contraception (see Chapter 20)?

This may influence the type of MHT provided.

Women using combined hormonal contraception (CHC) are unlikely to develop menopausal symptoms. Women using progestogen-only methods can do so.

Mirena has a license to provide endometrial protection in addition to contraception (and it also has a license for the management of heavy menstrual bleeding). This makes it an ideal solution to many of the issues in the perimenopause, especially providing the progestogenic component hormone therapy. Women using Mirena for endometrial protection can have a choice of estrogen delivery.

Recommendations

Take a good history especially about symptoms relating to the menopause.

Using the attached score sheet is a valuable way to record symptoms and their severity.

Take a detailed history with respect to risk factors for breast cancer, thromboembolic disorders and osteoporosis.

Ordering a series of expensive hormone tests (Estradiol, Progesterone, FSH, LH, androgens, sex binding globulin, etc.) is not indicated for women who are having a physiological menopause. Firstly, FSH levels are variable and a single raised level is not meaningful. Secondly, estrogen levels vary a lot from day to day, and the blood levels of the hormone bear no relationship to the symptoms experienced. Thirdly, the results of hormone tests will not change the management of the patient – this should be determined by the woman's symptoms.

The initial prescription of MHT should be a 'therapeutic trial'. If the woman's symptoms and quality of life improve, then she will continue with the prescribed treatment. If there is no improvement, a different preparation of MHT can be tried. Using the 'score sheet' from Table 2.1 will facilitate a more objective evaluation of any improvement in symptoms.

References

1. Sievert LL. Subjective and objective measures of hot flashes. *Am J Hum Biol* 2013;25:573–80.

2. Col NF, Guthrie JR, Politi M, Dennerstein L. Duration of vasomotor symptoms in middle-aged women; a longitudinal study. *Menopause* 2009;16:453–7.

3. Vilar-Gonzales S, Perez-Rozos A, Cabarillas-Farpon R. Mechanism of hot flashes. *Clin Transi Oncol* 2011;13:143–7.

4. Sassarini J, Fox H, Ferrell W, Sattar N, Lumsden MA. Hot flushes, vascular reactivity and the role of α-adrenergic system. *Climacteric* 2012;15:332–8.

5. Bourey RE. Primary menopausal insomnia: definition, review, and practical approach. *Endocr Pract* 2011;17:122–31.

6. Kaunitz AM. Should new-onset arthralgia be considered a menopausal symptom? *Menopause* 2013;20:591–3.

7. Tassorelli C1, Greco R, Allena M, Terreno E, Nappi RE. Transdermal hormonal therapy in perimenstrual migraine: why, when and how? *Curr Pain Headache Rep* 2012;16:467–73.

8. MacGregor EA. Headache and hormone replacement therapy in the postmenopausal woman. *Curr Treat Options Neurol* 2009;11:10–17.

9. Studd J. Personal view: hormones and depression in women. *Climacteric* 2014 Jul;21:1–3.

Chapter 3

The Ovarian Reserve
Predicting the Menopause

Richard A. Anderson

The essential cause of the existence of the menopause is that the ovary contains a finite number of follicles: these are progressively lost with time until insufficient remain to support menstrual cyclicity. Ovarian follicles are both the source of the female gamete, and the key site of reproductive hormone production. Depletion of follicle numbers therefore results in both loss of fertility and gonadal estrogen production, and thus differs substantially from the situation in the male where the two functions of the gonad are anatomically and functionally more independent, and loss of one does not necessitate loss of the other.

Establishment and Loss of the Ovarian Reserve

Ovarian follicles are formed during fetal life, with primordial follicles first seen in the ovary from about 18 weeks of gestation. Prior to this, the female germ cells have been specified, migrated to the gonadal ridge where they have proliferated before exiting mitosis and enter meiosis only to arrest at diplotene of meiosis. During this process they reorganize their interactions with surrounding somatic cells to form primordial follicles. This process is completed during later pregnancy and indeed some newly formed follicles start growing immediately so that during later fetal life and throughout childhood the ovary contains follicles at a range of stages of development up to small antral sizes. Subsequent development to ovulatory stages does not, of course, occur until after puberty when there is sufficient gonadotropic stimulation to support folliculogenesis through to completion of growth and maturation.

Ovaries from different women contain a very wide range of numbers of follicles. This is demonstrated in histologic studies, which have also led to the development of models showing the decline in the primordial follicle pool with age (Figure 3.1) [1]. These studies show that there is a range of at least 50-fold in the number of follicles in the ovaries of women of the same age. The various models that have demonstrated this have tended to present their data on a logarithmic scale which promotes the view that the decline in follicle number accelerates with age. While this may be true when presented as a percentage of the number of follicles present, a very different perspective is gained when the number of follicles is presented on a linear scale (Figure 3.2). This highlights how the vast majority of follicles are lost during the early years of life, even before reproductive maturity is achieved. These data can also be used to calculate the number of follicles being lost to either growth or atresia per month in women with a larger or smaller follicle complement. This analysis indicates that in the ovaries of the 'average' woman, with expected age of menopause of 51 years, some 900 follicles will start to grow

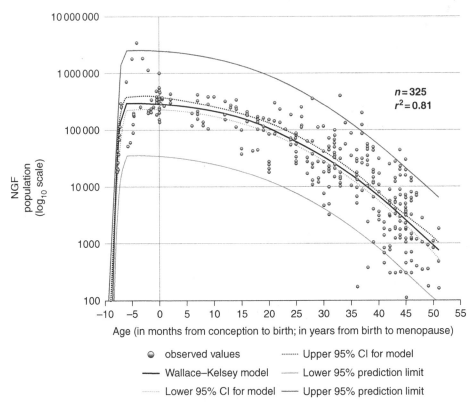

Figure 3.1 The number of non-growing follicles in women from conception to the menopause. The figure shows the data set (n = 325), the model (thicker line), the 95 per cent confidence interval for the model (dotted lines), and the 95 per cent prediction limits of the NGF population (outer solid lines). Reproduced from [1].

each month at the peak of this activity (which is at age 14 years), declining to 200 per month at age 35. In women with a high number of follicles, this number is approximately 1900 follicles a month at age 35, whereas in women at the lower end of the still normal range (i.e. with expected age of menopause 42 years) it is approximately 26 follicles a month at the same age, thus fewer than 1 per day. Many of these early growing follicles will then be lost across all stages of folliculogenesis. This has implications for understanding the range of normality across the major milestones of reproductive life. In this context it has been proposed that women become essentially sterile some 10 years before the menopause and subfertile a further 10 years before that [2]. If one considers the range of age at menopause, it will rapidly become clear that the age at which a women may become subfertile will also vary considerably, and this also highlights that the reproductive lifespan, i.e. the interval between puberty and this proposed time of subfertility, will be relatively brief in women destined to go through a menopause in their early forties.

Measurement of the Ovarian Reserve

From these considerations, the size of the remaining follicle pool is clearly a major determinant of age at menopause and indeed of time to menopause, although the rate

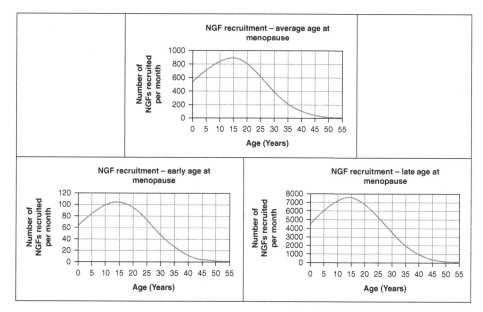

Figure 3.2 Rates of non-growing follicle (NGF) recruitment towards maturation. Each sub-figure describes the absolute number of NGFs recruited per month, for ages from birth to 55 years, based on population decline predicted by the model shown in Figure 2.1. The top panel denotes recruitment for "average" women with menopause aged 51; maximum recruitment of 880 follicles per month occurs at 14 years 2 months, falling to 221 per month at age 35. The lower panels denote recruitment for women who will have an early or late menopause, left and right respectively (42 and 58 years). These indicate maximum recruitment of 104 follicles vs 7,520 follicles per month, at 14 years 2 months, falling to 26 and 1,900 per month at age 35. Reproduced from [1].

of loss is also an essential consideration. The size of the ovarian reserve is starting to become clinically assessable. Analysis of the rate of loss cannot be determined from single measurements, although it can be extrapolated with repeated measures over time. Data are starting to emerge as to the value of measuring the ovarian reserve in the context of predicting the menopause, although this field remains in its infancy, due to the essential requirement for long-term follow-up. It is therefore not possible to predict 'how long a woman will be fertile for'.

Before addressing how one might measure the ovarian reserve, it is important to discuss what is meant by the term, as unfortunately it is used to mean two separate although related aspects of ovarian biology. Most commonly in the clinical literature, and generally in the context of studies involving assisted reproduction, the ovarian reserve is used to mean the number of follicles that can be recruited to grow by administration of supraphysiological doses of FSH, i.e. as administered during ovarian stimulation for IVF. This is a very valuable measure as it will predict (to some extent) the number of oocytes that will be obtained after ovarian stimulation. It can be used to identify women either at risk of over response and therefore ovarian hyperstimulation syndrome, or conversely those whose response is less than their age or other markers of ovarian function (notably FSH) would have otherwise predicted. The follicles identified through this usage are already at an advanced, antral stage of gonadotropin-dependent growth and will have been in the growth phase for many weeks already: they constitute what can be termed the *functional ovarian reserve*. The second usage of the term *ovarian reserve* is used to mean the size of the primordial follicle pool. This is a more accurate biological usage and thus while ultimately more correct, its value in clinical practice is limited as the primordial follicle pool can only be determined at present by histologic analysis, and not *in vivo*. The size of the two follicle pools is related under normal circumstances, although the relationship between the two may well vary in different physiological and pathological states, for example in adolescence versus later adulthood, and in women with disorders such as hypothalamic amenorrhea and polycystic ovary syndrome, as well as in a range of systemic illnesses. It may also be partially suppressed during hormonal contraceptive use.

The assessment of the ovarian reserve has long been a goal in reproductive medicine, particularly in assisted reproduction, to optimize the prediction of the response of an individual woman. It can be used to improve the safety and effectiveness of ovarian stimulation regimes, and in the development of new regimes. As the ovarian reserve declines with age, then age is itself a measure of the ovarian reserve. It also includes an aspect of the quality of the oocytes within that reserve, reflected clinically in the increasing risk of non-conception, miscarriage and chromosomally abnormal conceptions with age. It does not, however, allow much in the way of individualization and therefore a range of biochemical and biophysical tests have been explored over the years. It has long been recognized that serum FSH increases with age and a high FSH is one of the diagnostic tests of the menopause, i.e. loss of the ovarian reserve. The biological function of FSH, however, is to regulate antral stages, follicle growth and selection such that only a single follicle emerges as dominant and mono-ovulation occurs, and the early stages of follicle growth are gonadotropin independent. Follicle-stimulating hormone remains a useful screening test in that a high FSH predicts a poor ovarian response at IVF, but the accuracy of this prediction is poor and the marked cycle-to-cycle variation within a single woman (as well as variation through the menstrual cycle) has led to a search for more robust indices. Measuring a woman's FSH would be of little value in predicting her fertile life, although a high value (>10 IU/L, or more worrying >25 IU/L) would indicate that it is short, and that the menopause may be imminent. Estradiol is even less use as its production largely reflects the function of the single preovulatory follicle of that particular menstrual cycle and not any measure of the ovarian reserve. Inhibin B was identified as a product of the granulosa cells of smaller follicles and indeed is of predictive value in assisted reproduction. It also declines prior to the menopause although this decline is relatively late. The key physiological role of inhibin B is the negative regulation of FSH secretion particularly in the early follicular phase, so the two hormones are functionally interrelated. The identification of anti-Müllerian hormone (AMH) as a product of smaller preantral as well as early antral follicles has led to dramatic development in our ability to clinically assess the ovarian reserve and it has become of routine use in many IVF clinics around the world [3]. AMH is produced by granulosa cells of the follicles as soon as they start to grow, although not by primordial follicles (Figure 3.3). While the concentration of AMH in blood reflects the size of the true as well as the functional ovarian reserve, the relationship with the true ovarian reserve is therefore indirect. As it is produced by smaller and therefore less gonadotropin-dependent follicles, its concentration through the menstrual cycle

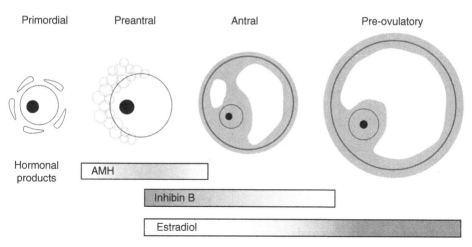

Figure 3.3 Illustration of changing hormone production by the developing follicle. AMH is produced by follicles as soon as they start to grow but declines sharply at approximately 8–10 mm diameter. Inhibin B is predominantly produced by smaller antral follicles, whereas estradiol production increases through the antral stages to ovulation.

is much less variable than that of the aforementioned reproductive hormones. While there is some variability, this is generally regarded as not clinically significant as relatively few women will be misclassified; this is a very substantial practical clinical advantage particularly where transvaginal ultrasound (to measure antral follicle count) is not immediately available.

Predicting the Menopause

There have now been several studies which have assessed the role of AMH in predicting the menopause. These initially demonstrated that AMH declines to undetectable concentrations some 5 years before the menopause and that it was a more accurate predictor of time to and age at final menstrual period than either FSH or inhibin B. Subsequent studies have confirmed and strengthened this finding and although they show a clear relationship between AMH measured at any adult age and subsequent age at menopause, the predictive ability is relatively modest [4, 5]. It has also been demonstrated that interpretation of AMH concentration is not independent of age, thus a given AMH concentration predicts different age at menopause according to the age of the woman. AMH therefore needs to be age adjusted (Figure 3.4). This relationship appears to be very clear on a population basis, but while the published studies are promising, the data show very substantial variability and do not appear sufficiently robust to allow an individual woman to have her AMH measured and derive from that a clear and accurate prediction of the age at which she will become menopausal. This may reflect variability in the relationship between AMH and the true ovarian reserve between individual women, but less explored is the impact of variation in the rate of decline of AMH (and indeed of the ovarian reserve) which may well vary with time within an individual woman, as well as between different women. The impact of the rate of loss (as reflected by the fall in

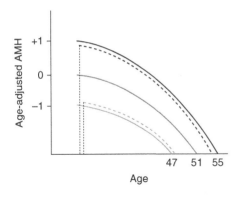

Figure 3.4 Schematic of the relationship between AMH and time to menopause. The lines represent the decline in age-adjusted AMH (depicted in standard deviations from the mean) with increasing age, with the menopause occurring when the line crosses the abscissa (indicative values only for mean ±1 SD). The black, grey and light grey lines indicate the trajectory of women with high, average and low age-adjusted AMH, respectively. The dotted lines represent two women of similar age but with different age-adjusted AMH: plotting their ages against age-adjusted AMH shows which lines they are predicted to follow and hence anticipated age at menopause.

AMH between two sampling time points) has recently been explored, but in women over the age of 25, the rate of decline did not add to the value of AMH measurement at a single time point [6].

An additional problem in this area has been the assays that are available. The initial generation of AMH assays were not sufficiently sensitive to detect AMH in the last 5 years before the menopause, although current assays (including those on automated platforms that are now in routine use) have an approximately 10-fold improved sensitivity. There are also issues of standardization, but although no internationally accepted calibration standard exists, in practical terms there is little difference between the most widely used assays. It is likely that technical improvements and further large prospective studies will clarify how accurately AMH can be used to predict the menopause, perhaps in combination with other information. Similar considerations have applied to the use of AMH in diagnosing the menopause: initial assays were unable to detect AMH in normal women for several years before the menopause, but recently an AMH assay has been approved by the FDA 'as an aid in the determination of menopausal status'. AMH has also been demonstrated to be an accurate diagnostic for postchemotherapy premature ovarian insufficiency (POI) in women treated for breast cancer [7]. Thus while measuring an individual woman's AMH would be indicative, its predictive accuracy is very unclear.

Biophysical, i.e. ultrasound, markers of the ovarian reserve have also been developed. Both ovarian volume and antral follicle count (AFC) decline with age and both predict the response in assisted reproduction. AFC in particular is of routine value in this context, promoted by its wide availability in the reproductive medicine clinic. Notwithstanding that, and particularly in general practice, ultrasound is less immediately available and biochemical tests may be more useful. There is a close relationship between AFC and AMH and indeed the two markers can be regarded as essentially measuring the same thing, i.e. the population/activity of the small antral follicle pool, as AMH is produced by the granulosa cells of the small follicles that are being counted by ultrasound. Although in skilled hands AFC is as accurate a predictor of ovarian response as AMH, there is much larger opportunity for interindividual variation and the results obtained are also dependent on the technical quality of the instrument, which is changing with time. Consequently an AFC count carried out by transvaginal ultrasound is of limited value in predicting the duration of a woman's reproductive life.

Prediction in Special Circumstances

The above discussion relates primarily to the value of currently available markers in normal healthy women. Specific considerations may apply in certain pathological states; these include women whose ovarian reserve may be damaged iatrogenically either by surgery or chemotherapeutic agents, or in other diseases. Of particular importance in the latter are women who are either identified as being at risk of POI, for example on the basis of family history or risk factors such as having anti-ovarian antibodies, and potentially in the future on the basis of identification of genetic susceptibility.

Anti-Müllerian hormone declines rapidly during chemotherapy, and recovery thereafter is dependent on the gonadotoxicity of the regimen administered. Thus, women treated with alkylating agent-based therapies show much less recovery than those with non-alkylating regimes [8]. More importantly, AMH measured before the administration of chemotherapy has been shown to predict long-term ovarian function postchemotherapy, thus women still menstruating several years after chemotherapy have markedly higher AMH concentrations pretreatment than those who become and remain amenorrheic after chemotherapy [9]. In this context AMH seems to add to the information provided by age (Figure 3.5) although larger studies are required to fully explore this relationship. These data therefore support the contention that AMH may become valuable in predicting the risk of menopause after cancer therapy. It may also have application in the pediatric oncology context. Prior to puberty, current reproductive hormones are very low but AMH is readily detectable in serum of all healthy girls, and indeed rises steadily through childhood [10]. As in adults, chemotherapy results in a marked decline in serum AMH in girls and adolescents, with very variable recovery reflecting the predicted gonadotoxicity of the administered regimen [11]. This may well be of use in identifying girls who have suffered POI at a very early age and in whom endocrine therapy to induce puberty can then be started at an earlier age than might previously have been the case. There are as yet no data linking pretreatment AMH with early menopause in childhood cancer survivors. Such a relationship would be expected, but will be complicated by the fact that AMH rises during childhood (as opposed to the steady fall during adulthood), with peak levels at approximately 24 years. During puberty AMH shows a plateau or even slight fall before rising further, thus there are changing

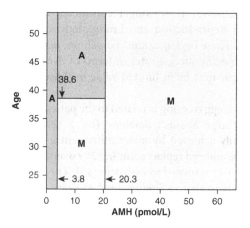

Figure 3.5 Classification mosaic chart for ongoing menses (M) or chemotherapy-related amenorrhea (A) using prechemotherapy serum AMH and chronological age as predictor variables, in women with early breast cancer. The primary cut-off values are both for AMH. Between these AMH levels is an age threshold, above which amenorrhea is predicted and below which ongoing menses are predicted. The classification schema has a sensitivity of 98.2 per cent and specificity of 80.0 per cent. Reprinted with permission from [9].

relationships between AMH and the ovarian reserve during these periods of development, which are as yet incompletely understood.

Women at risk of POI provide a particularly challenging context in which to address these markers. While there are a wide range of genes that have been identified in animal studies to cause POI, with very few exceptions these have not entered clinical practice. Mother's age at menopause remains a guide, but although this is widely recognized, there are few data assessing its accuracy. Furthermore, in most cases the diagnosis of POI by definition indicates loss of the ovarian reserve that has already happened, and it is a much rarer situation when a woman is identified who is at risk of POI while still having a relatively normal ovarian reserve. AMH may be of value in identifying women whose ovarian reserve is very low, and in the presence of another factor indicating a risk of POI it would seem likely that this would be of clinical use. However, as discussed above, the predictive value of measurement of AMH under these circumstances is of unknown accuracy.

Insuring Against Oocyte Loss

The question arises as to whether one can effectively mitigate against the inevitable age-related loss of oocyte quality and quantity. For a single woman deferring motherhood, this essentially means consideration of oocyte vitrification, often termed *social* or *elective* egg freezing. The other potential option would be embryo cryopreservation (of course requiring sperm from either a partner or a donor to fertilize the oocytes) or ovarian tissue cryopreservation. The latter is not used in this context, although it is becoming increasingly widely used for young women and indeed prepubertal girls facing chemotherapy-induced ovarian failure. Previously, slow oocyte cryopreservation was possible but relatively ineffective, but with modern vitrification techniques oocyte viability is essentially as good as that of unfrozen oocytes. Indeed vitrified oocyte banks are increasingly used in IVF centres with large oocyte donation programs. Vitrification involves the extremely rapid freezing of tissue by immersion in liquid nitrogen, with high concentrations of cryoprotectants. This is, however, a still-developing technology with many technical issues still potentially to be optimized, and very limited data on outcomes of infants born as a result of it [12]. Most of the literature refers to embryo outcome after oocyte vitrification in optimal circumstances, i.e. from oocytes donated by young women, and the most important determinant will be the woman's age. Oocyte vitrification is, however, no longer considered experimental by the European Society of Human Reproduction and Embryology and the American Society of Reproductive Medicine. These organizations' guidelines, however, highlight the limited published data on age-specific success rates in terms of live births achieved and the possibility that this technique may be of limited value in those older women who are most interested in it.

Calculating the probability of live birth after egg freezing is related to the patient's age and freezing method. Recent data from a large Spanish database (i.e. a centre of excellence, with results that are not necessarily achieved by many other centres) have recently reported on warming and fertilization/embryo replacement in 5289 women who had electively vitrified their oocytes, of whom 641 returned to use them [13]. The results again highlight the importance of age, but suggest that in women aged 35 years or less, very high cumulative live birth rates can be achieved provided sufficient eggs are obtained: 10–15 oocytes yielded cumulative live birth rates (CLBR) of 42.8–69.8 per cent. However, in women aged over 35, 10 oocytes gave a CLBR of 25.2 per cent, and that number of oocytes may require more than one stimulation cycle to achieve. The term *insurance* in this context, while widely used especially in marketing literature, is clearly inappropriate, and any woman considering this should consider very carefully the success rates of the clinic she might choose, as well as all the costs involved.

References

1. Wallace WH, Kelsey TW. Human ovarian reserve from conception to the menopause. *PLoS ONE* 2010;5:e8772.

2. Broekmans FJ, Soules MR, Fauser BC. Ovarian aging: mechanisms and clinical consequences. *Endocr Rev* 2009;30:465–93.

3. Dewailly D, Andersen CY, Balen A, et al. The physiology and clinical utility of anti-Mullerian hormone in women. *Hum Reprod Update* 2014;20:370–85.

4. Freeman EW, Sammel MD, Lin H, et al. Anti-Mullerian hormone as a predictor of time to menopause in late reproductive age women. *J Clin Endocrinol Metab* 2012;97:1673–80.

5. Tehrani FR, Solaymani-Dodaran M, Tohidi M, et al. Modeling age at menopause using serum concentration of anti-Mullerian hormone. *J Clin Endocrinol Metab* 2013;98:729–35.

6. de Kat AC, van der Schouw YT, Eijkemans MJC, et al. Can menopause prediction be improved with multiple AMH measurement? Results for the prospective Doetinchem Cohort Study. *J Clin Endo Metab* 2019; doi 10.21210/jc.2018-02607.

7. Anderson RA, Mansi J, Coleman RE, Adamson DJA, Leonard RCF. The utility of anti-Mullerian hormone in the diagnosis and prediction of loss of ovarian function following chemotherapy for early breast cancer. *Eur J Cancer* 2017;87:58–64.

8. Anderson RA, Remedios R, Kirkwood AA, et al. Determinants of ovarian function after response-adapted therapy in patients with advanced Hodgkin's lymphoma (RATHL): a secondary analysis of a randomised phase 3 trial. *Lancet Oncol* 2018;19:1328–1337.

9. Anderson RA, Rosendahl M, Kelsey TW, et al. Pretreatment anti-Mullerian hormone predicts for loss of ovarian function after chemotherapy for early breast cancer. *Eur J Cancer* 2013;49:3404–11.

10. Kelsey TW, Wright P, Nelson SM, et al. A validated model of serum anti-Müllerian hormone from conception to menopause. *PLoS ONE* 2011;6:e22024.

11. Brougham MF, Crofton PM, Johnson EJ, et al. Anti-Mullerian hormone is a marker of gonadotoxicity in pre- and postpubertal girls treated for cancer: a prospective study. *J Clin Endocrinol Metab* 2012;97:2059–67.

12. Argyle CE, Harper JC, Davies MC. Oocyte cryopreservation: where are we now? *Hum Reprod Update* 2016;22:440–9.

13. Cobo A, García-Velasco J, Domingo J, Pellicer A, Remohí J. Elective and onco-fertility preservation: factors related to IVF outcomes. *Hum Reprod* 2018;33:2222–31.

Premature Ovarian Insufficiency
Fertility Options

Anthony J. Rutherford and Gab Kovacs

Although in vitro fertilization (IVF) was developed for the treatment of tubal infertility, [1], it soon became apparent that human IVF had many other applications such as male factor subfertility [2], unexplained subfertility [3] and restoring fertility in women without functioning ovaries using ovum [4] or embryo donation. Although ovum donation was originally used to treat women with Turner's syndrome [5], it has also been successfully applied to women with other causes of premature ovarian insufficiency (POI) over the last 35 years. The concept of gamete donation is not new, with sperm donation (DI) having been utilized, initially with fresh sperm and subsequently with stored frozen sperm for several decades [6]. In DI the woman's partner becomes the social father but is not the genetic father, whereas in oocyte donation the woman who has the child is the birth and social mother, but not the genetic mother. Although the child is not directly genetically linked, egg donation allows the patient to carry and deliver her husband's genetic child. The woman is responsible for the child's existence, playing an essential role in epigenetic programming in prenatal development and nurturing the embryo from conception to delivery [7]. Furthermore, legally, in the United Kingdom, the birth mother's name is recorded as the mother on the child's birth certificate.

The use of egg donation has increased substantially as a treatment option in Europe, increasing four-fold from 13 609 in 2008 [8] to 56 516 egg donation cycles in 2014 [9]. In the UK, the use of egg donation doubled over a decade, from 1912 egg donation cycles in 2006 to 3924 cycles in 2016 according to data from the Human Fertilisation and Embryology Authority (HFEA) [10].

Although IVF technology is now readily available around the world and women with POI can be treated successfully, the availability of oocyte donors remains a significant challenge for those needing oocyte donation.

Source of Donated Oocytes
Excess IVF Oocytes

Before embryo freezing was developed, in most units a maximum of three embryos were replaced. As a consequence, some couples who had many oocytes collected were happy to donate some of their oocytes to other couples, to mitigate the risk that their embryos would potentially be wasted [11].

Historically, Monash IVF limited the number of oocytes inseminated to eight at one attempt, to avoid discarding many potentially viable embryos. Oocytes in excess could either be discarded without being inseminated, or donated to approved research, or to another couple (for the use of oocyte donation). This gave a ready supply of donated oocytes and enabled the world's first donor egg program to be established, under the care of John Leeton [4]. However, with the development of embryo freezing, couples could utilize all their oocytes for their own use, and the supply of donated oocytes became scarce. Women who required donated oocytes then depended on altruistic oocyte donors.

Altruistic Oocyte Donors

Women who donate altruistically principally do so to help others, either friends or family who have had difficulty conceiving, or in response to stories in the media. In known donation, the recipient can use a family friend or relative directly, such as a sister donating to another sister. At times, this at can prove difficult, as ovarian insufficiency may unknowingly be unearthed in the sibling [12]. Women who donate altruistically may also provide oocytes to women they do not know in response to media campaigns promoting the need for egg donors. Whilst these donations were initially anonymous, changes in regulation in many countries (including the United Kingdom and Australia) now allow identifying information on the donor to be released to the offspring when he or she reaches adulthood.

Ethically, altruistic donors show an unselfish concern for the welfare of others, and make the donation voluntarily without payment in return, other than receipted expenses or minimal compensation. The donor's motives are hugely relevant from the child's perspective [13]. It could also be argued that those donating altruistically are more likely to be committed, rather than those donors who potentially donate for monetary gain, who are less likely to think about the long-term consequences. Interestingly, 'altruistic' donors accounted for less than half (43 per cent) of all UK donors in 2010, but, following the 2012 HFEA rule change on compensation, which allowed UK donors to be paid reasonable expenses up to the value of £750, more potential donors came forward [14].

Altruistic Donor 'Pool'

This is a unique system where a potential recipient introduces a known donor to the pool, who is happy to donate to others, specifically to gain access to other donors in the pool in a crossover arrangement. This is applicable where the donor does not want to know the outcome, and does not want to be involved with her offspring, but is willing to help a friend or relative.

Egg Sharing

The second, and largest group of donors in the UK are those who receive 'benefit in kind', where they receive free or subsidized fertility treatment by donating a proportion of their gametes during their own fertility treatment. This so-called egg sharing arrangement started over 20 years ago [15]. In 2013, 533 patients registered as egg sharers [10]. These patients, who require either IVF or ICSI treatment, donate a set number of their oocytes to a recipient. Careful selection is essential to ensure that the donor will produce sufficient oocytes to make the process worthwhile for both parties. Should the donor not produce enough oocytes for her own and the recipient's use, it is not allowed in UK law for the cycle to continue with the aim to give all the oocytes to the recipient, then for her to start a fresh cycle for her own use. This process, known as 'egg giving', was outlawed by the HFEA in 2003 [10]. The HFEA expects clinics to have a clear policy of whether a charge will apply to the donor under these unusual circumstances.

Egg sharers mainly consist of women not eligible for NHS-funded treatment, often as they or their partners have had children in previous relationships. Research has shown that in comparison to altruistic donors the chance of a successful outcome is similar, and that the donor and the recipient both have an equal chance of a live birth [16]. Nevertheless, there is evidence that the occasional unsuccessful egg-sharing donor feels regret in the knowledge that another couple may become the parents of a child genetically related to her [17]. In many countries the concept of 'egg sharing' does not exist as it is considered commercialization of human tissues.

Commercial Oocyte Donation

Those countries that perform the majority of egg donation in Europe pay their donors a financial incentive to donate. Recent data from the Spanish Fertility Society demonstrate that in Spain (the largest exponent with around 50 per cent of all egg donation activity), approximately one-third of all their ART cycles are oocyte donation. Other countries within Europe performing a large number of oocyte donation cycles include Czech Republic 2365, Russia 2147, the UK 1891 and Belgium 1412. There are potential concerns about paid oocyte donation, as there is a risk that where money is involved donors may be encouraged to donate several times, which may ultimately have an impact on their own health and fertility [18].

In 2007 the American Society of Reproductive Medicine recommended a limit on the payment to donors to US$5000, and no more than US$10 000 could be justified as financial compensation of oocyte donors [19].

A recent survey of agencies and clinics offering egg donor matching and donation in the US demonstrated that these guidelines are being flouted. Furthermore, many of these agencies and clinics are paying additional amounts for certain characteristics [20]. There is evidence that the community does not have concerns about oocyte donors being rewarded, although they undervalue the effort and inconvenience associated with the process. A recent Australian community opinion poll carried out by GTK [21] found two-thirds of respondents supported the payment of egg donors. However, oocyte donation was grossly undervalued with 21 per cent of those surveyed suggested less than US$500 per donation, with 13 per cent suggesting A$500–1000.

'Cross-Border' Oocyte Donation

Recruitment of donors overseas is variable, and some countries like Sweden manage almost entirely on altruistic donation. However, because of the shortfall of egg donors in the UK with long waiting lists many patients now choose to travel overseas. In other countries, such as Turkey, where egg donation is not permitted on religious grounds, services have developed across the borders in neighbouring states or provinces where the rules permit, such as Northern Cyprus, which now has a flourishing egg donation program. Across the globe in North America egg donation programs are well developed, with payment of donors an established practice.

Oocyte/Embryo Banking

If there was a way of predicting whether a girl or woman will undergo POI (Chapter 3) it would be possible for these individuals to consider fertility preservation. This could be achieved by either collecting and cryopreserving oocytes, or if they have a life partner, creating embryos to be cryopreserved. In prepubertal girls, ovarian cortical ovarian tissue containing immature oocytes could potentially be harvested laparoscopically and cryopreserved for subsequent grafting. Unfortunately, in the majority of situations currently POI cannot be predicted, and once diagnosed, none of these techniques are applicable.

Screening of Oocyte Donors

Egg donors in the UK have to be under the age of 36, unless there are exceptional documented reasons to use older women, such as a known donation. Donors are encouraged to allow the clinic to verify their medical and psychological history with their general practitioner. When selecting donors, clinics need to take into account the implications of the donation for the donor's family and her future fertility.

Assessment of donors includes a very careful medical and social history with specific reference to any current or past physical conditions that may have a bearing on a future child. People with a known gene, chromosomal or mitochondrial abnormality that may cause serious physical or mental disability, and those who have a personal history of a transmissible infection are excluded. Clearly lifestyle issues such as diet, weight and smoking are important in those considering donating. A thorough psychological assessment, with implications counselling, is essential, and considered mandatory in the UK. Only those who successfully complete this phase of the assessment are then subject to laboratory testing.

Laboratory testing focuses on three aspects: the donor's natural fertility, a transmissible infection screen and a simple genetic screen. The latter will be modified according to their ethnicity. In some countries, a more extensive genetic screening test is offered screening for up to 600 genetic diseases [22]. The infection screen is performed contemporaneously with the time the donor will donate and will be repeated should the donation process happen on more than one occasion. When a fresh embryo transfer takes place there is a small but largely hypothetical risk of a donor being infected with HIV despite screening negative for HIV antibody (if they are still in the immune window period). However, modern fourth-generation tests, which test for both the antibody and antigen, minimize this potential issue [23].

Counselling

Although donors in the UK can put conditions on the use and storage of their gametes, these need to be compatible with the Equality Act 2010. Both donors and potential recipients need to be aware that the donors can withdraw their consent to the use of their gametes and to the use of embryos created from their gametes at any stage in the treatment process. It is therefore mandatory that all gamete donors and recipients are provided with the opportunity to receive appropriate implications counselling. In the UK, couples are encouraged to reveal to their donor-conceived child their genetic origins. The emphasis placed on telling the child following egg donation comes from the extensive psychological literature outlining the experiences of adopted children and their perceived need to find out about their genetic origins. However, we need to understand that like sperm donation, egg donation cannot be equated to adoption, and the same conclusions cannot be drawn.

Regulation

The regulations governing egg donation vary substantially around the world. In the UK, where IVF treatment has been closely regulated by the HFEA since 1991, information on donors, including a description of themselves, their ethnic group, marital status, the number and gender of their current children, their physical characteristics, details of screening tests and medical history as well as a 'goodwill message' for potential children, is held by the HFEA. A change in the HFEA Act saw anonymity removed from all gamete donations from 1 April 2005. Since that time, at the age of 18 a child can contact the HFEA and be provided with identifying information about their genetic origins including contact information. The HFEA will inform the donor that a request has been received, prior to releasing information.

This loss of anonymity did not receive uniform approval, and there was a decline in those coming forward as egg donors in 2006, although this has now recovered almost completely. Furthermore, in a recent survey up to a 34 per cent of recipients travel overseas for egg donation, mainly to avoid the rules about identifying information being recorded [24]. Donors who donated prior to 2005 can apply to the HFEA to add their identifying information to the records. However, no donor has the legal right to contact their donor-conceived child, although they can find out how many children were born as a result of their donation.

Donor Matching

When donor gametes are employed, most couples are keen to have a donor that matches their physical characteristics and their ethnicity. Physical features such as height, build, hair, skin and eye colour of both partners are recorded. Blood group is often matched such that the conceived child's blood group could have arisen from the parents, to preserve the desire for anonymity, though with current regulations and the availability of relatively cheap genetic testing this is becoming less relevant. In the UK, where most clinics offering egg donation perform less than 100 cycles per annum, the choice is extremely limited, particularly for certain ethnic groups.

The advent of successful oocyte cryopreservation using vitrification techniques has led to the development of egg donor banks, which potentially offer greater choice of matching for prospective donors, similar to sperm banking, which has been available for 50 years. These include some large egg donation programs in Southern Europe and the commercial North American egg banks. The World Egg Bank (TWEB) is the first and largest international frozen egg bank. Located in Phoenix, Arizona, TWEB is unique because it does everything from recruitment, to retrieval, to shipping all under one roof.

Recipients are carefully screened for common transmissible infections, similar to the donor infection screening. Cytomegalovirus is a relatively common infection that can cause a mild flu-like illness in an adult, but if a woman is infected in early pregnancy, it can cause a similar spectrum of fetal abnormalities to rubella infection. Recipients found to be CMV negative are generally matched with donors that are CMV negative. However, the risk of reactivation of a CMV infection using donor eggs is theoretical only, and where all other parameters match, an informed couple may select to use a CMV-positive donor.

Cycle Programming

In the majority of egg donor programs the aim is to perform a fresh embryo transfer, usually achieved using freshly obtained oocytes. When the donor has her oocytes collected the recipient needs to have a well-developed endometrium completely in phase to maximize the chance of implantation. The best way of achieving synchrony is to ensure that once the donors are screened, they are kept on the oral contraceptive pill, which in combination with a short antagonist stimulation cycle makes the process of donor–recipient coordination relatively straightforward. Programming the recipient simply involves manipulating her hormone replacement therapy, ceasing the HRT 7–10 days before starting her endometrial stimulation.

Endometrial Development

The options for stimulating endometrial development include oral, transdermal, vaginal and intramuscular estrogen, with the majority of clinicians (86 per cent) choosing the oral route as reported in the oocyte donation survey [25]. The recipient restarts estrogen a couple of days before the donor starts ovarian stimulation, with the dose increased gradually to mimic the rise in estrogen seen in natural cycles (from 2 mg going up to 8 mg). Endometrial development is assessed by ultrasound around day 10–12 of stimulation. The thickness of the endometrium does have a bearing on outcome, with optimal clinical pregnancy rates where the endometrium has a trilaminar appearance and measures between 9 and 13 mm. Nevertheless, acceptable pregnancy rates are achieved where the endometrium is between 5–8 mm and 13–18 mm. If endometrial thickness remains less than 8 mm, the dose of estrogen is commonly increased and/or changed to a transdermal preparation. In addition, Tocopherol, Pentoxyphyline and Viagra have also been used, but none of these as adjunct therapies have been shown to have convincing evidence of benefit [26]. Progesterone is started on the day the of the donor's oocyte recovery, administered either orally, trans-vaginally, intramuscularly (IM) or using a subcutaneous route. Surprisingly, according to the survey (oocyte donation survey) [25], the intramuscular route is favoured by most clinicians (74 per cent), compared to the trans-vaginal (23 per cent) and oral alternatives (3 per cent). Despite this preference there is limited evidence that one preparation is better than the other in terms of clinical pregnancy or live birth rates. From a patient perspective, the transvaginal route would appear kinder. The dose of progesterone is generally higher than that used to support the luteal phase after conventional IVF, from 100 mg daily by IM injection to 800–1200 mg transvaginally. The time the progesterone is started in relation to the donor's oocyte recovery is important and does influence outcome. Starting the progesterone on the day of the egg collection or the day after gives better pregnancy rates than starting the progesterone the day before the egg collection.

Egg Collection and Embryo Transfer

The number of oocytes each recipient will receive will vary dependent on the number of oocytes produced by the donor, and whether those are split with other recipients. This will usually be between five and 10. On the day of the donor's oocyte recovery the recipient's partner produces his sperm sample. Under normal circumstances, the method of fertilization employed should reflect the quality of the semen sample, as there is no evidence that intracytoplasmic sperm injection (ICSI) improves the live birth rates where the sperm sample is normal. However, in reality because of the unjustified fear of unexpected failed fertilization, ICSI is employed in over 55 per cent of cases [27]. Fertilization rates are generally around 70 per cent, providing the recipient with between three and seven early cleavage-stage embryos.

The timing of the embryo transfer and the number of embryos transferred are important in determining the outcome. As the implantation rate per embryo transferred is likely to be high due to the young age of the donor, transferring two embryos will substantially increase the risk of multiple births. To reduce this risk, many countries have adopted a policy of selecting the single best embryo for transfer. Statistical modelling has shown that replacing a single embryo on day 3 will reduce the overall clinical pregnancy rate, whereas this fall is not as evident when a single embryo is selected for transfer at the blastocyst stage, on day 5. Today almost all reputable programs transfer a single blastocyst. Surplus good-quality embryos that reach the blastocyst stage are cryopreserved for future use, to give the couple the chance of a genetically similar sibling. Unlike sperm donation, where sperm can be stored to help expand the family in the future, most egg donors will not go through the process of donation again, and therefore the frozen embryos may be the couple's only chance of a child with similar genetic lineage.

As the recipient has no functioning corpus luteum the pregnancy has to be sustained by hormone replacement until the placental tissue is functional, which usually occurs around 8 weeks' gestation. However, most clinicians continue both estrogen and progesterone supplements until between 10 and 12 weeks' gestation.

Success Rates

Live birth rates throughout the world mirror the success rates seen in infertile populations and vary between 30 and 50 per cent. In the UK there has been a steady improvement in live birth rates following egg donation with the HFEA statistics showing a rate of 30.8 per cent [10].

The Australian figures for 2016 show that of the 3276 initiated oocyte/embryo recipient cycles undertaken in 2016, 77.5 per cent resulted in an embryo transfer; 25.3 per cent resulted in a clinical pregnancy and 20.3 per cent in a live delivery [28].

Repeat treatment cycles offer a similar chance of conception, such that cumulative pregnancy rates after three attempts of 87 per cent are possible [29].

Although high success rates are available to those travelling to overseas programs, many of these countries have no restrictive regulation, and as such often multiple embryos are transferred increasing the likelihood of multiple gestation. Unfortunately, in Britain this has translated to a substantial increase in higher-order multiple pregnancy births in women over 40, which is almost certainly as a result of overseas egg donation programs [30].

It is imperative for those clinicians thinking about referring or helping women to travel overseas that there is a clear dialogue outlining a commitment to reduce the number of embryos transferred, to minimize multiple births.

Cost

Rules and regulations vary so much across the world that it is impossible to give an accurate assessment of the cost of treatment to the patient. In the UK, a nulliparous 35-year-old presenting with POI could attract NHS funding for up to three full treatment cycles [31]. If no state funding was available, the cost of self-funding treatment varies considerably, ranging from around €8000 to €12 000 in Europe, to between US$17 000 to US$30 000 in North America.

Possible Future Options

Ovarian Stem Cells

A new possibility for women with POI was the emergence of a publicly traded biotechnology company OvaScience. It was founded in 2011 based on scientific work done by Tilly concerning mammalian oogonial stem cells. Tilly, having pioneered the retrieval of oogonial stem cells from the ovaries of mice [32], was working on a procedure to retrieve stem cells from the ovaries of sterile women. This experiment, he hoped, would prove that ovaries have the potential to make eggs indefinitely. This defies the long-held belief that female mammals are born with all the oocytes (precursors to eggs) they will ever produce and that this population dwindles with age and the ovary is exhausted of all oocytes at the menopause [33].

Tilly's work was controversial, with some groups unable to replicate it [34].

The technique was to be commercialized by OvaScience with a process called 'OvaTure', where it would harvest oogonial stem cells from a woman, mature them into oocytes *in vitro*, and then utilize IVF technology to produce embryos for these sterile postmenopausal women.

OvaScience was unable to successfully commercialize its other product 'Augment' where mitochondria from ovarian stem cells was to be isolated and injected into the oocytes of older women during the ICSI procedure, and was absorbed by Millendo Therapeutics, in a reverse merger. The new company has no plans to proceed with the 'OvaTure' project [35], so it is unlikely that this possibility will be developed for women with POI in the foreseeable future.

References

1. Steptoe PC, Edwards RG. Birth after the reimplantation of a human embryo. *Lancet* 1978 Aug 12;2(8085):366.

2. deKretser DM, Yates C, Kovacs GT. The use of in vitro fertilization in the management of male infertility. *Clin Obstet Gynecol* 1986;12:767–73.

3. Trounson AO, Leeton JF, Wood C, Kovacs GT. The investigation of idiopathic infertility by in vitro fertilization. *Fertil Steril* 1980;34:431–8.

4. King CM, Kovacs GT. Oocyte donation: review of results. *Reprod Fertil Develop* 1992;4:719–24.

5. Trounson A, Leeton J, Besanko M, Wood C, Conti A. Pregnancy established in an infertile patient after transfer of a donated embryo fertilised in vitro. *Br Med J (Clin Res Ed)* 1983;286(6368):835–8.

6. Kovacs GT, Lording DW. Artificial insemination with donor semen – a review of 252 patients. *Med J Aust* 1980;2:609–11.

7. Conradt E, Adkins DE, Crowell SE, Raby KL, Diamond LM, Ellis B. Incorporating epigenetic mechanisms to advance fetal programming theories. *Dev Psychopathol* 2018;30(3):807–24.

8. Ferraretti AP, Goossens V, de Mouzon J, Bhattacharya S, Castilla JA, Korsak V, Kupka M, Nygren KG, Nyboe Andersen A, European IVF-Monitoring (EIM), Consortium for European Society of Human Reproduction and Embryology (ESHRE). Assisted reproductive technology in Europe, 2008: results generated from European registers by ESHRE. *Hum Reprod* 2012;27(9):2571–84.

9. De Geyter C, Calhaz-Jorge C, Kupka MS, Wyns C, Mocanu E, Motrenko T, Scaravelli G, Smeenk J, Vidakovic S, Goossens V. The European IVF-monitoring Consortium (EIM) for the European Society of Human Reproduction and Embryology (ESHRE) ART in Europe, 2014: results generated from European registries by ESHRE. *Hum Reprod* 2018;33(9):1586–1601.

10. www.HFEA.gov.uk

11. Wood C, Downing B, Trounson A, Rogers P. Clinical implications of developments in in vitro fertilisation. *Br Med J (Clin Res Ed)* 1984 Oct 13;289 (6450):978–80.

12. Sung L, Bustillo M, Mukherjee T, Booth G, Karstaedt A, Copperman AB. Sisters of women with premature ovarian failure may not be ideal ovum donors. *Fertil Steril* 1997;67(5):912–16.

13. Rodino IS, Burton PJ, Sanders KA. Donor information considered important to donors, recipients and offspring: an Australian perspective. *Reprod BioMed Online* 2011;22:303–11.

14. Kupka MS, Ferraretti AP, de Mouzon J, Erb K, D'Hooghe T, Castilla JA, Calhaz-Jorge C, De Geyter C, Goossens V, European IVF-Monitoring Consortium, for the European Society of Human Reproduction and Embryology. Assisted reproductive technology in Europe, 2010: results generated from European registers by ESHRE the European IVF-monitoring (EIM), Consortium, for the European Society of Human Reproduction and Embryology (ESHRE). *Hum Reprod* 2014;29(10):2099–113.

15. Ahuja KK, Simons EG, Fiamanya W. Egg sharing in assisted conception: ethical and practical considerations. *Human Reprod* 1996;11:1126–31.

16. Oyesanya OA, Olufowobi O, Ross W, Sharif K, Afnan M. Prognosis of oocyte donation cycles: a prospective comparison of the in vitro fertilization – embryo transfer cycles of recipients who used shared oocytes versus those who used altruistic donors. *Fertil Steril* 2009;92 (3):930–6.

17. Ahuja KK, Simons EG, Mostyn BJ, Bowen-Simpkins P. An assessment of the motives and morals of egg share donors: policy of 'payments' to egg donors requires a fair review. *Hum Reprod* 1998;13(10):2671–8.

18. Kovacs G. Oocyte collection. In: Gardner DK, Weissman A, Howles CM, Shoham Z, eds., *Textbook of Reproductive Technologies*, 5th ed. 2018. CRC Press pp. 594–601.

19. Ethics Committee of the American Society for Reproductive Medicine. Financial compensation for ovum donors. *Fertil Steril* 2007;88(2):305–9.

20. Keehn J, Holwell E, Abdul-Karim R, Chin LJ, Leu CS, Sauer MV, Klitzman R. Recruiting egg donors online: an analysis of in vitro fertilization clinics and agency websites' adherence to American Society for Reproductive Medicine guidelines. *Fertil Steril* 2012;98 (4):1995–2000.

21. www.roymorgan.com

22. www.Igenomix.com

23. Seem DL, Lee I, Umscheid CA, Kuehnert MJ, United States Public Health Service. PHS Guideline for Reducing Human Immunodeficiency Virus, Hepatitis B Virus, and Hepatitis C Virus Transmission through Organ

Transplantation. *Public Health Rep* 2013;128:247–304.

24. Shenfield F, de Mouzon J, Pennings G, Ferraretti AP, Andersen AN, de Wert G, Goossens V, ESHRE Taskforce on Cross Border Reproductive Care. Cross border reproductive care in six European countries. *Hum Reprod* 2010;25:1361–8.

25. www.IVF-Worldwide.com/survey/oocyte-donation/results-oocyte-donation.html

26. Gutarra-Vilchez RB, Bonfill Cosp X, Glujovsky D, Urrútia G. Vasodilators for women undergoing assisted reproduction. *Cochrane Database Syst Rev* 2012;7: CD010001.

27. Bhattacharya S, Hamilton MP, Shaaban M, Khalaf Y, Seddler M, Ghobara T, Braude P, Kennedy R, Rutherford A, Hartshorne G, Templeton A. Conventional in-vitro fertilisation versus intracytoplasmic sperm injection for the treatment of non male factor infertility: a randomised controlled trial. *Lancet* 2001;357 (9274):2075–99.

28. Fitzgerald O, Paul RC, Harris K, Chambers GM. *Assisted Reproductive Technology in Australia and New Zealand 2016*. 2018. National Perinatal Epidemiology and Statistics Unit, University of New South Wales Sydney.

29. Budak E, Garrido N, Soares SR, Melo MA, Meseguer M, Pellicer A, Remohí J. Improvements achieved in an oocyte donation program over a 10-year period: sequential increase in implantation and pregnancy rates and decrease in high-order multiple pregnancies. *Fertil Steril* 2007;88(2):342–9.

30. Roberts SA, McGowan L, Hirst WM, Vail A, Rutherford A, Lieberman BA, Brison DR. Reducing the incidence of twins from IVF treatments: predictive modelling from a retrospective cohort. *Hum Reprod* 2011;26(3):569–75.

31. NICE Guidelines 2013.

32. Woods DC, Tilly JL. Isolation, characterization and propagation of mitotically active germ cells from adult mouse and human ovaries. *Nat Protocol* 2013 May;8(5):966–88.

33. Gura T. Reproductive biology: fertile mind. *Nature* 2012;491:318–20.

34. Grieve KM, McLaughlin M, Dunlop CE, Telfer EE, Anderson RA. The controversial existence and functional potential of oogonial stem cells. *Maturitas* 2015;82(3):278–81.

35. https://endpts.com/once-a-multibillion-dollar-company-ovascience-ends-a-pennystock

Premature Ovarian Insufficiency

Optimizing Quality of Life and Long-Term Effects

Vujovic Svetlana, Miomira Ivovic, Milina Tančić-Gajić, Ljiljana V. Marina and Svetlana Dragojevic-Dikic

Quality of life is defined as the psychological and physical well-being depending on influences of genetic and environmental factors.

Reproduction represents the biological key point necessary for the existence of humankind during 20 million years on this planet. Adaptive mechanisms of women's bodies, influenced by many stressors, are trying to maintain homeostasis and reproductive potential. Stress develops when adaptive mechanisms are broken under the influences of too strong stressors or of too long duration [1]. Gonadal steroids, estradiol, progesterone, testosterone and others represent very important factors for maintaining homeostasis equilibrium. 'Natural' decreasing of gonadal steroids in the menopause represents the hallmark for braking mechanisms of defence and initiating many diseases leading to increased mortality rate. According to our definition, stress develops when adaptive mechanisms are broken under the influences of too strong stressors or stressors of long duration. Menopause is the 'physiological process' but, at the same time, untreated hypogonadal status triggers diseases. So, the question is: 'Shall we stand like the innocent bystanders doing nothing and waiting for consequences?!' Whenever the hypofunction of the endocrine gland exists it has to be treated immediately. Low levels of gonadal and other steroids have to be treated in order to avoid diseases. It is necessary to add all deficient hormones, not only estrogens, in order to keep homeostasis.

Definition, Aetiology

Premature ovarian insufficiency (POI) is characterized by oligo/amenorrhoea with high gonadotropin and low estradiol levels in women before 40 years of age. Follicle-stimulating hormone (FSH) cut-off value is above 40 IU/L [2] or over 25 IU/L [3] on two occasions more than 4 weeks apart. It is not 'the loss or cessation' of ovarian activity but a significant decrease. Some significantly decreased level of ovarian activity is present for the whole life and an extremely low number of follicles always remain. Possible initiation of ovarian activity depends of the complete endocrine milieu. Our goal will be to diagnose ovarian insufficiency in the very beginning, with FSH over 15 IU/L in order to initiate therapy on time.

The etiology of POI still remains an enigma for many cases. There are well-known chromosomal abnormalities, enzyme changes, autoimmune diseases, FSH receptor gene polymorphism, inhibin B mutations, rare infection diseases, etc. However, in our study on 1500 POI patients, stress was a triggering factor in 56 per cent cases. Among many stressors divorce or separation from the partner was the most prominent one.

POI and AGING

In 2009, the Nobel Prize in Physiology or Medicine was awarded to Drs Blackburn, Szostak and Greider for the explanation of how chromosomes are protected by telomere and the enzyme telomerase. Telomerase is responsible for the synthesis of chromosomal DNA ends. A significant association was found between shortening of telomerase repeats upon successive cell division, limiting viability and ending with cell death and a reduction of the replicative life span of cultured human cells, consistent with the early genetic evidence that short telomeres induce senescence. Introduction of telomerase into the normal human cells extends life span [4]. Mutations in genes encoding components of the telomerase complex cause hereditary disease characterized by defects in the stem cell renewal and tissue maintenance. Stressors triggering POI can influence telomerase and accelerate the biological clock.

In such an imbalance of homeostasis and loss of adaptive mechanism, resistance and resilience, POI is in the correlation with the inflammatory aging. Oxidative stress refers to an imbalance between oxidation and antioxidation leading to neutrophil infiltrations. Increase in interleukin 6, interleukin 8, interleukin 1 β, interleukin 10, tissue growth factor beta, interferon γ, prostaglandin E2 and decrease of tumour necrosis factor α, interleukin 2 were detected in POI. Antioxidants help organisms to fight against free radicals. They can be divided into two groups:

Enzymatic: superoxide dismutase, catalase, glutathione peroxidase, transferase, tiol disulphid oxidoreductase;

Non-enzymatic: transferin, ferritin, lactoferin, haemoglobin, lactoferrin, albumin, glutathione, ascorbic acid, A-tocopherol, ubihinon, beta-carotene, uric acid, bilirubin.

Decreased gama-glutaril transpeptide and diacron reactive oxygen metabolites were found, while C-reactive protein was increased. In POI patients DNA damage continues to accumulate leading to cell death. Autophagic cleansing capacity declines gradually. Dysfunctional protein accumulation in mitochondria increases levels of reactive oxygen species and oxidative stress [5]. Resveratrol restores ovarian function by increasing AMH and decreasing inflammation through upregulation of expression of the peroxisome proliferator-activator receptor and SIRT1 (sirtun) inhibiting interferon γ-induced inflammatory cytokines [6].

Hypoestrogenism, hypoprogesteronism and hypoandrogenism lower DHEA-S in POI and induce detrimental life events leading to increased mortality rates and premature death. Typical symptoms and signs of POI are hot flushes (narrower thermo-ventral zone), mood swings, anxiety, depression, loss of concentration, insomnia, loss of libido, dyspareunia, etc. Late complications of untreated POI are cardiovascular diseases, osteoporosis, cognitive impairment, depression, Alzheimer's disease, Parkinson's disease, etc., thus significantly decreasing quality of life and life expectancy.

Cardiovascular Diseases

William Harvey's discovery that the heart pumps blood and the blood circulates (1628) was fundamental for later understanding that gonadal steroids influence all blood vessels and organ functions, creating optimal quality of life.

Tao XY [7] found 48 per cent higher risk for ischaemic heart disease in POI patients, compared to the risk in women with the last menstruation around the age of 50 years.

Table 5.1 Mortality of cardiovascular disease in POI

Author	Location	Number	Follow-up (years)
Amagai [9]	Japan	3824	9.2
Gallagher [10]	China	267 400	9–11
Jacobsen [11]	Norway	1973	20

Ten observational studies (1966–2012) on 190 588 women with 9440 events showed that POI is an independent risk factor for ischaemic heart disease and coronary vascular disease [8]. It has been well documented that untreated women have a higher mortality rate [9, 10, 11] (Table 5.1).

Wu X in Shanghai Women's Health Study in a group of 1003 POI patients found increased risk of mortality with hazard ratio (HR) of 98 per cent, confidence interval of 1.29 [12].

Women with POI are at increased risk of cardiovascular diseases and should be informed about risk factors which they can modify through behavioural changes (stopping smoking, regulating body weight, limiting alcohol intake, controlling stressors, etc.).

Hypoestrogenism exerts effects on many levels: lipids, insulin resistance, obesity, inflammation, hypertension, vasoconstriction, endothelial dysfunction, autonomic nervous system dysfunction, nitric oxide disturbances, impaired flow-mediated dilatation [13]. Benefits of early initiation of estrogens and progestogens and menopausal hormone therapy (MHT) have been confirmed in many recent trials and in meta-analysis. The dose and type of hormones at initiation of therapy appeared crucial to obtaining coronary heart disease benefits [14].

Estrogen reduces cholesterol levels, decreases low-density lipoproteins (LDL) cholesterol levels and upregulates apolipoprotein B_{100} receptor. Small dense LDL particles, prone to oxidative damage, clear through scavenger mechanisms and become embedded in the subendothelial space. Estradiol increases high-density lipoprotein, particularly HDL_2 subfraction. It inhibits hepatic lipase activity and increases the hepatic synthesis of apolipoprotein A1, the main protein component of HD_1 and HDL_2. Oral estrogens increase triglycerides, while androgenic progestogens reduce or reverse them. Transdermal estradiol reduces triglycerides, reducing the risk of coronary heart disease (CHD). Matrix metalloproteinase normalizes vascular remodelling by estradiol therapy. Oral and transdermal estrogens and progestogens reduce activity of angioconverting enzyme (ACE) reducing cardiovascular disease. Progestogen drospirenone has antimineralocorticoid effects and influences the renin–angiotensin–aldosterone system by blocking the effects of aldosterone [15].

Estradiol therapy has antioxidative effects, by increasing levels of endothelial nitric oxide synthase and production of nitric oxide regulating blood pressure, platelet function, vascular smooth muscle proliferation and the expression of adhesion molecules. It reduces the release of endothelin 1, a potent vasoconstrictor exerting anti-inflammatory effects on blood vessels. Calcium channels are inhibited and BKCa channels stimulated by estradiol therapy inducing vasodilatation and improving arterial function, heart rate variability, baroreceptor sensitivity. It modulates arrhythmia vulnerability. Slopes are

Table 5.2 Some favourable effects of estradiol therapy in POI patients

Increased	Decreased
Vasodilatation	Vascular inflammation
Insulin sensitivity	Endothelin
Fibrinolysis	Angiotensin II, angioconverting enzyme
Hepatic excretion of apolipoprotein and LDL	Oxidative stress
Natrium excretion	Vascular hypertrophy
Lypolitic adrenalin effects	Myocardial hypertrophy
	Ventricular ectopic activity
	Adipocyte proliferation
	Orexigene peptides
	Cholesterol, LDL, Lipoprotein a, apo B
	Lipoprotein lipase transcription
	PAI
	CRP
	Cytokine, Interleukin 6
	Mitochondrial reactivity
	Oxygen species in cardiomyopathy
	Glomerular filtration rate

steeper and QT dynamics are impaired in POI. Canpolat and colleagues showed that therapy with 17 β estradiol could exert an antiarrhythmic effects by inhibition of Ca 2^+ channels [16]. In Table 5.2 most prominent effects of estradiol therapy are presented. Vascular effects show beneficial changes in vasodilation and vasoconstriction mechanisms, vascular remodelling and inflammatory cytokines. Data obtained with ambulatory blood pressure monitoring and with transdermal estradiol and drospirenone are concordant with definitively positive effects on blood pressure compared to control group.

MHT is strongly recommended and has to be initiated early, at the onset of symptoms in an adequate dose. Therapy should be continued until the average age of the natural menopause at least. According to International Menopause Society (IMS) statements, there is no time limiting for menopause hormone therapy. It has to be individually tailored, with appropriate dosages and routes of administration.

Metabolic Changes

Estradiol regulates many of the key enzymes involved in mitochondrial bioenergetics including glucose transporters, required for the regulation of glucose uptake in cells and tissues. GLUT4 is regulated by insulin receptor Akt/Tor signalling network. Disturbances in insulin metabolism in the endometrium decrease endometrium receptivity and fertility rate and trigger obesity, insulin resistance and diabetes mellitus later in life [17]. Adipocyte hypertrophy, adipose tissue inflammation, fat liver, changes of glucose uptake from the circulation, without changes in 'de novo' free fatty acid synthesis create redistribution of body fat to centripetal, metabolic type. Kulaksizoglu and colleagues found increased serum glucose, insulin homeostatis model of assessment insulin resistance (HOMA) in POI patients with hypoestrogenism [17].

Tissue resistance to insulin increases the risk of developing coronary heart disease and type 2 diabetes mellitus. Estrogen has beneficial effects on the metabolism of glycose and insulin improving insulin sensitivity. Oral estrogens have greater effects compared with transdermal estrogen. These effects can be impaired by addition of androgenic progestogens (norgestrel, medroxyprogesterone acetate), while non-androgenic progestogens do not have this unwanted effect.

Hypoestrogenism leads to weight increase of 5 kg, and redistribution of fatty tissue to more central type, leading to metabolic syndrome. MHT reverses this change of body fat distribution by increasing levels of endothelial nitric oxide synthase and production of nitric oxide.

Decreased dehydroepiandrosterone (DHEA) and dehydroepiandrosterone sulphate (DHEA-S) in POI patients result in increased ratio of cortisol to DHEA creating 'cortisol potentiated diseases': obesity, insulin resistance, diabetes mellitus type 2, osteoporosis, neurodegeneration.

Hyperinsulinism increases LH directly in the pituitary. Treating insulin resistance with metformin alters energy metabolism in cells. It lowers glucose levels by inhibiting hepatic gluconeogenesis and opposing the actions of glucagon. The primary site of metformin action is at the mitochondria. The inhibition of mitochondrial complex I of the electron transport chain induces a drop in energy charge, resulting in adenosine triphosphate (ATP) decrease. Adenosine monophosphate (AMP) increases binding of P-site adenylate cyclase enzyme and inhibition of activity leading to defective cAMP protein kinase A (CAMPK) signalling on glucagon receptors. AMPK is an energy sensor and a master coordinator of an integrated signalling network that comprises metabolic growth pathways acting in synchrony to restore cellular energy balance. It switches on the catabolic pathway that generates ATP and switches off anabolic pathways. Stimulation of 5'-AMP activated protein kinase confers insulin sensitivity, mainly by modulating lipid metabolism. Metformin increases glucose uptake in skeletal muscles. It blocks insulin receptor /R/3 K/Akt/mTOR signalling in the hyperplastic endometrial tissue inducing GLUT4 expression and inhibits AR expression [18].

Metformin suppress food intake by increasing levels of glucagon-like peptide1, interaction with ghrelin and leptin on the T-cell memory by altering fatty acid metabolism [19]. Insulin resistance with increasing LH in the menopause plays a role in adrenal tumorigenesis showing us that early detection and treatment of insulin resistance can be protective for many diseases [20].

Osteoporosis

Hypoestrogenism in POI induces excess production of the cytokine receptors activator of nuclear factor kappa β ligand (RANKL) by osteoblasts, which stimulates osteoclastogenesis and bone resorption leading to osteoporosis. Therapy with estradiol increases osteoproctogerin (OPG), secreted by osteoblasts, which inhibits RANKL [21]. The incidence of hip fracture in POI was was 9.4 per cent compared to 3.3 per cent in those starting menopause at age of 48 years [22]. Meczekalski and colleagues found that hypoestrogenism and hypoandrogenism have a deleterious effects on peak bone mass formation and bone mineral density [23]. FSH is in positive correlation with skeletal bone density. In Popat's study of 32-year-old POI patients, a significantly decreased BMR was found. In 21 per cent of patients, Z-score was −2.8, and in 67 per cent, femoral BMD Z-score was less than −1.0 [24]. Therapy with 100 ug/day of transdermal estradiol and 10 mg MPA for 10 days monthly over 3 years made no difference compared to bone mineral density in a normally cycling control group. Prompt treatment of POI with MHT prevents osteoporosis and fractures. Bisphosphonates are not indicated in POI patients.

Brain Function

Two-thirds of the brain's weight is blood vessels with receptors for estradiol, progesterone and androgens. Estradiol is involved in all brain functions and studies were done at the level of hippocampus, striatum, prefrontal cortex controlling language abilities, verbal influences, memory, sleeping, learning and evaluation processes. POI patients complain of nervousness, depression, irritability, lack of concentration, insomnia and restlessness. Luine FN and colleagues found that estradiol promotes neuronal growth, survival, transmission, myelination, neural plasticity, dendritic branching, function, synaptogenesis and improved cognitive function [25]. Bove and colleagues found cognitive decline and increased incidence of Alzheimer's diseases in women with early age at surgical menopause [26]. MHT reduces the possible risk of cognitive impairment.

Urogenital Function, Sexuality, Fertility

Vaginal dryness, painful intercourse, vulvar pruritus, burning and discomfort, recurrent urogenital infections are induced by hypoestrogenic effects on vagina, vulva, bladder, urethral epithelium and changes in pH [27].

POI patients showed worse sex performance with more pain and poorer lubrication than controls, suggesting that estrogen and testosterone therapy re-establishes epithelium cells, vaginal pH and microflora.

Changes in body shape, body image concerns, gaining weight and psychological changes may impair the sense of attractiveness. The young age and distressing impact of such a life-changing as well as symptomatic vulvo-vaginal atrophy and hypoactive sexual desire modulate central and peripheral sexual response [28]. Adequate MHT is fundamental in POI patients for normalizing sexual function. Estrogen therapy maintains vaginal elasticity and optimal length. Testosterone has an initiating role on desire and central arousal, acting on the dopaminergic tone and modulating peripheral actions as permitting factor for nitric oxide, the main mediator of clitoral and cavernosal body's congestion.

Information that oocyte donation is the only option for fertility in women with POI can make them feel shocked, devastated, worthless and confused. Is it really the truth? It is not always the only truth and we have to be more empathetic to POI patients. They should be informed that there is a small chance of spontaneous pregnancy. As well, they have to be reassured that their pregnancy will not show any higher obstetric or pathological risk than in the general population.

In menopausal women 1 year after the last menstruation about 1000 oocytes are still present in the ovaries. Some of them are of good quality but most are not. The Success rate of oocyte donation is not so high and in vitro fertilization (IVF) has to be repeated due to underdiagnosed endometrial endocrine, immunological and haematological disorders.

Van Kesteren and colleagues showed that nearly three out of four women with POI have ovarian follicles remaining in the ovary [29]. A study by Letru-Konirsch and colleagues showed that endometrium previously prepared with adequate dosages of estradiol and progesterone combined with pentoxifilline and tocopherol resulted in 30–50 per cent pregnancies with fresh embryos and 15–25 per cent with frozen-thawed embryos [30]. Conventional substitution of estradiol in POI is not sufficient for inducing dominant follicle growth and adequate endometrial responsiveness. Estradiol actions are mediated via genomic and non-genomic pathways. Estradiol receptor alfa promotes mitogenic activation and proliferation while ER β protects endometrium from undesired action of ERα.

Estradiol down-regulates FSH receptors and luteinizing hormone receptors. It increases response of FSH and the number of LH receptors previously induced by FSH. One of the important goals of estradiol therapy is to decrease the high endogenous FSH. Chronic elevation of FSH down-regulates granulosa FSH receptors. Premature ovarian insufficiency is not a failure but rather intermittent and unpredictable ovarian function that can persist for decades. Tonic elevation of LH causes premature luteinization of growing antral follicles [31]. MHT may restore FSH receptors and may enhance the ability of ovarian follicles to avoid premature luteinization.

Estradiol improves vascularization and endometrial flow, sensitizes and differentiates granulosa cells, stimulates endometrial proliferation, myometrium receptivity, production of the cervical mucus and directly influences the immune response. Estradiol receptors are expressed in various lymphoid tissue cells, lymphocytes, macrophages and dendritic cells. It decreases activated T-lymphocytes, improves autoimmunity, activates effector helper T-lymphocytes and macrophages, facilitates the maturation of pathogenic autoreactive B cells. Releasing of a few FSH receptors may diminish the autoimmune process and possibly lower the levels of autoantibodies.

The main principle of endocrinology is to replace insufficient hormones. In order to create optimal endocrine milieu for remaining follicle growth we suggested higher doses of estradiol trying to decrease FSH to 10–15 IU/L [32]. Optimal concentrations of estradiol and progesterone are crucial for early steps of embryo implantation and development. Clinical experience and higher pregnancy rates allowed us to suggest the following: In cases where for 6 months no dominant follicles were obtained with day 2 FSH 10–15 IU/L the best solution would be oocyte donation. Well-estrogenized brains of POI women allowed them to accept this solution even more bearing in mind that all other tissues are well prepared, especially the endometrium.

Bearing in mind important multiorgan effects of hyperinsulinism and especially detrimental effects on endometrium receptivity we suggest that an oral glucose tolerance test has to be routinely performed by 75 mg of glucose and glucose and insulin levels have to be measured at 30 min interval for 2 hours. HOMA index is less sensitive and specific, but the area under the curve has to be calculated in order to test insulin values during a longer period. In a case of hyperinsulinism specific diet habits and metformin therapy have to be added during the 6 month period at least prior to conception. Insulin resistance and hyperinsulinism induce obesity, increase androgen and plasminogen activator inhibitor, and decrease glycodelin, an insulin-like growth factor binding protein 1 (IGFBP 1) and uterine vascularity, decreasing endometrium receptivity.

Also, thyroid function has to be tested. Suggested TSH value is 1–2.5 mmol/L in order to prepare endometrium for embryo implantation. During any kind of therapy for the thyroid gland (hyper or hypothytroidism) TSH has to be detected once monthly. Detection of thrombophilia (Leiden V, FII, MTHFR, PAI mutations) is suggested in order to improve endometrial receptivity and prevent miscarriages. Depending on the type of thrombophilia methilfolat, aspirin is suggested. During pregnancy, depending on D-dimer, Fraxiparin has to be added.

Therapy of POI

Patients with POI must be provided with adequate information about the therapy. They should maintain a healthy lifestyle, balanced diet, physical activity, sleeping habits and avoid smoking.

Unfortunately, a study by Hipp and colleagues showed that 52 per cent of young POI patients have never taken MHT. Some of them initiated therapy many years after the diagnosis was confirmed and /or discontinued therapy before the age of 40. Such an inappropriate lack of treatment leads to complications, including increased mortality rate [33].

The aim of MHT is to achieve typical mean serum estradiol level of 100 pg/ml or 400 pmol/L. Depending on the route of administration, the following dosages are suggested: 17 β estradiol 2 mg/day; 1.25 mg of conjugate equine estrogens; ethynyl estradiol 10 μg or transdermal estradiol 75–100 μg/day. Ethynyl estradiol has a more potent effect on bone markers. It suppresses gonadotrophins profoundly. Combined oral contraceptives may be used until the expected time of the menopause [34].

The role of progestogens in POI therapy is very often limited to the effect at the level of the uterus in women with ovaries. We would like to accentuate that progesterone receptors A and B are present in all blood vessels inducing many changes from the brain to all other tissues. It balances with estrogens and imitates 'natural cycles'. The confusion was due to testing various kinds of progestogens. Today, we prefer to use natural progestogens vaginally, orally and transdermally. The National Institute of Health's study of transdermal estrogens 100 μg/day with medroxyprogesterone acetate 10 mg/day during 12 days a month showed cardiovascular risk factors decreased, including LDL levels, fibrinogen and blood pressure [35]. Micronized progesterone is superior for insulin resistance and HDL improvement.

A special issue represents adding testosterone to therapy of POI women. In reproductive years endogenous production of testosterone is 300 μg daily (50 per cent by ovaries and 50 per cent by adrenal glands). It is advised in women with hypoactive sexual desire and bilateral oophorectomy. In Europe we have 30 years' experience with testosterone gels, but the FDA has not approved such preparations in the past. After measuring serum-free testosterone, DHEA-S, it is possible to add an appropriate dose of transdermal testosterone (gel or patch). It is very important for feelings of well-being, energy and sexuality.

Other types of therapy include melatonin, DHEA and other hormones. An individualized approach is necessary and yearly hormone-level assessment is recommended in order to optimize dosages. Hormone therapy is not age limited. Previously, it was suggested to continue therapy until the age of 50 or 55 years. But, there are no rational explanations except that studies were only done until that period of life. Stopping MHT after the age of 55 sharply increases cardiovascular diseases in the first year of discontinuation. After the age of 60 transdermal therapy is preferable.

Bearing all these scientific facts in mind, POI patients receiving therapy and taking care of their lifestyle can live long, with the best quality of life.

References

1. Slijepcevic D, Stozinic S, Vujovic S. Stres i somatizacija. In: *Strucna knjiga*. 1994. Ur Vlahovic Z. Beograd.

2. Vujovic S, Brincat M, Erel T, et al. EMAS position statement: managing women with premature ovarian failure. *Maturitas* 2010;67:91–3.

3. ESHRE guideline: management of women with premature ovarian insufficiency. *Human Reprod Embriol* 2016;5:926–37.

4. Bodnar AG, Quekkette M, Frolkis AM, et al. Extension of life-span by introduction of telomerase into normal human cells. *Science* 1998;16:349–52.

5. Huang Y, Hu C, Yehaifeng, et al. InflammAging: a new mechanism affecting premature ovarian insufficiency. *J Immunol Res* 2019;2019:8069898.

6. Said S, el-Demerdash J, Tuohy VK. Autoimmune targeting disruption of pituitary-ovarian axis causes premature ovarian insufficiency. *J Immunol* 2006;3:1988–98.

7. Tao XY, Zuo AZ, Wang JQ, Tao FB. Effects of primary ovarian insufficiency and early natural menopause on mortality: a meta analysis. *Climacteric* 2016;19:27–36.

8. Van Lennep JER, Heida KV, Bots ML, Hoek A. Cardiovascular disease in women with premature ovarian insufficiency: a systematic review and meta analysis. *Eur J Prevent Cardiol* 2016;23:178–86.

9. Amagai Y, Ishikawa S, Gotoh T, et al. Age at menopause and mortality in Japan: the Jichi Medical School Cohort Study. *J Epidemiol* 2006;16:161–8.

10. Gallagher LG, Davis LB, Ray RM, et al. Reproductive history and mortality from cardiovascular diseases among women textile workers in Shangai, China. *Int J Epidemiol* 2011;40:1510–18.

11. Jacobsen BK, Heuch I, Kvale G, et al. Age at natural menopause and all-cause mortality: a 37 year follow up of 19 731 Norwegian women. *Am J Epidemiol* 2003;1(57):923–9.

12. Wu X, Cai H, Kallianpur A. Impact of premature ovarian failure on mortality and morbidity among Chinese women. *PloS ONE* 2014;9:e89597.

13. Gianini A, Genazzani AR, Simoncini T. The long-term risks of premature ovarian insufficiency. In: Genazzani AR, Tarlatszis B, Genazzani AR, eds. *Frontiers in Gynecological Endocrinology*, vol. 3, *Ovarian Function and Reproduction – from Need to Possibilities*. 2016. Springer pp. 61–6.

14. Gerval MO, Stevenson J. Establishing the risk related to hormone replacement therapy and cardiovascular disease in women. *Clin Pharm* 2017;5:7–24.

15. Archer DF, Thorneycroft IH, Foegh M. Long term safety of drospirenone – estradiol for hormone therapy: a randomized, double blind multicenter trial. *Menopause* 2005;12:716–27.

16. Canpolat U. The association of premature ovarian insufficiency with ventricular repolatization dynamics by QT dynamicity. *Europace* 2013;15:1657–63.

17. Kuylaksizoglu M, Ipeka S, Kebapcilar L, et al. Risk factors for diabetes mellitus in women with premature ovarian insufficiency. *Biol Trace Elim Rep* 2013;154:313–20.

18. Pernicova I, Korbonis M. Metforin – mode of action and clinical implications

for Diabetes and cancer. *Nat Rev Endocrinol* 2014;10:577–86.

19. Pearce EL. Enhance CD-8 T-cell memory by modulating fatty acid metabolism. *Nature* 2009;460:103–7.

20. Marina LJ, Ivovic M, Vujovic S, et al. Luteinizing hormone and insulin resistance in menopausal patients with adrenal incidentalomas: the cause–effect relationship? *Clin Endocrinol* 2018;4:541–8.

21. Boyle WJ, Simonet WS, Lacey DL. Osteoclast differentiation and activity. *Nature* 2003;423:337–42.

22. Vega EM, Egoa MA, Mautalen CA. Influence of menopausal age on the severity of osteoporosis in women with vertebral fractures. *Maturitas* 1994;19:117–24.

23. Meczekalski B, Podfigurna-Stopa A, Genazzani AR. Hypoestrogenism in young women and its influence on bone mineral density. *Gynecol Endocrinol* 2010;26:625–57.

24. Popat VB, Calis KA, Vanderhoot VH. Bone mineral density in estrogen deficient young women. *J Clin Endocrinol Metab* 2006;54:2777–83.

25. Luine VN. Estradiol and cognitive function: past, present, future. *Horm Behav* 2014;66:602–18.

26. Bove R, Secor E, Chibnik LB. Age at surgical menopause influences cognitive decline and Alzheimer pathology in older women. *Neurology* 2014;82:222–9.

27. Pacello PC, Yelc PA, Rabelo C. Dyspareunia and lubrication in premature ovarian failure using hormone therapy and vaginal health. *Clin Endocrinol* 2014;17:342–7.

28. Nappi RE, Cucinella L, Martini E, et al. Sexuality in premature ovarian insufficiency. *Climacteric* 2019;22:289–95.

29. Van Kesteren YM, Schoemaher J. Premature ovarian failure: a systematic review on therapeutic interventions to restoring ovarian function and achieve pregnancy. *Hum Reprod Update* 1999;5:483–92.

30. Letru-Kornish H, Delaian S. Successful pregnancy after combined pentoxyphilline tocopherole treatment in women with premature ovarian failure. *Fertil Steril* 2003;79:439–41.

31. Hubayler ZR, Popat V, Vanderhoof VH, et al. A prospective evaluation of antral follicle function in women with 46,XX spontaneous premature ovarian insufficiency. *Fertil Steril* 2010;94:1769–74.

32. Vujovic S, Ivovic M, Tancic Gajic M, Genazzani AR, et al. Endometrium receptivity in premature ovarian insufficiency – how to improve fertility rate and predict diseases? *Gynecol Endocrinol* 2018;12:1011–15.

33. Hipp HS, Claren KH, Spencer JF. Reproductive and gynecological care of women with fragile X premature ovarian insufficiency. *Menopause* 2010;23:993–9.

34. Baber R, Pannay N. Tenton and International menopause society writing group: IMS recommendations in women's midlife health and hormone replacement therapy. *Climacteric* 2016;2:109–50.

35. Sullivan SP, Sarrel PM, Nelson LM. Hormone replacement therapy in young women with premature ovarian insufficiency and early menopause. *Fertil Steril* 2016;100:1588–99.

Natural Hormone Replacement Therapy after Menopause by Ovarian Tissue Transplantation

Jacques Donnez and Marie-Madeleine Dolmans

The Ovary from Birth to Menopause

During fetal life, 100–2000 primordial germ cells enter a massive proliferation process and, by mid-gestation, there are several million potential oocytes. However, most (85 per cent) of them are lost prior to birth [38] (Figure 6.1). Indeed, of around 1 million oocytes per ovary at birth, only 450 go on to be used. The decline in follicle numbers extends from birth until puberty and continues throughout reproductive life, during which time around 450 monthly ovulatory cycles occur. The majority of follicles undergo atresia during their growth phase. Cyclic folliculogenesis and ovulation, associated with massive follicle atresia and aging-induced apoptosis, subsequently result in ovarian atrophy and reduced fertility [13, 38]. Poor oocyte quality, characterized by abnormalities in the meiotic spindle, chromosome misalignment and shortened telomeres, are among various mechanisms put forward to explain decreased fertility in women over 40 years of age [13, 22, 23].

Depletion of the ovarian reserve at a young age may be the consequence of medical therapy. Indeed, some cancers as well as certain benign diseases are treated by chemotherapy, often with alkylating allografting agents, considered to be the most gonadotoxic drugs [13, 15]. Ovarian surgery for severe and recurrent endometriosis is also a common cause of ovarian reserve decline, as are known risk factors for premature menopause (Turner syndrome, family history) [12, 13, 15].

At menopause, follicular density is very low. Although around 1500 primordial follicles remain, the vast majority are caspase-positive and resistant to stimulation by gonadotropins [16, 38]. According to Lobo, Amundsen and Diers, the age of menopause has changed very little over the centuries, while life expectancy has continued to climb [2, 3, 24, 27].

The Facts: Menopause and Its Symptoms

At the dawn of humanity, life expectancy rarely exceeded 35 years, so the ovary was designed to work for an entire lifetime. However, women now commonly live beyond 80 years, which somewhat changes the picture and begs the question: is it possible for natural ovaries, each containing several million oocytes at mid-gestation, to continue functioning until death? [15–16]

A better standard of living and improved health care have boosted life expectancy markedly over the last 100 years or so, from 48.3 years in 1900 to 80 years in 2000, essentially thanks to advances in public health measures and efforts. In the course of the

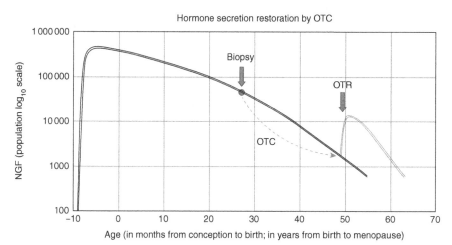

OTC: ovarian tissue biopsy and cryopreservation; OTR: ovarian tissue reimplantation;
NGF: non-growing follicles

Figure 6.1 The ovarian reserve throughout a woman's life, from conception to 55 years of age. Only around 1000 follicles remain at menopause. Donnez and Dolmans [13] propose ovarian tissue re-implantation when women reach the menopause. Ideally, their tissue should have been harvested and frozen at the age of 20–25 years. Adapted from [38], published under an open-access license by PLoS.

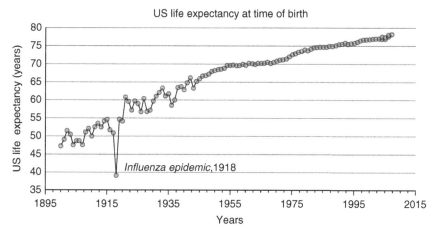

Figure 6.2 Life expectancy in the US. Based on *National Vital Statistics Reports* 58 [33].

twentieth century, despite a brief dip caused by the 1918 flu pandemic (Figure 6.2) [33], the average lifespan increased by more than 30 years (in the US and the Western world). It is predicted that 50 per cent of all girls born today will live to over 100 years of age in many parts of the world [4,5]. The consequence of this extended longevity is that much greater numbers of women will spend substantial portions of their lives in the menopause, exposing them to a high risk of diseases linked to the absence of estrogens, like cardiovascular disease and bone mineral density loss [24, 27]. Indeed, around 30–50 per cent of women aged greater than 50 years will suffer an osteoporosis-related fracture in their remaining lifetime. The medical costs of treating broken bones from osteoporosis amounts to US$18 billion a year, and loss of work adds billions more [4,5].

From an economic perspective, preventing disease is vastly preferable to having to treat it. With many major chronic diseases occurring after the menopause, the goal should be to combat them not only to extend life but also enhance its quality [24, 27]. Individualization and tailor-made medical approaches remain the key.

Does Menopause Hormone Therapy (MHT) Alleviate Menopausal Symptoms?

In the 1980s, a number of studies (including meta-analyses) suggested that MHT could be beneficial for prevention of osteoporosis, coronary heart disease and dementia, thereby cutting mortality rates. In 1992, the American College of Physicians actually recommended MHT for prevention of coronary heart disease [1]. In the early 2000s, however, several randomized trials (Women's Health Initiative [WHI] [31], Million Women Study [MWS]) indicated that the risks, including for breast cancer, outweighed any benefits. This unfortunately led to the introduction of new guidelines, resulting in a 50 per cent drop in MHT use [24]. In 2013, 10 years after the WHI, Lobo wanted to revisit the question. Reanalysing data from the original MHT trials, he concluded that women aged 50–59 years or those within 10 years of menopause showed lower rates of coronary heart disease and all-cause mortality and, notably, no increase in perceived risks, including for breast cancer [24–27]. Indeed, the relative risk for coronary heart disease was 0.65 (0.44–0.96), for breast cancer 0.76 (0.52–1.11), and for total mortality 0.78 (0.59–1.03) [25, 27] in the 50–59-year age group taking part in the conjugated equine estrogen-alone trial of the WHI. MHT is also known to decrease the incidence of menopausal symptoms and risk of bone fractures, improving quality of life. Thus, despite an increased incidence of breast cancer in women receiving estrogen-progestin therapy, overall mortality was found to be reduced, with deaths related to cardiovascular disease or osteoporosis [9].

The risk–benefit balance therefore remains positive for MHT use, with risks considered rare in healthy women aged 50–60 years, something known as the 'timing hypothesis' [25, 27]. As suggested by Lobo [26] (Figure 6.3), having already come full circle with MHT since its introduction, it is now time to implement a general prevention strategy for women approaching menopause.

Could Ovarian Tissue Re-implantation Be Considered a Form of MHT?

The literature on this topic is of course very scarce. A first paper by Callejo and colleagues [8] described a series of three patients undergoing hysterectomy and bilateral oophorectomy, followed by immediate re-implantation of ovarian cortical tissue in the abdominal wall. In this series, ovarian secretion had only a short reproductive span, so the authors concluded it was unlikely that heterotopic grafts would have the longevity to serve as an adequate substitute for MHT after natural menopause. Their conclusion was

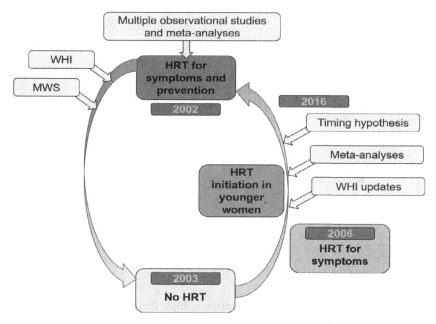

Figure 6.3 Lobo's full circle, giving rise to the timing hypothesis. Adapted from [27].

clearly wrong, because of the group of women involved, aged 45–49 years, as their ovarian reserve was already extremely depleted.

The second paper, by Kiran and colleagues, was a case report. A 44-year-old patient operated on for uterine fibroids had ovarian tissue (10 cortical strips) implanted above the rectus abdominis fascia [19]. Folliculogenesis was confirmed by ultrasound 18 months later, as were low luteinizing hormone and follicle-stimulating hormone (FSH) levels. No further details on this case could be found, however, so no conclusions could be drawn.

Duration of Ovarian Activity after Re-implantation of Frozen-Thawed Ovarian Tissue in Case of Iatrogenic Menopause

Series of Donnez and Dolmans

In this series, restoration of ovarian activity with recovery of menses occurred in 100 per cent of cases [14]. In an earlier series, ovarian function had failed to resume in three patients who were found to have no follicles in their grafted tissue [13, 14], emphasizing the importance of an intact follicular reserve. Figure 6.4 shows long-term ovarian activity in a series of five women who underwent ovarian tissue cryopreservation before the age of 22 years, followed by re-implantation some years later. Ovarian function was restored for a period of 6–7 years, as evidenced by estradiol and FSH values similar to those observed during reproductive life.

The ovaries of a newborn girl contain an average of 1 million primordial follicles, dropping to 100 000 by 20 years of age and 65 000 by 25 years [38]. Ideally, ovarian

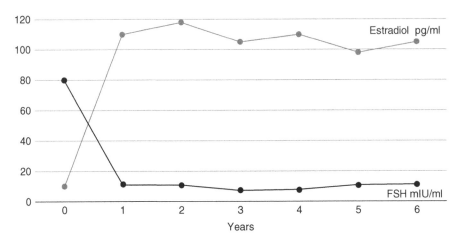

Figure 6.4 Mean estradiol and FSH values following grafting of ovarian tissue that had been biopsied and frozen when the women were less than 22 years of age. At that age, follicle density is still very high, which explains the long-term duration of ovarian function restoration.

biopsies should be taken when follicular density is high (between 20 and 25 years) because, as demonstrated by our team, ovarian function can then be restored for longer periods of time [14].

Series of Andersen and Kristensen

In a recent paper, Andersen and Kristensen reported that four patients underwent their first tissue transplantation procedure more than 10 years ago in their centre [5]. Two of the women subsequently experienced ovarian activity for a period of 6–7 years.

Series of Kim

In Kim's series, four patients aged 27–37 years had their ovarian tissue cryopreserved between 1999 and 2004 with re-implantation performed between 2001 and 2011 [17]. Ovarian tissue slices were grafted to a heterotopic site (between the rectus muscle and rectus sheath) and long-term follow-up was initiated. While recovery of ovarian function was achieved, its duration was relatively short (3–6 months), so the patients underwent a second transplantation. In one woman, low FSH and high estradiol levels proved that the graft was still functioning 7 years later. This clearly shows that if the goal is restoring ovarian function rather than fertility, a heterotopic location (forearm, abdominal wall) could be an easily accessible and effective site for re-implantation [18]. According to Kim [17, 18], there was progesterone secretion from the heterotopic grafts.

Progesterone secretion has also been documented in animal models [10, 21, 36] after autografting of vitrified ovarian tissue to heterotopic sites.

The Future

Taking biopsies from the ovary has little if any impact on fertility or age at menopause. Even removal of a whole ovary has been demonstrated to have a negligible effect, and it is now widely known that women with one ovary remain as fertile as women with both [20].

Table 6.1 Advantages of heterotopic transplantation for ovarian function restoration

Advantages
Less invasive procedure
Repeat transplantations possible
Feasible even with severe pelvic adhesions
Preferred method for restoration of ovarian function (not fertility)
Allows close monitoring for potential recurrence of malignancy in grafts

Onset of menopause is also only marginally affected in these women, who tend to start their menopause around 1 year earlier [7, 39]. We may therefore state with some degree of certainty that removal of less than 30 per cent of one ovary has a minimal impact on the ovarian reserve [15, 16].

Long-term endocrine function could well persist for more than 7 years (12 years with a repeat procedure) after frozen-thawed ovarian tissue re-implantation [16] (Figure 6.4), and consequently prevent menopause-related conditions like osteoporosis and other symptoms of estrogen deficiency [16].

Thus, having proved that ovarian tissue re-implantation is able to restore ovarian activity after induced menopause, why not use it to re-establish sex steroid secretion after natural menopause? As the goal in this case is not fertility restoration, the graft site can be heterotopic, namely outside the pelvic cavity (such as the forearm or rectus muscle) (Figure 6.5). Moreover, the procedure is potentially achievable under local anaesthesia (Table 6.1). When the implants stop working surgery may be repeated and endocrine function restored for longer. Thanks to improvements in new techniques serving to hasten revascularization, follicle loss rates may be reduced, with the benefits of grafting felt sooner and for longer periods [28].

There is no doubt that this application will become increasingly widespread in the future [15, 16].

Risks and Uncertainties

Questions surrounding possible risks and uncertainties will naturally be raised and must be adequately addressed [4, 15, 16], but some remain unresolved at present. Is progesterone actually secreted by ovarian tissue grafted to a heterotopic site? Is the endometrium adequately protected by progesterone secretion? Kim [17, 18], who has the most extensive experience in heterotopic grafting, has confirmed that progesterone secretion is similar to that observed after orthotopic grafting. Furthermore, a progesterone value of 5 mg/ml sustained for 10 days is enough to induce differentiation of the endometrium to the secretory phase, and this level is easily achieved even after heterotopic grafting. Heterotopic transplantation is not optimal for oocyte quality, but corpora lutea may still develop in heterotopic sites, as reported in several papers [11, 17, 30, 34, 35]. However, other issues are of even greater concern and need to be fully investigated [16].

Is there an increased risk of cancer after tissue re-implantation? There is no clear-cut response at this stage, but the debate should at least be opened, taking into account the

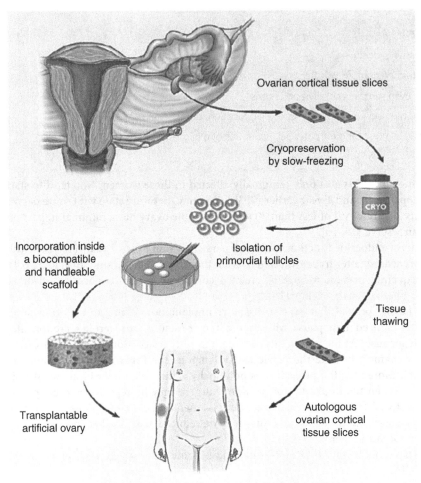

Ovarian cortical tissue slices

Cryopreservation
by slow-freezing

CRYO

Incorporation inside
a biocompatible
and handleable
scaffold

Isolation of
primordial tollicles

Tissue
thawing

Transplantable
artificial ovary

Autologous
ovarian cortical
tissue slices

Reimplantation in the forearm or abdominal cavity
for hormone restoration

Figure 6.5 Ovarian tissue freezing followed by re-implantation upon reaching menopause. Ovarian tissue may be grafted to a heterotopic site in the form of ovarian tissue strips or inside an artificial ovary containing isolated primordial follicles. Adapted from [14].

widely acknowledged benefits of HRT. Would postponing the age of menopause increase the risk of **breast cancer**? The question is certainly pertinent, but the risks attributed to HRT have been somewhat overestimated [16, 26, 32]. According to a very recent paper, the risk–benefit balance of HRT use in healthy young women aged 50–59 years or within 10 years of menopause shows lower rates of all-cause mortality, and no increase in breast cancer [27].

Ovarian neoplasms originating from ovarian tissue grafted beneath the skin or in the rectus muscle are the subject of the most heated debate related to the procedure. When evaluating the cancer risk of transplanted tissue, it is logical to compare values with those of normal intra-abdominal ovaries. However, if the biopsy was taken at the age of 20–25 years, the risk of developing ovarian cancer over a 10-year period is very low, since this risk generally increases after the natural menopause when the ovary is more than 50 years old [16]. Moreover, isolating follicles, transferring them inside a specially created scaffold (artificial ovary), and then re-implanting this scaffold in the forearm or abdominal wall (Figure 6.5) is a further strategy for avoiding the threat of ovarian cancer [16].

The Debate

If ovarian tissue freezing and re-implantation can restore ovarian hormone function in case of iatrogenic menopause, why not consider it for naturally occurring menopause [15, 16]? In response to the opinion paper by Andersen and Kristensen[4], von Wolff et al. [37] question whether it is really more advantageous for women's health than menopausal HRT. They argue that women without a uterus should be given conventional estrogen therapy, while frozen-thawed ovarian tissue transplantation may benefit patients with an intact uterus, as there is a need for progesterone. They also claim there are no studies supporting grafting of ovarian tissue as a way of postponing menopause [37].

In their subsequent response, Andersen and Kristensen [5] reiterate their central message, maintaining that an individualized approach is key and that new diagnostic tools should always be considered when choosing the type of HRT and avoiding menopausal effects. Strong family predisposition to osteoporosis, previous hysterectomy, age at menopause and a range of other factors need to be taken into account in such individually tailored therapy. There is clearly a need for clinical trials to investigate this approach, but we should bear in mind that the majority of natural estrogens are produced by the ovary itself, and not by a pharmaceutical company [15, 16].

In another letter to the editor, Patrizio and Caplan [29] reason that both medical and ethical issues must be fully addressed before this alternative can be offered as potential treatment for menopause. They stress the key moral challenge with respect to efficacy, querying the capacity of ovarian tissue harvested at a young age to maintain its 'youth' and not adapt to the actual age of the patient, ceasing to function much sooner than anticipated. We can allay such misgivings, having proved that ovarian function can be maintained for 6–7 years or more, and that the procedure, being easily repeatable (at least once), can extend ovarian activity for over 12 years [4, 14, 16].

Using of ovarian tissue transplants to provide hormones is an intriguing and exciting opportunity to both increase available options for women who require HRT and **research** some still unanswered questions. We must explore issues like minimum hormone levels needed for the ovary to maintain normal physiological functions in the uterus, bone, cardiovascular system and brain [6]. We look forward to **carefully designed and rigorously conducted studies** investigating these potential benefits and risks in the many women who have ovarian tissue stored, are on the road to recovery or in remission from their cancer, and wish to use their tissue [6].

It would indeed be very useful to have **robust** predictors of the anticipated duration of endocrine function in re-implanted, warmed cryopreserved ovarian tissue [6].

Our Reply

1. We have data proving that endocrine function can persist for more than 6 years if follicular density is high.

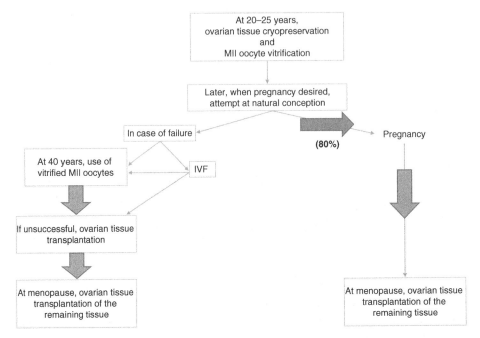

Figure 6.6 Proposal for an algorithm to preserve fertility for future conception and restore ovarian hormone secretion upon reaching menopause [16] MII: metaphase II.

2. Last year, the world celebrated the fortieth anniversary of Louise Brown's birth, the first ever IVF baby.

   PLEASE remember:

   If we had waited **for robust studies and predictors** before embarking on IVF in human beings, nobody knows if we would today be celebrating the lives of millions of babies born thanks to this technique.

Conclusion

We do of course acknowledge that there are still numerous issues that need to be satisfactorily addressed, and that animal research and human investigations should be conducted according to morally responsible and ethical standards. Nevertheless, we feel it is now time to ascertain, once and for all, whether ovarian tissue freezing at a young age followed by re-implantation at menopause could indeed be the anti-aging therapy of the future. We now have enough evidence to initiate a meaningful debate on this subject and advance further in this important field of study (Figure 6.6) [16].

References

1. American College of Physicians. Guidelines for counseling postmenopausal women about preventive hormone therapy. *Ann Intern Med* 1992;117: 1038–41.

2. Amundsen DW, Diers CL. The age of menopause in classical Greece and Rome. *Hum Biol* 1970;42:79.

3. Amundsen DW, Diers CL. The age of menopause in medieval Europe. *Hum Biol* 1973;45:605.

4. Andersen CY, Kristensen SG. Novel use of the ovarian follicular pool to postpone menopause and delay osteoporosis. *Reprod Biomed Online* 2015;31:128–31.

5. Andersen CY, Kristensen SG. Response: transplantation of ovarian tissue to postpone menopause – is it really more advantageous for women's health than menopause hormone therapy? *Reprod Biomed Online* 2015;31:828.

6. Anderson RA, Fauser B. Ovarian tissue transplantation for hormone replacement. *Reprod Biomed Online* 2018;37(3):251–2.

7. Bjelland EK, et al. Is unilateral oophorectomy associated with age at menopause? A population study (the HUNT2 Survey). *Hum Reprod* 2014;29:835–41.

8. Callejo J, et al. Long-term ovarian function evaluation after autografting by implantation with fresh and frozen-thawed human ovarian tissue. *J Clin Endocrinol Metab* 2001;86:4489–94.

9. Clemons M, Goss P. Estrogen and the risk of breast cancer. *N Engl J Med* 2001;344:276–85.

10. Damásio LC, et al. Heterotopic ovarian transplantation results in less apoptosis than orthotopic transplantation in a minipig model. *J Ovarian Res* 2016;9:14.

11. Demeestere I, et al. Orthotopic and heterotopic ovarian tissue transplantation. *Hum Reprod* 2009;15:649–55.

12. Donnez J, et al. Live birth after transplantation of frozen-thawed ovarian tissue after bilateral oophorectomy for benign disease. *Fertil Steril* 2012;98:720–5.

13. Donnez J, Dolmans MM. Fertility preservation. *Nat Rev Endocrinol* 2013;9:735–49.

14. Donnez J, Dolmans MM. Fertility preservation in women. *N Eng J Med* 2017;26:1657–65.

15. Donnez J, Dolmans MM. The ovary from conception to death *Fertil Steril* 2017;108:594–595.

16. Donnez J, Dolmans MM. Natural hormone replacement therapy with a functioning ovary after the menopause: dream or reality? *Reprod Biomed Online* 2018;37:359–66.

17. Kim SS. Assessment of long-term endocrine function after transplantation of frozen-thawed human ovarian tissue to the heterotopic site: 10 year longitudinal follow-up study. *J Assist Reprod Genet* 2012;29:489–93.

18. Kim SS. Revisiting the role of heterotopic ovarian transplantation: futility or fertility. *Reprod Biomed Online* 2014;28:141–5.

19. Kiran G, et al. Ovarian cortical transplantation may be an alternative to hormone therapy in patients with early climacterium. *Fertil Steril* 2005;84:1509.

20. Lass A. Women with one ovary have decreased response to GnRHa/HMG ovulation protocol in IVF but the same pregnancy rate as women with two ovaries. *Hum Reprod* 1997;12:298–300.

21. Lee DM, et al. Subcutaneous ovarian tissue transplantation in nonhuman primates: duration of endocrine function and normalcy of subsequent offspring as demonstrated by reproductive competence, oocyte production, and telomere length. *J Assist Reprod Genet* 2017;34:1427–34.

22. Liu L, Keefe DL. Ageing-associated aberration in meiosis of oocytes from senescence-accelerated mice. *Hum Reprod* 2002;17:267–85.

23. Liu JP, Li H. Telomerase in the ovary. *Reproduction* 2010;140:215–22.

24. Lobo RA. Where are we 10 years after the Women's Health Initiative? *J Clin Endocrinol Metab* 2013;98:1771–80.

25. Lobo RA. Reproductive endocrinology: don't be so quick to stop hormone-replacement therapy. *Nat Rev Endocrinol* 2016;12:11–33.

26. Lobo RA, et al. Back to the future: hormone replacement therapy as part of

a prevention strategy for women at the onset of menopause. *Atherosclerosis* 2016;254;282–90.

27. Lobo RA. Hormone-replacement therapy: current thinking. *Nat Rev Endocrinol* 2017;13:220–31.

28. Manavella DD, et al. Adipose tissue-derived stem cells in a fibrin implant enhance neovascularization in a peritoneal grafting site: a potential way to improve ovarian tissue transplantation. *Hum Reprod* 2018;1(33):270–9.

29. Patrizio P, Caplan AL. Forever young? The ethical challenges of using ovarian tissue transplants to treat menopause. *Reprod Biomed Online* 2015;31:132–3.

30. Rosendahl M, et al. Biochemical pregnancy after fertilization of an oocyte aspirated from a heterotopic autotransplant of cryopreserved ovarian tissue: case report. *Hum Reprod* 2006;21:2006–9.

31. Rossouw JE, Writing Group for the Women's Health Initiative Investigators, et al. Risks and benefits of estrogen plus progestin in healthy postmenopausal women: principal results from the Women's Health Initiative randomized controlled trial. *JAMA* 2002;288:321–33.

32. Sitruk-Ware R. New hormonal therapies and regimens in the postmenopause:

routes of administration and timing of initiation. *Climacteric* 2007;10:358–70.

33. Smith DW, Bradshaw BS. Variation in life expectancy during the twentieth century in the United States. *Demography* 2006;43:647–57.

34. Stern CJ, et al. First reported clinical pregnancy following heterotopic grafting of cryopreserved ovarian tissue in a woman after a bilateral oophorectomy. *Hum Reprod* 2013;28:2996–9.

35. Stern CJ, et al. Delivery of twins following heterotopic grafting of frozen-thawed ovarian tissue. *Hum Reprod* 2014;29:1828.

36. Suzuki N, et al. Assessment of long-term function of heterotopic transplants of vitrified ovarian tissue in cynomolgus monkeys. *Hum Reprod* 2012;27:2420–9.

37. von Wolff M, et al. Transplantation of ovarian tissue to postpone menopause – is it really more advantageous for women's health than menopause hormone therapy? *Reprod Biomed Online* 2015;31:827.

38. Wallace WH, Kelsey TW. Human ovarian reserve from conception to menopause. *Plos ONE* 2010;5:e8772.

39. Yasui T, et al. Factors associated with premature ovarian failure, early menopause and earlier onset of menopause in Japanese women. *Maturitas* 2012;72:249.

Migraine in the Menopause

E. Anne MacGregor

Overview

Up to 43 per cent of women and 18 per cent of men are affected by migraine at some time in their lives [1]. This sex difference is accounted for by the influence of reproductive hormones in women, with notable effects of menarche, menstruation, pregnancy, lactation, menopause and hormonal contraception on migraine. In particular, the perimenopause is a time of worsening migraine [2–4]. Despite this, migraine is significantly under-reported by women seeking management of menopause who should routinely be asked about headache [4]. Too often such women are incorrectly advised that menopause hormone therapy (MHT) is contraindicated because of migraine and so do not receive effective treatment.

Migraine

Migraine is simply defined as attacks of moderate to severe headache associated with nausea, photophobia and phonophobia which usually last between 1 and 3 days [5]. It is a fluctuating disorder with periods of remission interspersed by relapse, with women less likely to experience episodes of remission than men [6]. Migraine is a disabling condition, recognized by the World Health Organization to be the second leading cause of years lived with disability (YLDs) in all women and the leading cause in women aged 15–49 years [7].

The two principal types of migraine differ only in their presence or absence of an 'aura'. About 70–80 per cent of people with migraine experience attacks of migraine *without* aura (formerly known as common or simple migraine); 10 per cent have migraine *with* aura (formerly known as classical or focal migraine); fewer than 1 per cent of attacks are aura alone, with no ensuing headache. These phenotypes are not mutually exclusive and 15–20 per cent of people with migraine experience more than one type.

Attacks of episodic migraine occur between once a week and once a year, with a median of one per month, and with complete freedom from symptoms between attacks [8]. There is also an uncommon chronic type affecting around 2 per cent of the population, defined as headache occurring on 15 or more days per month for more than 3 months, which on at least 8 days per month have the features of migraine headache [5].

Diagnosing Migraine

Migraine without Aura

The best predictive symptoms of migraine are throbbing unilateral headache associated with nausea and disability, lasting a day. The presence of these can diagnose migraine with

Table 7.1 Screening for migraine headache

P	Pulsatile quality (headache described as pounding or throbbing)
O	One-day duration (episode of headache lasts 4–72 hours if untreated)
U	Unilateral location
N	Nausea or vomiting
D	Disabling intensity (altered usual daily activities during headache episode)

Note. Three symptoms are predictive for migraine; four symptoms are highly predictive. From [9].

a sensitivity of 95 per cent and a specificity of 78 per cent [9]. These symptoms may be remembered more easily by the mnemonic 'POUND', as in 'pounding headache' (Table 7.1).

Migraine is commonly misdiagnosed as recurrent sinus headache because of sinus fullness and frontal or facial pressure but a careful history leads to the correct diagnosis [10]. Tension-type headache is sometimes misdiagnosed as migraine but is non-pulsating and typically described by patients as a 'band-like' constriction around the head. While mild photophobia or phonophobia may be present with tension-type headaches, they lack the characteristic symptoms of nausea and disability that define migraine.

Menstrual migraine, in which attacks of migraine without aura start on or between 2 days before menstruation and the first 3 days of bleeding, in which the association between migraine and menstruation is greater than chance, affects between 20–60 per cent of women [11].

Aura

Aura is characterized by any combination of visual, hemisensory or language abnormalities, with each symptom developing over at least 5 min and lasting a maximum of 60 min. Visual aura is typically scintillating scotoma, comprising an enlarging blank spot rimmed with a shimmering edge or jagged lines affecting the same hemifield in both eyes, spreading from central to peripheral vision (Figure 7.1) [12]. As the symptoms arise from the visual cortex, they are 'seen' even with the eyes closed [13]. Less common are non-visual auras, which include spreading unilateral numbness or tingling spreading up the arm into the face and disturbed thinking or speech. If present, headache usually occurs within one hour of aura symptoms resolving. Because visual aura is the most frequent symptom, its presence can be used to screen for migraine with aura (Table 7.2) [14].

Managing Migraine

Effective treatment is dependent on correct diagnosis of migraine [15]. Triggers and predisposing factors should be reviewed and treated appropriately. Simple factors like sleep hygiene, maintaining stable blood sugar levels and avoiding dehydration can easily

Table 7.2 Screening for typical migraine with aura

Do you have visual disturbances that . . .

Start before the headache?

Last up to one hour?

Resolve before onset of headache?

Persist with your eyes closed?

Note. From [14].

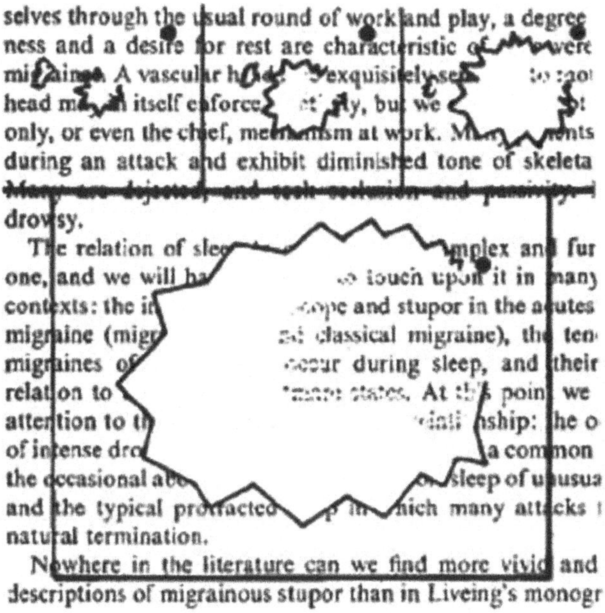

selves through the usual round of work and play, a degree
ness and a desire for rest are characteristic of ... were
migraine. A vascular head ... exquisitely se ... to not
head may in itself enforce ... ly, but we ... t
only, or even the chief, mechanism at work. M ... ents
during an attack and exhibit diminished tone of skeleta
...
drowsy.

The relation of sleep ... mplex and fur
one, and we will ha ... touch upon it in many
contexts: the i ... ope and stupor in the acutes
migraine (mig ... classical migraine), the ten
migraines of ... ccur during sleep, and their
relation to ... more states. At this point we
attention to t ... ship: the o
of intense dr ... a common
the occasional ab ... sleep of unusua
and the typical protracted ... hich many attacks
natural termination.
Nowhere in the literature can we find more vivid and
descriptions of migrainous stupor than in Liveing's monogr

Figure 7.1 Depiction of an expanding scintillating scotoma and fortification spectra by Sir William Richard Gowers [12].

be managed by lifestyle modification. Diaries are an essential aid to diagnosis and management and can help to identify any associations between migraine, menstruation, menopausal symptoms and MHT.

Symptomatic Treatment

For many women with migraine, effective attack therapy (Table 7.3) and an explanation about the probable cause of worsening migraine are sufficient [16]. Over frequent use of symptom medication, more than 2 days a week, can indicate medication overuse headache requiring drug withdrawal.

Preventive Treatment

If migraine attacks are frequent and/or acute treatment is inadequate, standard prophylactic strategies should be considered (Table 7.4) [16]. Women should be warned that complete

Table 7.3 Medication for acute treatment of episodic migraine

First line

Simple analgesics	Aspirin 900 mg
	Ibuprofen 400–600 mg
Triptans	Sumatriptan 50–100 mg

Second line (if no response to first line)

Other triptans	Almotriptan
	Eletriptan
	Frovatriptan
	Naratriptan
	Rizatriptan
	Zolmitriptan
Triptan plus NSAID combination	Sumatriptan 50–100 mg plus naproxen 500 mg

Early or persistent vomiting

Add antiemetic	Metoclopramide 10 mg
	Prochlorperazine 10 mg
Non-oral formulation of triptan	Intranasal zolmitriptan
	Subcutaneous sumatriptan

Note. Avoid codeine and other opiates. From [16].

Table 7.4 Medication for preventive treatment of episodic migraine

Drug class	Drug example	Route	Target dose
Beta blockers	Propranolol	oral	80 mg twice daily
Antiepileptic	Topiramate	oral	50 mg twice daily
	Sodium valproate[a]	oral	600 mg twice daily
Tricyclic antidepressant	Amitriptyline	oral	30–50 mg at night
Angiotensin II receptor antagonist	Candesartan	oral	16 mg daily
Calcitonin gene related peptide antagonists	Erenumab	subcutaneous injection	70–140 mg monthly
	Fremanezumab	subcutaneous injection	225 mg monthly or 675 mg three monthly
	Galcanezumab	subcutaneous injection	240 mg first month followed by 120 mg monthly

Note. From [16].
[a] Second line: contraindicated in women at risk for pregnancy.

response is unlikely; a more reasonable expectation is a 50 per cent reduction in frequency and/or severity of attacks.

Specific management strategies for continuous or perimenstrual prophylaxis are an option for women with a confirmed diagnosis of menstrual migraine. Perimenstrual prophylactic options include non-steroidal anti-inflammatory drugs (NSAIDs), estrogen, or triptans [11]. Hormonal options that inhibit ovarian activity such as continuous combined hormonal contraceptives are useful for women with menstrual migraine without aura needing contraception [11]. The desogestrel progestogen-only pill may be an option for women with migraine aura, but does not fully suppress ovarian activity. Unscheduled bleeding is a common reason for discontinuation [17].

Relationship between Migraine and Menopause

Menopause transition is associated with loss of the regular premenopause hormone cycle as the follicles respond unpredictably to rising FSH resulting in unpredictable swings in hormone levels [18, 19]. Ultimately, the ovaries resist further stimulation and menstruation ceases as estrogen and progesterone levels finally decline [20]. Evidence from several studies supports the clinical impression that these hormone changes parallel an increase in migraine prevalence during perimenopause [2]. Migraine predicts risk of vasomotor symptoms, particularly during late perimenopause, further increasing the burden of disability (Figure 7.2) [21]. Following menopause, migraine prevalence decreases over time, with low estradiol and high FSH levels predictive of lower migraine prevalence [22, 23].

Clinical observations indicate that estrogen levels affect migraine without aura and migraine in different ways. Estrogen 'withdrawal' migraine, one of the mechanisms associated with menstrual migraine, is almost invariably without aura, even in women who have attacks with aura at other times of the cycle [22]. Women with a history of menstrual migraine may be more vulnerable to exacerbation of migraine during the hormonally unstable perimenopausal period [23].

In contrast, high levels of estrogen as occur during pregnancy, with use of combined hormonal contraception, and with MHT, increase the risk of migraine aura [22]. Estrogen levels across the natural menstrual cycle also affect the phenotype of migraine, with one study finding twice the average levels of estradiol in women with migraine with aura, compared to women with migraine without aura and women without migraine [24].

Few studies have addressed differences in endogenous testosterone levels in women with and without migraine. A case control study of postmenopausal women participating in a mammography screening program matched each of 15 women with migraine to three controls by body mass index and by time since menopause [25]. None of the women were taking estrogen replacement therapy. No statistically significant differences were found in serum levels of androstenedione, total testosterone or free testosterone between women with and without migraine.

However, while hormone fluctuations play a significant role in migraine in women, non-hormonal triggers are still the most important factors initiating migraine attacks, with hormonal factors either being additional or altering the 'threshold' to migraine

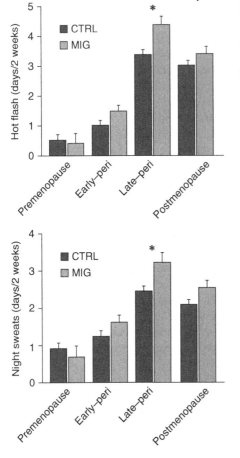

Figure 7.2 Vasomotor symptoms and migraine according to menstrual status. Adjusted mean vasomotor symptoms. Displayed are the mean values predicted by the fixed effects of the model for the migraine groups (control [CTRL] vs migraine [MIG]) at different menstrual status stages for frequency of hot flashes and night sweats. These are covariate adjusted means, specifically means estimated at the grand means of other covariates in the model. Asterisks indicate $p < 0.05$ (p-values are adjusted for multiple pairwise post hoc tests using the Tukey method). The bar heights represent the average estimated values, and the error bars represent the standard error associated with each estimate. Peri = perimenopause. Reproduced with permission from [21].

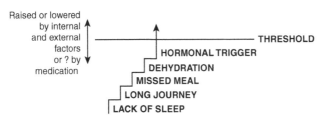

Figure 7.3 The threshold theory of migraine. Reproduced from [26].

(Figure 7.3) [26]. This is relevant in managing expectations of treatment since, even in women with a strong hormonal pattern of migraine, effectively managing the hormonal trigger is unlikely to eliminate migraine as non-hormonal factors remain unaffected.

Type of Menopause

Improvement in migraine is more likely to occur following spontaneous menopause while surgical menopause can result in worsening migraine [27, 28].

In a cross-sectional study, 1436 Chinese women aged 40–54 years with migraine were classified into five categories of menopausal status: premenopause, early perimenopause, late perimenopause, natural menopause, and surgical menopause [23]. Women were classified as: premenopause if they had regular menstruation; early perimenopause if menstrual cycles were irregular (cycles less than 23 days or more than 35 days) or varied by more than 5 days during the preceding 3 months; late perimenopause if menstrual bleeding had occurred between 3 and 12 months prior to the study; natural menopause if last menstruation was more than 12 months prior to the study; surgical menopause if they had undergone hysterectomy and/or bilateral oophorectomy before natural menopause. The prevalence of migraine was similar in premenopausal and perimenopausal women (16.7 per cent) and lower in the spontaneous menopausal women (10.5 per cent) (OR 0.6; [95 per cent CI 0.4 to 0.9], $p = 0.03$). Among all menopausal groups, the highest migraine prevalence was seen in women who had had hysterectomies (27 per cent). Low estradiol levels and high FSH levels predicted lower migraine prevalence.

Hysterectomy appears to have an adverse effect on migraine even when the ovaries are retained. A Dutch cross-sectional population questionnaire survey of 986 hysterectomized women with one or both ovaries and 5636 non-hysterectomized women with both ovaries present found that 15.1 per cent of hysterectomized women with ovarian retention reported moderate to severe migraine compared with 8.8 per cent of the non-hysterectomized women ($p < 0.001$) [29].

Effect of Systemic MHT on Migraine

Two large studies have reported increased prevalence of migraine in women using MHT compared to non-users (Table 7.5) [30, 31]. Both suggest that overall, women using MHT have a higher risk of migraine compared to never-users. Limited data suggest that tibolone has a more favourable effect on migraine than estrogen-progestogen HRT (Table 7.6) [32].

Estrogen

Regimen

Sequential estrogen, 21 days of treatment followed by a 7-day break, increases the risk of migraine (Table 7.6) [33]. Such breaks can result in estrogen 'withdrawal' migraine, which is more likely to affect postmenopausal women with a history of menstrual migraine [22, 34]. As the break is also associated with return of vasomotor symptoms, sequential estrogen regimens should be abandoned in favour of continuous estrogen.

Route of Delivery

Oral estrogen replacement therapy is associated with greater risk of migraine than non-oral routes of delivery [35, 36]. Peak plasma estradiol levels vary considerably with dose and route of delivery, with large inter- and intraindividual variations in serum concentrations [37]. Such fluctuations in exogenous estradiol levels increase the risk of migraine, particularly when coupled with the fluctuating endogenous estrogen levels associated with the perimenopause [18, 19]. Transdermal or percutaneous routes are associated with more stable estrogen levels at physiologic doses.

Table 7.5 The effect of menopausal hormone therapy on migraine: users versus never-users

Study	Study design	Sample size	Migraine prevalence	HRT use	Odds ratio (95% CI) current vs never-users
Women's Health Study [30]	Population-based questionnaire	17 107 postmenopausal women	11.2% reported migraine headaches within the preceding year, of which 73% fulfilled modified IHS diagnostic criteria for migraine	38.5% never-users 61.5% current users	All HRT 1.42 (1.24–1.62); estrogen-only 1.39 (1.14–1.69); estrogen-progestogen 1.41 (1.22–1.63)
Nord-Trøndelag Health Study [31]	Cross-sectional questionnaire	5507 postmenopausal women	12.5% never-users, 14.4% past users, 18.3% current (local or systemic) users	57% never-users 43% current users (26% past use, 20% current local estrogen, 54% current local systemic HRT)	All HRT 1.6 (1.4–1.9); estrogen-only 1.7 (1.4–2.0); combined estrogen-progestogen 1.7 (1.2–2.4)

Note. IHS = International Headache Society.

Table 7.6 The effect of different types of HRT on migraine following natural menopause

Study	Study design	No. of women	Age (years)	Duration of observation	HRT	Outcome
Nappi et al. [36]	Open-label, randomized, parallel group study comparing transdermal E2 vs oral CEE cyclical combined HRT	30	50.7 ± 3.1	7 months: 1 month run-in; 6 months treatment	Cyclical combined transdermal: 50 mcg E2 patches weekly plus 10 mg MPA days 15–28	No change
					Cyclical combined oral: 0.625 mg CEE daily plus 10 mg MPA days 15–28	Increased frequency of attacks ($p < 0.000$) Increased days with headache ($p < 0.000$) Increased analgesic use ($p = 0.001$)
Facchinetti et al. [33]	Open-label, non-randomized, parallel group study comparing oral regimens of continuous combined vs cyclical combined vs sequential combined	33	51.1 ± 1.9	7 months: 1 month run-in; 6 months treatment	Continuous combined oral: 1 mg E2 plus 0.5 mg NET daily	In all three subgroups: increased attack frequency ($p < 0.001$), severity ($p < 0.001$), days with headache ($p < 0.001$), and analgesic use ($p < 0.001$); shorter attack duration ($p = 0.005$)
					Cyclical combined oral: 0.625 mg CEE daily plus 10 mg MPA days 15–28	
					Sequential combined oral: 2 mg E2 days 1–21 plus 1 mg cyproterone acetate days 12–21; no treatment days 22–28	Continuous combined regimen best tolerated; sequential combined worst tolerated

Table 7.6 (cont.)

Study	Study design	No. of women	Age (years)	Duration of observation	HRT	Outcome
Nappi et al. [32]	Open-label, randomized, parallel group study oral continuous combined vs tibolone	40	E2/NET group: 52.4 ± 1.3 Tibolone group: 52.8 ± 1.4	7 months: 1 month run-in; 6 months treatment	Continuous combined oral: 1 mg E2 plus 0.5 mg NETA daily 2.5 mg tibolone daily	Increased days with migraine headache ($p < 0.001$) Increased analgesic use ($p < 0.001$) No change in days with migraine headache Reduced severity ($p < 0.001$) Reduced analgesic use ($p < 0.001$)

Note. E2 = estradiol. CEE = conjugated equine estrogens. MPA = medroxyprogesterone acetate. NA = not applicable. NETA = norethisterone acetate.

These differences likely account for the increase in migraine seen in women using oral versus transdermal estrogen replacement therapy (Table 7.6) [36]. Hence transdermal estrogen preparations are preferred for women with migraine.

Type and Dose of Estrogen

In the Women's Health Study, univariate analyses suggested that conjugated equine estrogens in doses of 0.625 mg/day or higher were significantly associated with increased reporting of migraine compared to lower doses but this association was lost with multivariate and age-adjusted analyses [30].

Tailoring treatment is particularly difficult for perimenopausal women as too high a dose, coupled with surges of endogenous estrogen, can trigger migraine aura, as well as causing symptoms of estrogen excess including nausea, fluid retention, breast tenderness and leg cramps. A study of 10 women starting 50 μg transdermal estrogen patches reported that six women with a history of migraine (three migraine with aura, three migraine without aura) prior to using MHT developed increased headache severity and accompanying visual aura [38]. One patient with no previous history of migraine developed aura without headache. Withdrawal of estrogens and additional prophylactic migraine therapy led to marked improvement in all women, with complete resolution of migraine in four patients. A similar development of aura associated with use of MHT was reported in a series of case studies with no further aura following reduction in estrogen dose [39].

Progestogen

Regimen

The regimen of progestogen is also important, as migraine appears to be more of a problem with cyclical progestogens than with continuous combined regimens (Table 7.6) [33].

Route of Delivery

There are no published studies regarding the effects of route of delivery of progestogens on migraine.

Type and Dose of Progestogen

Headache is commonly reported as an unwanted side effect of progestogen treatment, particularly with testosterone derivatives such as norethisterone [40]. There are no data specifically regarding the effects on migraine of either oral, transdermal or intrauterine progestogens or of oral or vaginal progesterone used adjunctively with estrogen for MHT. From a practical perspective, women using estrogen patches needing progestogen may find it easier to use combined estrogen-progestogen patches than patches with daily oral or vaginal progestogens. For perimenopausal the levonorgestrel intrauterine system has obvious advantages providing contraception with endometrial protection and management of bleeding.

Testosterone

Only three studies have addressed the effects of testosterone replacement on women with migraine.

Table 7.7 Preferred MHT for women with migraine

Hysterectomy		Continuous estrogen patches or gel
Uterus intact		
	Premenopause	Continuous estrogen patches or gel plus LNG-IUS
	Postmenopause	Continuous combined estrogen/ progestogen patches
		Continuous estrogen patches or gel plus micronized progesterone

Note. Use lowest dose of estrogen to control vasomotor symptoms.

Moehlig, writing in 1955, noted that 49/60 (81 per cent) of women with migraine (age not reported) reported 'relief' from migraine following treatment with methyltestosterone 10 mg daily for the first 4 weeks, followed by 10 mg alternate days for 8 weeks and subsequently 10 mg every third day [41].

In 1974, Greenblatt and Bruneteau recognized the benefits of stable hormone levels achieved with hormone implants [42]. They reported that more than twice as many of their patients responded to an androgen-estrogen (150 mg testosterone plus 25 mg estradiol) than to estrogen-androgen regimen (75 mg testosterone plus 50 mg estradiol), estrogen only (50–100 mg estradiol) or androgen only (150–225 mg testosterone) implant regimens.

Only one study is recent, a pilot study of 100–160 mg testosterone implants in 16 pre- and 11 postmenopausal (natural or surgical) women [43]. By 3 months of treatment, 92 per cent of women reported a significant improvement in migraine, with no difference between premenopausal and postmenopausal groups. None of the postmenopausal women were using estrogens.

Implications for Practice

The preferred regimen for women with migraine is transdermal estrogens in the lowest dose to control vasomotor symptoms, taken continuously (Table 7.7). Progesterone or progesterone derivatives are the preferred progestogens, also used continuously. Limited data are suggestive of testosterone benefit on migraine.

Management of Vulvo-vaginal Atrophy

In the Head-HUNT study, in contrast to systemic combined or estrogen-only MHT, local estrogen was not associated with a significant increased risk of migraine (OR, 1.3; 95 per cent CI, 0.9–1.7) [31]. This is anticipated, since low doses of vaginal estrogens are not absorbed systemically. There are no data regarding oral Ospemifene or intravaginal prasterone (dehydroepiandrosterone) on migraine.

Migraine and Ischemic Stroke

Meta-analyses conclude that migraine without aura is not associated with an increased risk of ischemic stroke in women, while migraine with aura is associated with an

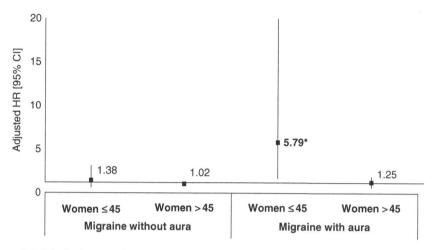

Figure 7.4 Risk of ischemic stroke in women based on age and type of migraine. Migraine ($n = 119\,017$) vs no migraine control ($n = 119\,017$). *$p < 0.01$. Based on data from [46].

approximately 2–fold increased risk [44]. Smoking and use of contraceptive estrogens further increase the risk [45].

Risk also appears to be modulated by age, with the highest risk in young women with migraine with aura (Figure 7.4), decreasing with increasing age as other major risk factors for stroke such as hypertension, hypercholesterolemia and diabetes increase in prevalence [46].

Two studies have addressed the risk of ischemic stroke in women with migraine using MHT. The Women's Health Initiative study did not detect increased risk of ischemic stroke [47], while the Oxford Vascular Study (OXVASC), a population-based cohort study found a non-significant trend towards increased risk of cryptogenic events [48].

Hence, in contrast to contraceptive estrogens, migraine aura does not contraindicate use of estrogen replacement therapy [49].

Alternatives to MHT for Women with Migraine

For women in whom estrogen is contraindicated, a number of alternative treatment option are available (Table 7.8). Clonidine is licensed for both migraine prophylaxis and management of menopausal hot flushes. There is also evidence to support the efficacy of the selective serotonin reuptake inhibitors (SSRIs) escitalopram and paroxetine, and the selective noradrenaline reuptake inhibitor (SNRI) venlafaxine for management of migraine and vasomotor symptoms but women should be warned that these drugs must be tapered slowly to reduce the risk of withdrawal symptoms [50]. Non-drug strategies with evidence to show benefit on both migraine and vasomotor symptoms include weight loss, exercise and cognitive behavioural therapy.

Table 7.8 Non-hormonal management of migraine and vasomotor symptoms

Prescription medication			
Alpha-adrenergic agonist	Clonidine	50–150 mcg/day	Licensed for migraine prophylaxis and menopause flushing
			Antihypertensive
SNRI	Venlafaxine	37.5–150 mg/day	Unlicensed
			More evidence of efficacy for migraine
SSRIs	Escitalopram	10–20 mg/day	Unlicensed
			Better tolerated than venlafaxine
	Paroxetine	20–40 mg/day	Unlicensed
			Better tolerated than venlafaxine
			Avoid concomitant use with tamoxifen

Note. SNRI = selective noradrenaline reuptake inhibitor. SSRI = selective serotonin reuptake inhibitor.

Conclusions

Women should be informed that while the menopause transition can be a time of worsening migraine, it is likely to improve with increasing time following menopause. Both women with and without migraine aura can use menopausal hormone therapy, preferably continuous transdermal estrogens in the lowest dose to control vasomotor symptoms. If progestogens are necessary, progesterone or derivates are the preferred oral hormone, otherwise transdermal patches or, if contraception is required, the levonorgestrel intrauterine system. Limited data suggest testosterone may have a favourable effect on migraine. If hormone therapy is contraindicated, non-hormonal medication and lifestyle changes can be recommended.

References

1. Stewart WF, Wood C, Reed ML, et al. Cumulative lifetime migraine incidence in women and men. *Cephalalgia* 2008;28 (11):1170–8.

2. Ripa P, Ornello R, Degan D, et al. Migraine in menopausal women: a systematic review. *Int J Women's Health* 2015;7:773–82.

3. Martin VT, Pavlovic J, Fanning KM, et al. Perimenopause and menopause are associated with high frequency headache in women with migraine: results of the American Migraine Prevalence and Prevention Study. *Headache* 2016;56 (2):292–305.

4. MacGregor EA, Barnes D. Migraine in a specialist menopause clinic. *Climacteric* 1999 Sep;2(3):218–23.

5. Headache Classification Committee of the International Headache Society (IHS). The International Classification of Headache Disorders, 3rd edition. *Cephalalgia* 2018 Jan;38(1):1–211.

6. Bille B. A 40-year follow-up of school children with migraine. *Cephalalgia* 1997;17:488–91.

7. Vos T, Abajobir AA, Abate KH, et al. Global, regional, and national incidence, prevalence, and years lived with disability for 328 diseases and injuries for 195 countries, 1990–2016: a systematic analysis for the Global Burden of Disease Study 2016. *Lancet* 2017 Sep 16;390 (10100):1211–259.

8. Steiner TJ, Scher AI, Stewart WF, et al. The prevalence and disability burden of adult migraine in England and their relationships to age, gender and ethnicity. *Cephalalgia* 2003 Sep;23 (7):519–27.

9. Michel P, Dartigues JF, Henry P, et al. Validity of the International Headache Society criteria for migraine. GRIM. Groupe de Recherche Interdisciplinaire sur la Migraine. *Neuroepidemiology* 1993;12(1):51–7.

10. Schreiber CP, Hutchinson S, Webster CJ, et al. Prevalence of migraine in patients with a history of self-reported or physician-diagnosed 'sinus' headache. *Arch Intern Med* 2004 Sep 13;164 (16):1769–72.

11. MacGregor EA. Migraine management during menstruation and menopause. *Continuum* 2015 Aug;21(4):990–1003.

12. Gowers WR. Subjective sensations of sight and sound, abiotrophy, and other lectures. In: *Lectures on Diseases of the Nervous System*, 2nd series. 1904. J & A Churchill pp. 18–41.

13. MacGregor EA. Diagnosing migraine. *J Family Plann Reprod Health Care* 2016 Oct 1;42(4):280–6.

14. Russell MB, Olesen J. A nosographic analysis of the migraine aura in a general population. *Brain* 1996 Apr;119(Pt 2):355–61.

15. Steiner TJ, Jensen R, Katsarava Z, et al. Aids to management of headache disorders in primary care (2nd edition): on behalf of the European Headache Federation and Lifting the Burden: the Global Campaign against Headache. *J Headache Pain* 2019 May 21;20(1):57.

16. Network SIG. Pharmacological management of migraine. SIGN Publ 155. 2018. www.sign.ac.uk

17. Sacco S, Merki-Feld GS, Aegidius KL, et al. Effect of exogenous estrogens and progestogens on the course of migraine during reproductive age: a consensus statement by the European Headache Federation (EHF) and the European Society of Contraception and Reproductive Health (ESCRH). *J Headache Pain* 2018 Aug 31;19(1):76.

18. Hale GE, Hughes CL, Burger HG, et al. Atypical estradiol secretion and ovulation patterns caused by luteal out-of-phase (LOOP) events underlying irregular ovulatory menstrual cycles in the menopausal transition. *Menopause* 2009 Jan–Feb;16(1):50–9.

19. Miro F, Parker SW, Aspinall LJ, et al. Sequential classification of endocrine stages during reproductive aging in women: the FREEDOM study. *Menopause* 2005 May–Jun;12(3):281–90.

20. Su HI, Freeman EW. Hormone changes associated with the menopausal transition. *Minerva Ginecol* 2009 Dec;61 (6):483–9.

21. Maleki N, Cheng YC, Tu Y, et al. Longitudinal course of vasomotor symptoms in perimenopausal migraineurs. *Ann Neurol* 2019 Jun;85 (6):865–74.

22. MacGregor EA. Oestrogen and attacks of migraine with and without aura. *Lancet Neurol* 2004 Jun;3(6):354–61.

23. Wang SJ, Fuh JL, Lu SR, et al. Migraine prevalence during menopausal transition. *Headache* 2003 May;43 (5):470–8.

24. Nagel-Leiby S, Welch KM, Grunfeld S, et al. Ovarian steroid levels in migraine with and without aura. *Cephalalgia* 1990;10(3):147–52.

25. Mattsson P. Serum levels of androgens and migraine in postmenopausal women. *Clin Sci (Lond)* 2002 Nov;103 (5):487–91.

26. MacGregor EA. 'Menstrual' migraine: towards a definition. *Cephalalgia* 1996 Feb;16(1):11–21.

27. Cupini LM, Matteis M, Troisi E, et al. Sex-hormone-related events in migrainous females: a clinical comparative study between migraine with aura and migraine without aura. *Cephalalgia* 1995 Apr;15 (2):140–4.

28. Neri I, Granella F, Nappi R, et al. Characteristics of headache at menopause: a clinico-epidemiologic study. *Maturitas* 1993 Jul;17(1):31–7.

29. Oldenhave A, Jaszmann LJ, Everaerd WT, et al. Hysterectomized women with ovarian conservation report more severe climacteric complaints than do normal climacteric women of similar age. *Am J Obstet Gynecol* 1993 Mar; 168(3 Pt 1):765–71.

30. Misakian AL, Langer RD, Bensenor IM, et al. Postmenopausal hormone therapy and migraine headache. *J Womens Health (Larchmt)* 2003 Dec;12(10):1027–36.

31. Aegidius KL, Zwart JA, Hagen K, et al. Hormone replacement therapy and headache prevalence in postmenopausal women: the Head-HUNT study. *Eur J Neurol* 2007 Jan;14(1):73–8.

32. Nappi RE, Sances G, Sommacal A, et al. Different effects of tibolone and low-dose EPT in the management of postmenopausal women with primary headaches. *Menopause* 2006 Sep–Oct;13 (5):818–25.

33. Facchinetti F, Nappi RE, Tirelli A, et al. Hormone supplementation differently affects migraine in postmenopausal women. *Headache* 2002;42(9):924–9.

34. Lichten EM, Lichten JB, Whitty A, et al. The confirmation of a biochemical marker for women's hormonal migraine: the depo-estradiol challenge test. *Headache* 1996 Jun;36(6):367–71.

35. MacGregor A. Effects of oral and transdermal estrogen replacement on migraine. *Cephalalgia* 1999;19:124–5.

36. Nappi RE, Cagnacci A, Granella F, et al. Course of primary headaches during hormone replacement therapy. *Maturitas* 2001 Apr 20;38(2):157–63.

37. Kuhl H. Pharmacokinetics of oestrogen and progestogens. *Maturitas* 1990;12:171–97.

38. Kaiser HJ, Meienberg O. Deterioration or onset of migraine under oestrogen replacement therapy in the menopause. *J Neurol* 1993;240(3):195–6.

39. MacGregor A. Estrogen replacement and migraine aura. *Headache* 1999;39:674–8.

40. Palacios S, Mejia A. Progestogen safety and tolerance in hormonal replacement therapy. *Expert Opin Drug Saf* 2016 Nov;15(11):1515–25.

41. Moehlig RC. Methyl testosterone for migraine of women; report of sixty cases. J Mich *State Med Soc* 1955 May;54 (5):577–9.

42. Greenblatt RB, Bruneteau DW. Menopausal headaches – psychogenic or metabolic? *J Am Geriatr Soc* 1974 Apr;22 (4):186–90.

43. Glaser R, Dimitrakakis C, Trimble N, et al. Testosterone pellet implants and migraine headaches: a pilot study. *Maturitas* 2012 Apr;71(4):385–8.

44. Kurth T, Chabriat H, Bousser MG. Migraine and stroke: a complex association with clinical implications. *Lancet Neurol* 2012 Jan;11(1):92–100.

45. Sacco S, Merki-Feld GS, Ægidius KL, et al. Hormonal contraceptives and risk of ischemic stroke in women with migraine: a consensus statement from the European Headache Federation (EHF) and the European Society of Contraception and Reproductive Health (ESC). *J Headache Pain* 2017 Oct 30;18 (1):108.

46. Peng KP, Chen YT, Fuh JL, et al. Migraine and incidence of ischemic stroke: A nationwide population-based study. *Cephalalgia* 2017 Apr;37(4):327–35.

47. Pavlovic J, Hedlin H, Yang J, et al. The relationship between migraine, cardiovascular disease (CVD) and hormone therapy (HT) in

postmenopausal women in the Women's Health Initiative study (WHI) [abstract]. *Menopause* 2017;12:1429.

48. Li L, Schulz UG, Kuker W, et al. Age-specific association of migraine with cryptogenic TIA and stroke: population-based study. *Neurology* 2015 Oct 27;85(17):1444–51.

49. Stuenkel CA, Davis SR, Gompel A, et al. Treatment of symptoms of the menopause: an Endocrine Society Clinical Practice Guideline. *J Clin Endocrinol Metab* 2015 Nov;100(11):3975–4011.

50. MacGregor EA. Migraine, menopause and hormone replacement therapy. *Post Reprod Health* 2018 Mar;24(1):11–18.

Psychological Aspects of the Menopause

Myra S. Hunter

The menopause – the last menstrual period – takes place within a gradual process of physiological change, but also concurrently with age and developmental changes, and within varied psychosocial and cultural contexts. Psychological perspectives on menopause include the meanings of menopause, appraisals and attributions of symptoms to menopause, as well as cognitive, affective and behavioural reactions to the menopause. Assessment and psychological interventions will be described with particular reference to depression, anxiety, sleep and vasomotor symptoms – hot flushes and night sweats.

The relationships between menopause, hormone changes and psychological distress have troubled clinicians and researchers alike over the centuries, and women have been subject to a range of generally unhelpful and sometimes punitive treatments, including prolonged bed rest, application of leaches and gynaecological surgery. Polarized views and theories from psychoanalytic (bereavement of loss of reproductive capacity) to biomedical (estrogen deficiency) have resulted in very different treatments being offered to women depending upon where they seek help. Fortunately, today, the accumulation of anthropological and epidemiological research and prospective studies provide clear evidence that a biopsychosocial understanding provides the way forward in understanding these complex mind–body relationships. A biopsychosocial perspective will be described in relation to understanding menopausal depression in the following sections on assessment and treatment, but first what does the literature tell us about the roles of psychological and social factors on women's experience during the menopause?

The Psychosocial Context

Anthropological and cross-cultural studies have challenged the concept of the menopause as a universal phenomenon with wide variations in the symptom perception and reporting in women from different ethnic origins, living in different countries. Cultural explanations of these differences need to include lifestyle (diet, exercise), social factors, as well as reproductive patterns, which can affect biological processes, population differences in biology, as well as beliefs and attitudes to the menopause and the social status of mid-aged and older women. In other words, this is a bio-psycho-socio-cultural process, which may vary within and between cultures and change over time.

The menopause is generally perceived as a time of poor emotional and physical health in Western societies, and attitudes to the menopause are influenced by social and cultural assumptions about older women. Nevertheless, anthropological studies show how menopause can be a neutral or positive event, particularly when it signifies a change in social status and /or circumstances. Much of the early research that influenced the Western view of the menopause was based on clinic samples of women who had actively sought treatment for health problems. Women attending menopause clinics have more health problems, life stresses and low mood than those who do not, as well as differing beliefs about the menopause, so it is important not to generalize these presentations to the experience of women in general. Cultural attitudes and meanings of menopause may also influence women's expectations and perceptions of symptoms. For example, menopause in many developing countries tends not to be regarded as a medical problem and thus might be accepted, with less focus on 'symptoms' and more as a natural part of life. There are cultural differences in the attributions of different types of symptoms to the menopause. For example, in a study of Asian women living in the UK and in Delhi, visual changes (becoming short sighted in middle age) were often attributed to the menopause, as well as weight gain and high blood pressure. Such attributions could result in these women not receiving the most appropriate health care.

In Western societies women tend to be valued for their physical and sexual attractiveness, reproductive capacity and youthfulness, and the menopause is often associated with emotional and physical symptoms, ageing and uncertainty. In a systematic review of the evidence, Ayers and colleagues [1] concluded that there is a relationship between beliefs and attitudes held before the menopause and actual experience. For example, two prospective studies show that overly negative attitudes before menopause predict depressed mood and hot flushes during the menopause, suggesting that negative attitudes towards menopause can affect symptom experience – a self-fulfilling prophecy.

Menopause and Mood

Determining the precise relationship between menopause and mood has been a difficult area to research because of methodological challenges (defining menopausal stages, measurement of mood and confounding factors of age and social changes). Longitudinal studies have been designed in order to address these issues. The main findings from these studies suggest that the menopause transition is not necessarily associated with psychological symptoms in healthy women. Therefore, depressed mood should not be attributed automatically to the menopause transition. Past depression is the main predictor of depressive symptoms and depressive disorder [2] during the menopause and psychosocial factors are also highly relevant. Age is another strong predictor in that low mood is more prevalent during mid-age; psychological distress tends to rise during adulthood to middle age before declining and levelling off in old age, and after the menopause women generally report improvements in mood.

Two studies demonstrate the relationships between mood, life-stage, psychosocial factors and menopause. First the 'Household Survey for England Study' of men and women ($N = 94\,879$) investigated age bands from 16 to 84 and assessed the prevalence of psychological distress (using the 12-item General Health Questionnaire) as well as psychiatric diagnosis and use of psychiatric medications [3]. The authors examined the impact of age and gender on prevalence of common mental illness, and then studied these relationships by socioeconomic status (income).

The results show the increase during mid-life and also the expected gender differences – women reporting more distress and common mental illness than men (Figure 8.1); however, when the sample was divided on the basis of income a different picture emerged. For both men and women, the mid-life increases in distress applied only to the lower

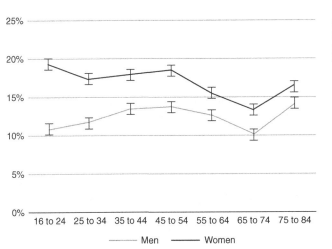

Figure 8.1 Midlife peak in common mental disorders: prevalence of high GHQ scores by gender and age.

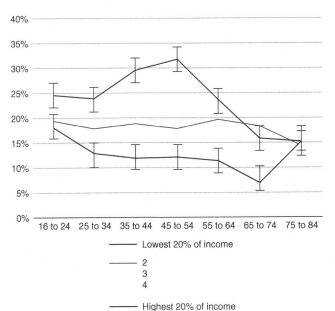

Figure 8.2 Prevalence of high GHQ scores for women by age and income.

income groups (bottom 20 per cent of the income groups) (the results for women are shown in Figure 8.2). These findings are consistent with other data showing that financial and social pressures may lead to increased stress in other areas of life.

The second study by Mishra and Kuh [4] reported provides detail on specific changes that occur for women across the menopause transition. For most women psychological symptoms generally tend to stay the same, with some increases and decreases, across the menopause transition (Figure 8.3). However, there is a proportion of women, estimated to be about 9–10 per cent, who may be at a higher risk of mood changes during the transition to menopause. However, this increase in psychological symptoms tends to

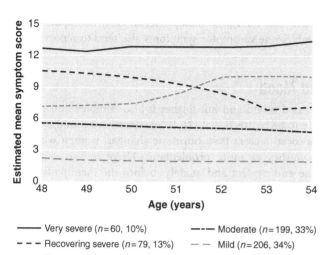

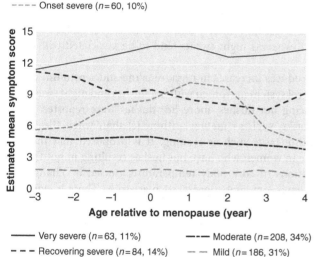

Figure 8.3 Profiles of psychological symptoms across midlife and according to age relative to menopause. Reproduced with kind permission from BMJ Group from [4].

decrease during the postmenopause, i.e. for most, it is relatively short-lived. Factors found to be associated with psychological symptoms and depressed mood during the menopause transition include: past history of psychological problems, social factors, educational and occupational status, poor health, stressful life events, body mass index (BMI), cigarette smoking, attitudes to menopause and ageing, and early life circumstances and experiences. Psychological symptoms may also be associated with beliefs about menopause, which can affect self-esteem, vasomotor symptoms, as well as coincidental psychosocial stresses and changes. There is no clear evidence that hormonal changes predict psychological symptoms during the menopause transition, but some women present to clinics with tension, anxiety and low mood, which appears to be similar to premenstrual symptomatology; premenstrual symptom reporting is also a predictor of psychological distress reported during menopause. These women may have a sensitivity to hormonal changes which renders them to be more at risk of psychological distress during the perimenopause. Women who have had a surgical menopause, an early menopause and those who have chronic and troublesome vasomotor symptoms also tend to report more psychological symptoms.

Vasomotor Symptoms and Mood

The relationship between depressed mood and hot flushes is also complex and recent evidence suggests that it is likely to be bidirectional [2]. While depressed mood is more strongly associated with psychosocial factors than hormone changes, women who are depressed tend to report hot flushes as more problematic. There is also evidence suggesting that childhood abuse and neglect and anxiety, before the menopause, are associated with the presence and the severity of hot flushes – women with moderate or high anxiety levels being three to five times more likely to report hot flushes than women in the normal anxiety range. There is likely to be an interaction whereby vasomotor symptoms can lead to sleep problems, tiredness and low self-esteem, which can in turn result in low mood; conversely feeling depressed or overly anxious might lead to overly negative appraisals of vasomotor symptoms and unhelpful coping strategies. Hot flushes are also associated with general stress and anxiety and can themselves result in social embarrassment and discomfort, whereas night sweats tend to be associated with sleep problems and tiredness.

We also know that stress produces increases in noradrenaline and serotonin, which may affect the temperature control system in women with hot flushes and night sweats. In one study of women experiencing hot flushes, more hot flushes were reported when women were doing stressful tasks, such as mental arithmetic, than when they were involved in calm or non-stressful tasks such as reading. It is proposed that there is a narrowed thermoneutral zone in women who have hot flushes resulting in hot flushes being triggered by small elevations in core body temperature, caused by changes in ambient temperature or other environmental triggers, such as stress. There is evidence from animal research that the thermoneutral zone is narrowed by elevated brain nor-epinephrine. This physiological model provides a framework with which to understand the role of hormonal and psychological factors upon hot flushes and night sweats.

A biopsychosocial model of hot flushes and night sweats, developed by Hunter and Mann [5], describes how a range of psychological factors might influence the perception and appraisal of hot flushes and night sweats, as well as behavioural reactions to them. Day to day, if we are occupied or our attention is focused on something specific, we are usually less likely to notice physical symptoms. Conversely, if we closely monitor or focus on a part of the body, we tend to notice sensations that we would normally be unaware of. Depressed mood and negative beliefs about hot flushes and night sweats (e.g. 'when I have a hot flush every one will stare at me', or 'if I have a night sweat I'll never get back to sleep') are associated with problematic or bothersome hot flushes and night sweats. Interestingly, it is this 'problem-rating', rather than frequency of hot flushes, that is strongly associated with quality of life and help-seeking, and consequently a measure of hot flush problem-rating is recommended as an important clinical outcome measure in clinical trials [5].

A Biopsychosocial Approach

What do we need to know to understand the factors that might be important in an individual case?

Assessment

A clinical interview should include a full medical and psychosocial history, including past history of depression, psychological symptoms, help-seeking, etc. However, a key aspect of a biopsychosocial assessment is to understand the patient's beliefs and understandings of the causes and influences on her symptoms. 'You must have thought a lot about this – what factors do you think have influenced why you feel this way?' Explore what was happening around the time that the symptoms started – prompting for hot flushes, night sweats, menstrual changes, but also looking out for psychosocial changes. Commonly women say 'nothing was happening really', but stresses accumulate during mid-life and if explored in more detail it is not uncommon that women will describe numerous roles, and stresses (family relationships, work worries, financial problems are common); if then menopausal symptoms are added to the list they can be the last straw that tip the balance into depressed mood or anxiety. It can be useful to draw a time line of the onset of depression, hot flushes and night sweats and any other events in order to make sense of their possible interactions. Writing down possible influences on the biopsychosocial model (Figure 8.4) can be helpful, acknowledging that stress and biological factors often interact. Diaries can be useful to record hot flushes and night sweats and mood so that any patterns can be discussed at a subsequent appointment.

Personality factors, typically used coping strategies, and past depression can be explored by asking if/when she has felt this way before and how does she generally cope when she feels low. For example, a woman might respond to these questions as follows:

> I was depressed about five years ago when I had an accident and had back pain for two months – I was frustrated and found it difficult not being able to do things and not being in control. I first noticed feeling low this time when the night sweats started – I couldn't sleep and it was a time when my job was really demanding so it was hard to cope. Over time I kept trying to put on a brave face and pretended that everything was fine but I started to be irritable with my husband and work colleagues, as I just felt more out of control and tired. When I woke at night I began to have thoughts that I was useless. I've always been the life and soul of the party and people won't like me if I'm miserable. I cope now by avoiding people and staying out of the way in bed. I catch up on sleep in the day, but feel very alone and hopeless about life.

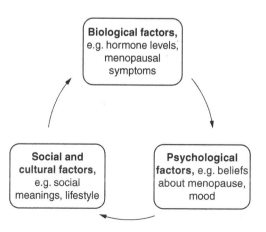

Figure 8.4 A biopsychosocial model of factors influencing experience of the menopause.

When asked about her thoughts about menopause in general, she said that she had tended to think that after the menopause women were in danger of 'letting themselves go', and that anything could happen, so she was concerned about the impact of menopause upon her own well-being and ability to function.

From this interview the biopsychosocial model could be completed by inserting:

- Night sweats into the biological section;
- Self-critical thoughts (beliefs that she should be in control and life and soul of the party or otherwise people won't like her), worries about the menopause, and unhelpful behaviours (avoidance and sleeping in the day) in the psychological section, and
- Work stress in the social section.

The possible influences and the relationships between her mood, sleep and night sweats and her thoughts and feelings would be discussed. Evidence-based treatment options for depression would include exercise (for mild to moderate depression), cognitive behaviour therapy, and antidepressants [2, 6]. Hormone therapy could also be offered to treat troublesome night sweats. Our patient may opt for non-medical treatment because she is wary of side effects and wants to be in control. She may be offered a course of cognitive behaviour therapy (CBT) for her mood and to help her to manage her sleep and night sweats.

Cognitive Behavioural Interventions for Menopausal Symptoms

What Is CBT?

Cognitive behaviour therapy, literally thinking (cognitive) and behaviour therapy, is a structured, collaborative and time-limited intervention. CBT was initially developed in the 1960s and 1970s by Aaron Beck, who noticed that emotional distress and unhelpful behaviours in his anxious and depressed patients were preceded by specific patterns of thinking. CBT offered a pragmatic and practical approach to emotional problems, such as anxiety and depression, and over the past few decades CBT has been applied to range of mental health and physical health problems with positive outcomes.

CBT for Depression

CBT is currently one of the major treatments for depression. When people are depressed, they tend to think more negatively about themselves and the world in general – it is as if their mood state takes them into a depressive and more negative thinking state. This can also happen to people who would normally think quite differently when they are not depressed. CBT can help people to identify overly negative thoughts, so that they can gain a perspective on their concerns and gradually learn how to manage these thoughts. Depressive thinking and behaviour can lead to a cycle of self-criticism and hopelessness, and many people often withdraw and avoid situations and feel worse as a result. To combat this tendency, early on in CBT treatment patients are encouraged to gradually reengage in activities that they previously valued and enjoyed but which they have withdrawn from since becoming depressed. This 'behavioural activation' and developing a structure to the day can help to initially lift mood. However, the overall aims of CBT are led by the patient, in order to be consistent with the individual's beliefs and values; an important part of the therapy is to enable people to value their own qualities, strengths and competencies.

CBT for Anxiety

The CBT model of anxiety disorders identifies 'anxious thinking', such as predicting the worst possible outcomes or viewing situations as unnecessarily threatening, as contributing to and maintaining anxiety. For people with social anxiety, this can mean assuming that others will have negative thoughts about them in social situations and, as a result, sufferers are likely to avoid these social occasions. People with panic disorder tend to misinterpret anxiety symptoms, such as hyperventilation and increased heart rate, as being signs of imminent disaster. They believe that they might have a heart attack or faint, and this belief leads to increased arousal. People with *health anxiety* (a term that replaced *hypochondriasis*) tend to misinterpret benign or normal physical sensations as signs of serious disease and become overly worried about their health. If health anxiety becomes chronic, people can repeatedly undergo hospital investigations or even unnecessary treatments. CBT approaches anxiety by examining how anxious thinking tends to 'catastrophize' or overestimate the likelihood of the worst-case scenario happening. CBT includes cognitive therapy for these beliefs and encouragement to systematically approach feared situations to learn that the expected consequences do not arise. Anxiety is a normal reaction, but it becomes problematic when benign and non-dangerous situations and events are regularly perceived as threats.

CBT for Sleep Problems

There is consistent evidence that CBT can help people to develop better sleeping habits (behaviours) and to tackle the worries about sleep and daytime performance that can keep people lying awake at three in the morning. Essentially, worry about not sleeping increases physiological arousal and therefore wakefulness. As a result, sleep is less likely to occur. Keeping a regular sleep schedule and not sleeping in the daytime is encouraged, as is a wind-down period before bed-time. In general, CBT delivered in groups or on a one-to-one basis has helped people to understand these patterns of thinking and behaviour, and to make changes, which reduce wakening as well as increase sleep time, sleep efficiency and sleep quality; and these improvements tend to be maintained. In a recent study, telephone-delivered CBT was found to reduce sleep problems in peri-and postmenopausal women with hot flushes and insomnia [7].

CBT for Vasomotor Symptoms

A cognitive behavioural intervention for hot flushes and night sweats, which includes relaxation, paced breathing and cognitive behaviour therapy, has been developed and evaluated in different formats (one-to-one with a psychologist, in groups of six to eight women, as a self-help booklet, and online) by comparing these forms of CBT with no treatment or usual care [8–12]. The CBT is based on the theoretical model [5] and has been found to be effective in randomized controlled trials for women going through the menopause transition (MENOS2 [8] and MENOS@Work [12] trials). CBT is also effective for women who have hot flushes and night sweats following breast cancer treatment (MENOS1 [9] and EVA [10, 11] trials of group and online CBT), for whom few effective treatment options exist that are safe and free from side effects.

The main elements of the CBT for hot flushes and night sweats include:

- Psycho-education about hot flushes and menopause
- Monitoring HFNS, identify precipitants
- Calm diaphragmatic breathing for stress and hot flushes and night sweats
- Cognitive therapy for stress and beliefs about hot flushes and menopause
- Behavioural experiments and strategies
- CBT for night sweats and sleep.

Group and self-help formats (book and CD) of the CBT were both equally effective in reducing problematic hot flushes and night sweats [8] and had additional benefits to mood and quality of life. The self-help guide (booklet format) used over a 4-week period was found to be as effective as four 2-hour weekly sessions of group CBT. In a recent study of working women [12] it was effective without health professional support, which makes the intervention more widely available for women. The treatment has been recommended by the North American Menopause Society as an effective non-hormonal treatment option for women with troublesome vasomotor symptoms [13]. It is available as a self-help book [14] and is manualized so that trained health professionals can deliver the group CBT [15]. The effect of CBT tends to be mediated mainly by changes in beliefs, and to a lesser extent by improvements in mood and sleep [16]. After treatment women typically report improved coping (using information, calm breathing and strategies) and a restored sense of control, and experienced beneficial changes, such as increased confidence, which extended beyond their menopausal symptoms [17].

Returning to the example above, a course of CBT for depression, night sweats and sleep might include:

- Behavioural activation to help her to structure her day and to start to engage in more (pleasant or neutral) activities
- CBT and problem-solving for managing and reducing stress at work
- CBT for sleep and night sweats – learning to schedule sleep times, to deal with problems in the day, to have a wind-down time, not nap and take exercise in the day time, and to manage night sweats using paced breathing, calm thoughts and an automatic routine to cool down and return to bed
- Cognitive therapy focusing on depressive thoughts, on her self-beliefs (I should be the life and soul of the party; I must be in control), her beliefs about others (people won't like me if I am not the life and soul of the party) and her beliefs about menopause

Summary

Women's experience of the menopause transition is influenced by psychosocial factors, such as past depression, past anxiety, life stresses, negative beliefs and expectations about menopause, as well as socioeconomic factors. There are bidirectional relationships between vasomotor symptoms and mood, and some common causal pathways for these symptoms. A biopsychosocial model is advocated for assessment as is a multidisciplinary approach to treatment for women with troublesome symptoms during the menopause transition. Cognitive behaviour therapy is an effective non-medical treatment option for depression, anxiety, sleep problems and for hot flushes and night sweats.

References

1. Ayers B, Forshaw M, Hunter MS. The impact of attitudes towards the menopause on women's symptom experience: a systematic review. *Maturitas* 2010;65:28–36.

2. Maki PM, Kornstein SG, Joffe H, et al. Guidelines for the Evaluation and Treatment of Perimenopausal Depression: summary and recommendations. *J Women's Health* 2019;28(2). doi 10.1089/jwh.2018.27099.

3. Lang IA, Llewellyn DJ, Hubbard RE, et al. Income and midlife peak in common mental disorder prevalence. *Psychol Med* 2011;41 :1365–72.

4. Mishra GD, Kuh D. Health symptoms during midlife in relation to menopausal transition: British prospective cohort study. *BMJ* 2012;344:e402.

5. Hunter MS, Mann E. A cognitive model of menopausal hot flushes. *J Psychosom Res* 2010;69:491–501.

6. National Institute for Health and Clinical Excellence (NICE). Depression: the treatment and management of depression in adults (update). 2009. www.nice.org.uk/guidance/CG90

7. McCurry SM, Guthrie KA, Morin CM, et al. Telephone-based cognitive behavioral therapy for insomnia in perimenopausal and postmenopausal women with vasomotor symptoms: a MsFLASH randomized clinical trial. *JAMA Internal Med* 2016;176:913–20.

8. Ayers B, Smith M, Hellier J, et al. Effectiveness of group and self-help cognitive behavior therapy in reducing problematic menopausal hot flushes and night sweats (MENOS 2): a randomized controlled trial. *Menopause* 2012;19:749–59.

9. Mann E, Smith MJ, Hellier J, et al. Cognitive behavioural treatment for women who have menopausal symptoms after breast cancer treatment (MENOS 1): a randomised controlled trial. *Lancet Oncol* 2012;13:309–18.

10. Duijts SF, van Beurden M, Oldenburg S, et al. Efficacy of cognitive behavioral therapy and physical exercise in alleviating treatment-induced menopausal symptoms in patients with breast cancer: results of a randomized, controlled, multicenter trial. *J Clin Oncol* 2012;30:4124–33.

11. Atema V, van Leeuwen M, Kieffer JM, et al. Efficacy of internet-based cognitive behavioral therapy for treatment-induced menopausal symptoms in breast cancer survivors: results of a randomized controlled trial. *J Clin Oncol* 2019;37:809–22.

12. Hardy C, Griffiths A, Norton S, Hunter MS. Self-help cognitive behavior therapy for working women with problematic hot flushes and night sweats (MENOS@ Work): a multicenter randomized controlled trial. *Menopause* 2018;25:508–19.

13. North American Menopause Society (NAMS). Position statement: non-hormonal management of menopause-associated vasomotor symptoms. *Menopause* 2015;22:1–20.

14. Hunter MS, Smith M. *Managing Hot Flushes and Night Sweats: A Cognitive Behavioural Self-Help Guide to the Menopause*. 2014. Routledge.

15. Hunter MS, Smith M. *Managing Hot Flushes with Group Cognitive Behaviour Therapy: An Evidence Based Treatment Manual for Health Professionals*. 2014. Routledge.

16. Norton S, Chilcot J, Hunter MS. Cognitive behaviour therapy for menopausal symptoms (hot flushes and night sweats): moderators and mediators of treatment effects. *Menopause* 2014;21(6):274–8.

17. Balabanovic J, Ayers B, Hunter MS. Cognitive behaviour therapy for menopausal hot flushes and night sweats: a qualitative analysis of women's experiences of group and self-help CBT. *Behav Cogn Psychother* 2013;41(4):441–5.

Memory and Mood in the Menopause

Michael C. Craig

Previous studies have reported that the menopause is associated with deterioration in memory and mood in some women. Also, a significant body of research suggests that hormone 'replacement' therapy (HRT) – now referred to as menopausal hormone therapy (MHT) – specifically with estrogen, may act as a *prophylaxis* against the risk for developing Alzheimer's disease (AD) and a *treatment* for perimenopausal depression. The precise nature, and biological basis, of this relationship is still not fully understood. However, it probably involves a complex interaction between genes, the environment and the mode and timing of MHT prescription. Increasing our understanding of the interplay between these factors during the menopause may permit us to target more specific treatments to vulnerable individuals. Furthermore, it offers a window of opportunity to understand the putative role of estrogen in psychiatric disorders at other times of the reproductive cycle. The current chapter will focus on the role of estrogen on Alzheimer's disease and depression during the menopause.

Alzheimer's Disease

By the year 2050 it has been estimated that 30 per cent of the population in Western Europe will be over the age of 65 and as many as 10 per cent will have Alzheimer's disease (AD) [1]. Also, mild cognitive impairment (i.e. a preclinical stage of AD) has an estimated prevalence of 20–30 per cent in elderly people [2]. Dementia currently costs the UK health care system approximately £17 billion per year and is predicted to reach £35 billion within 20 years [3]. The social and economic implications of this are greatest among women because their life expectancy, and risk of developing AD, are greater than for men [4]. However, it has been calculated that *if* severe cognitive impairment could be reduced by 1 per cent per year, this would cancel out the estimated increases in the long-term health care costs [5], as well as reducing the significant emotional costs. Studies into the effects of HRT on AD risk and/or prevention have been conflicting.

Support for the protective effect of sex hormones on cognitive impairment and AD has come both from studies into the negative effects of early surgical oophorectomy, prior to the onset of menopause, and the positive effects of MHT prescribed post-menopause. In the former category it has been reported, for example, that oopherectomy before 49 years of age is associated with a significant increased relative risk of dementia, and this risk increased the earlier the age of oophorectomy [6]. Furthermore, the risk disappeared if women were prescribed MHT until at least 50 years of age. Case control and cohort studies have also reported a reduced relative risk of AD in postmenopausal women treated with MHT, compared with never-users. Meta-analyses of these studies suggested that the relative risk was reduced by up to 34 per cent [7]. Importantly, most of these studies were carried out in the US, at a time where typical clinical practice was to prescribe MHT from the perimenopause until around 60 years old [8]. More recently this practice has been postulated to be particularly significant. For example, a prospective observational study reported that although HRT initiated early postmenopause protected against AD, that hormonal treatment initiated after the age of 60 years did not [4]. Furthermore, in a large multicentre randomized controlled study (RCT) (the Women's Health Initiative Memory Study), women over 65 years old randomized to MHT (with medroxyprogesterone acetate) had an increased risk of 'all-cause' dementia compared with the placebo group [9]. This finding is supported by a recent nationwide case control study from Finland [10], which reported a 9–17 per cent increased risk of developing AD in women prescribed, respectively, estrogen-only or estrogen plus progestin HRT. However, there was no increased risk reported in women prescribed MHT prior to the age of 60 for less than 10 years and the absolute risk in all women was small (i.e. 9–18 extra cases per 10 000 women per year).

In summary, these studies suggest that MHT prescribed to older women may have a small neutral or negative effect, particularly if it is combined with a progestin. However, MHT prescribed at a 'critical period' around the time of menopause (particularly postsurgical menopause in younger women) may be associated with a neutral or reduced risk of dementia in later life. Larger, appropriately powered RCTs are still needed to test the 'critical period' hypothesis further. The primary difficulty in designing such studies is the long delay between randomization and development of (or protection against) symptoms of dementia.

A compromise to this obstacle is to study the effects of MHT on cognitive markers for subsequent AD, including *verbal episodic memory* [11]. However, two recent double-blinded, placebo-controlled clinical trials designed to analyse the effects of MHT on cognitive function following prescription during the critical period did not detect *any* significant cognitive benefits. The first was the ancillary arm of the Kronos Early Estrogen Prevention Study (KEEPS), the Cognitive and Affective Study (KEEPS-Cog). This analysed the cognitive (and mood) effects of *transdermal* 17β-estradiol (50 mcg/day) or low-dose *oral* CEE (0.45 mg/day) + cyclical *oral* progestogen started within the first 3 years of *natural* menopause (average age 53 years). The study reported the absence of treatment-related cognitive benefits following a mean length of follow-up of 2.85 years [12]. The second study, the Early versus Late Intervention Trial with Estradiol (ELITE), analysed the effects of *oral* 17β-estradiol (1 mg/day) ± cyclical *vaginal* progesterone on cognition in women <6 years (i.e. Early Intervention, average age 55 years old) or >10 years (i.e. Late Intervention) postmenopause. The trial reported the absence of an effect of HRT on verbal memory, executive function or global cognition in either group [13].

Currently, the likelihood of an adequately powered RCT being funded to study the relationship between AD risk following prescription of MHT to younger women is low [14]. However, current evidence suggests that those requiring short-term MHT to treat significant perimenopausal symptoms should, at the very least, be reassured that there are no longer-term risks of therapy on cognitive function.

Depression

Major depressive disorder is the leading cause of disease-related disability among women worldwide [15]. Furthermore, later life depression in women increases cardiovascular mortality by 50 per cent [16]. Also, there is increasing evidence that fluctuation in reproductive hormones, such as at the time of the perimenopause, increases the risk of a major depressive episode in some women [17–26]. The biological basis of this risk is probably multifactorial. However, most of the evidence, albeit not all, suggests that it is predominantly driven by effects of estrogen on the brain. Recently, a double-blind RCT involving euthymic women in perimenopause, or early postmenopause, found that only 17.3 per cent of those randomized to transdermal 17β-estradiol (100 µg), and intermittent micronized progesterone, developed clinically significant depressive symptoms, compared with 32.3 per cent of women in the placebo group [27]. In addition to a protective effect, some studies have also reported that estrogen may have an antidepressant effect in perimenopausal women. For example, a 6-week RCT of 34 women with perimenopausal depression (major and minor) reported that 17β-estradiol (50 µg daily) was associated with a significant improvement in mood compared with placebo [28]. These findings were replicated in a 12-week double-blind RCT of 17β-estradiol (100 µg daily) in 50 women with perimenopausal depression (major/minor) or dysthymic disorder [29]. Furthermore, these results were still significant at the 4-week follow-up. Consequently, some doctors in the UK prescribe sex hormones as the first line of treatment in women with reproductive depression [30–34]. Nevertheless, the biological evidence to support this approach is limited and prescription for clinical depression (i.e. as defined by the *Diagnostic and Statistical Manual of Mental Disorders, Fifth Edition* (DSM–V) or the *International Statistical Classification of Diseases and Related Health Problems, Tenth Revision* (ICD–10)) in this patient group remains controversial. Studies are required that directly compare the effects of estradiol, preferably in the form of an implant, patch or gel (i.e. to avoid the effects of first-pass metabolism) with antidepressant medication and/or cognitive behaviour therapy (CBT).

It is outside the scope of this chapter to comprehensively review earlier basic science and animal studies into these mechanisms, but these can be found elsewhere [35]. Instead the remainder of the chapter will focus on some of the recent *in vivo* techniques that have been used to study the neurobiological mechanisms that underpin estrogen's effects on the brain over the menopause.

Neurobiological Mechanisms

Estrogen is a steroid hormone synthesized by aromatization of androgenic precursors (i.e. androstenedione and testosterone). Naturally occurring estrogens include, in order of potency, 17β-estradiol, estrone and estriol. Estradiol is mainly produced by ovarian granulosa and theca cells and is the predominant form of estrogen found in premenopausal women. Research in ovarectomized rhesus monkeys has recently demonstrated that estradiol can also be produced *directly* by neurons [36]. This finding suggests a novel role for 'neuroestrogen' as a neurotransmitter.

Estradiol mainly exerts its effects by binding to two intracellular estrogen receptors (ERs), ERα and ERβ [37]. However, subsequent modulation of brain function includes an interaction with a number of neurotransmitter systems [38, 39]. This interaction has been studied *indirectly* using neuroendocrine challenge tests and, more recently, more *directly* using *in vivo* brain imaging.

Neuroendocrine Studies

This early *in vivo* technique provided an indirect method to explore the effects of estrogen on neurotransmitter systems important to memory, AD and mood in the menopause. Studies have reported modulatory effects on MHT on the cholinergic, serotonergic and dopaminergic systems.

Cholinergic System

Many different lines of research have highlighted the importance of the cholinergic system in learning and memory. Perhaps the oldest hypothesis into the cause of AD is the 'cholinergic hypothesis' [40, 41], which proposed AD is caused by reduced cholinergic system activity. The role of the cholinergic system in mood is less understood. However, depressed mood has been reported to be associated with hypercholinergic neurotransmission which, paradoxically, may be mediated through excessive neuronal nicotinic receptor activation [42]. We have reported that postmenopausal women on long-term MHT (i.e. initiated at around the time of menopause) had greater responsivity to pyridostigmine challenge of the cholinergic system (measured by growth hormone response) than never-users. Furthermore, amongst long-term MHT users there was a significant positive correlation between response and duration of estrogen exposure [43].

Dopaminergic System

Dopamine has an important role in mood [44] and memory [45]. Previous studies have reported that the response to dopaminergic challenge is increased in women taking the combined oral contraceptive pill [46], during phases of the menstrual cycle associated with high estrogen [47] and on the fourth day postpartum in women at risk of puerperal psychosis compared with controls [48]. We have also reported greater responsivity to dopaminergic challenge, with apomorphine, in postmenopausal women on long-term MHT compared with never-users [49]. Furthermore, most women in the MHT arm had commenced treatment immediately post-hysterectomy and bilateral oophorectomy during the 'critical period'.

Serotonergic System

The serotonergic system plays a key role in mood and memory [50]. Greater responsivity (relative to MHT never-users) to serotonergic challenge (e.g. to d-fenfluramine) has also been reported in young postmenopausal women (mean age 49 years old) following short-term MHT [51] and in older women (mean age 60 years old) following long-term MHT [43]. In the latter study, women had been prescribed MHT for a mean of 13 years (i.e. starting around the time of menopause), suggesting that in both studies women received treatment during the 'critical period' immediately postmenopause.

In summary, neuroendocrine challenge studies suggest that MHT prescribed around the time of menopause is associated with greater responsivity of several neurotransmitter systems that are central to memory, AD and mood. However, these studies have several shortcomings. First, they were all observational, cross-sectional studies and although groups were matched (e.g. for age and IQ), it is possible that findings were still confounded by other factors (e.g. the 'healthy user bias') [52]. Second, neuroendocrine studies only provide an indirect method for analysing the effects of MHT on receptor responsivity at the hypothalamic–pituitary axis. Thus, they are not informative about the effects of HRT on brain regions that are more critical to AD and mood (e.g. prefrontal cortex and hippocampus).

The development of *in vivo* brain imaging techniques, however, has led to a more direct approach to studying the effects of HRT on brain structure and function and contributed to significant recent advances in our understanding of the effects of HRT on the brain.

In Vivo Brain Imaging Studies

Early studies into structural integrity of neural tissue in postmenopausal women using structural magnetic resonance imaging (sMRI) reported that MHT had a neutral effect on grey and white matter volumes [53–55]. Others, including our group, have found that compared with never-users, MHT has positive effects on regional grey and white matter concentrations [56–58]. This has included modulation of brain regions that are known to be important in memory and mood. For example, studies have reported atrophy of the hippocampus, prefrontal cortex and medial temporal lobe regions (e.g. amygdala) following *chronic* depression and/or stress [59]. Furthermore, atrophy of these same regions is also associated with memory impairment. A consistent finding reported in sMRI studies postmenopause has been that HRT users had regional sparing of grey matter in prefrontal regions [56, 60] and the hippocampus [56, 58]. It has also been reported that MHT users had sparing of white matter in medial temporal lobe regions [56]. Furthermore, white matter hyperintensities (a putative marker of brain aging) have been reported to be less extensive in MHT users than non-users in cross-sectional [61] and longitudinal [62] studies. In summary, studies in postmenopausal women suggest that MHT either improves or has a neutral effect on the structural integrity of neural tissue in brain regions important to memory and mood.

The inconsistencies between findings in these studies are probably due to a variety of methodological factors. First, the effects of MHT may be limited to grey or white matter compartments within brain regions that are vulnerable to the effects of aging [63–65]. Thus studies that specifically focused on other brain regions [54] or whole brain grey and white matter volumes [53] may not detect significant between-group differences. Second, some studies failed to explicitly exclude ex-users of MHT among 'non-users' [53, 54] and/or may have included women that did not receive MHT around the time of menopause with current users [53, 54, 61]. The 'critical period' hypothesis, however, predicts that these factors would reduce between-group differences. Third, as described above, it is probable that factors such as the type of MHT used (e.g. CEE versus estradiol), whether MHT is opposed or unopposed by progestogens, and the mode of administration (e.g. oral or implant) may modulate the putative protective effects of MHT on brain aging [66]. Finally, the methodological technique applied to analysing brain structure may be important. Thus although brain morphometry of bulk regions (a combined measure of both white and grey matter of whole brain or lobes) can be examined using hand-tracing methods, subtle regional differences in grey and white matter may occur that are undetectable using this approach. This difficulty has largely been overcome by studies using voxel-based morphometry (VBM), which generate statistical parametric maps of the significant between-group differences in grey matter concentration [56, 60]. In summary, studies suggest that initiation of MHT at the time of menopause may modulate age-related differences in regional grey and white matter concentration in regions that are important to memory and mood. Further studies, using functional imaging, suggest that MHT may also modulate brain activity in these regions.

Functional magnetic resonance imaging (*f*MRI) and positron emission tomography (PET) techniques have permitted analysis of the effects of estrogen on brain function in peri- and postmenopausal women. Several observational studies have reported a significant effect of MHT on brain function in postmenopausal women. An early PET study [53] that compared long-term MHT users to non-MHT users reported significant differences in the relative regional cerebral blood flow (rCBF) in brain regions that included the frontal and parahippocampal gyri during verbal memory, and parietal and parahippocampal cortices during visual memory. Furthermore, these changes were associated with improved memory performance – suggesting that these functional differences had significant behavioural consequences. A subsequent PET study in postmenopausal long-term MHT+ users, MHT non-users and women with AD reported that MHT– women had metabolic ratios that were intermediate to HRT+ women and AD patients in brain regions characteristically hypometabolic in AD (including the dorsolateral prefrontal, middle temporal and parietal cortices) [67]. Although the behavioural performance did not differ between MHT+ and MHT women, it was suggested that the relative hypometabolism in MHT women might be an early indicator of future cognitive decline.

The above studies of *long*-term MHT use have been supported by research into the *short*-term effects of MHT in women closer to the 'critical period'. For example, a placebo-controlled, crossover *f*MRI study reported that MHT+ was associated with increased activation of frontal, prefrontal and inferior parietal regions during a verbal memory task [68].

In summary, studies of brain function in older women report that long-term MHT, if prescribed since around the time of menopause, and short-term MHT, if prescribed close to the time of menopause, probably have positive modulatory effects on brain function in brain regions that are important to memory. These findings have been supported by studies in younger, premenopausal women.

Pseudo-menopause

A useful model to research the effects of reduced ovarian function on the brain is to study the consequences of acute ovarian steroid suppression (i.e. post-GnRHa) in premenopausal women. One advantage of this approach is that it avoids confounding effects of the 'healthy user' bias. Studies using this approach by our group and others have reported a significant reduction in brain activity in similar regions reported postmenopause, including the dorsolateral prefrontal and parietal cortex [69, 70]. Furthermore, these changes have been reported to be reversed following estrogen (and progesterone) add-back [69] or the return of ovarian function [71].

In summary, studies into the effects of MHT on brain function in younger and older women suggest that it modulates brain function in regions critical to memory and mood, including the prefrontal cortex and hippocampus. However, these studies do not provide insight into putative biological mechanisms that might underpin these actions. One mechanism indirectly suggested by neuroendocrine challenge studies is that HRT might modulate specific neurotransmitter systems in these regions.

To study this we extended our earlier findings and analysed the interaction between GnRHa and a muscarinic antagonist, scopolamine. We used a verbal memory task to probe specific brain regions important to memory and mood. We reported that scopolamine reduced activation in the left inferior frontal gyrus (LIFG) during encoding, which was attenuated further by GnRHa [39]. Furthermore, using a visual working memory task we also found an interaction at the parahippocampus [72]. These findings were also associated with significant behavioural effects. Following pseudo-menopause with GnRHa, cholinergic antagonism produced a more significant deficit in response accuracy and response time, respectively. In summary, these findings suggest that one mechanism via which acute loss of ovarian hormones might modulate brain function is via an interaction with the cholinergic system in frontotemporal brain regions. Another putative mechanism via which sex hormones could modulate brain function in these regions is by a direct effect on the neuronal and glial function. This effect can be studied using proton magnetic resonance spectroscopy (1H-MRS).

Magnetic Resonance Spectroscopy

In vivo 1H-MRS is a magnetic resonance imaging (MRI) technique that can measure the biochemical composition within specific brain regions. Using this technique in premenopausal women we found that ovarian suppression, with GnRHa, was associated with a significant increase in choline (Cho) concentration in the dorsolateral prefrontal cortex (DLPFC). We also found a significant trend in the increase in Cho concentration in the hippocampus. Choline is a marker of membrane metabolism and turnover [73] that has been reported to increase with age [74]. Therefore, our findings suggest that sex hormone concentration may be associated with increased neuronal/glial membrane turnover (i.e. less neuronal stability) in brain regions associated with memory and mood.

An earlier *in vivo* 1H-MRS study in postmenopausal women supported these findings. In this study we reported a significant reduction in Cho concentration in the hippocampus and parietal lobe of women prescribed long-term MHT+ compared with MHT naive (MHT−) women [75]. Other groups have also reported changes in brain chemistry in specific brain regions using 1H-MRS findings. For example, reduced myoinositol concentration has been reported in basal ganglia, frontal and hippocampal regions in women prescribed MHT compared with never-users [76]. This finding is significant as myoinositol increases with age [77] and has been reported to be particularly high in people with Alzheimer's disease [78].

In summary, studies suggest that the effects of estrogen on brain function may be biologically underpinned by direct modulation of neuronal function or via an interaction with neurotransmitter systems such as the cholinergic. A further technique that has been used to study the effects of MHT at the neurotransmitter *receptor* level is single photon emission computed tomography (SPECT).

Single Photon Emission Computed Tomography (SPECT)

Single photon emission computed tomography studies into *short-term* effects of MHT on postmenopausal women reported increased cortical $5-HT_{2A}$ receptor availability in the prefrontal cortex and anterior cingulate [79, 80]. We also found that *long-term* MHT was associated with lower $5-HT_{2A}$ receptor availability in the hippocampus, compared with never-users [81]. Furthermore, hippocampal $5-HT_{2A}$ receptor availability correlated negatively with verbal memory. This was consistent with previous studies, which reported total cortical 5-HT_{2A} binding potential was negatively correlated with delayed verbal memory [82]. These findings suggest that upregulation of postsynaptic 5-HT_{2A} receptors is associated with short-term use; but chronic use may lead to down-regulation.

Previous SPECT studies in healthy postmenopausal women have also reported an increased index of cortical cholinergic nerve terminal concentrations in multiple cortical regions (e.g. anterior and posterior cingulate, prefrontal and temporal cortex) with increasing years of HRT use [83]. In another SPECT study we investigated the relationship between m1/m4 muscarinic receptor density (using a novel ligand (R,R)[123I]-I-QNB) in premenopausal and postmenopausal women who were either long-term users of MHT, following prescription around the time of menopause, or never-users. We found that premenopausal women had more m1/m4 receptors than postmenopausal women and that MHT users had a higher density of m1/m4 receptors than never-users [84]. Thus, these data add to the evidence suggesting an important relationship between estrogen and neurotransmitters, such as the serotonergic and cholinergic system, in postmenopausal women.

Summary and Conclusion

Studies suggest that women requiring short-term MHT to treat significant perimenopausal symptoms should, at the very least, be reassured about the lack of longer-term risks on cognitive function. Furthermore, prescription of estrogen around the time of the menopause may reduce the risk of longer-term memory impairment and improve mood in some women. Research to date has suggested that this may be modulated by the effects of estrogen on the structure and function of brain regions that are central to mood and memory. However, there is still a significant need for better-designed studies to determine the clinical significance of these effects. In particular, studies are required that (a) test the 'critical period hypothesis', and (b) directly compare the effects of MHT with antidepressants and/or CBT in perimenopausal women suffering from clinical depression. It is hoped that future research in this area will address these important issues.

References

1. Evans D, Ganguli M, Harris T, Kawas C, Larson EB. Women and Alzheimer disease. *Alzheimer Dis Assoc Disord* 1999;13:187–9.

2. Lopez OL, Jagust WJ, DeKosky ST, et al. Prevalence and classification of mild cognitive impairment in the Cardiovascular Health Study Cognition Study: part 1. *Arch Neurol* 2003;60:1385–9.

3. McCrone P, Dhanasiri S, Patel A, Knapp M, Lawton-Smith S. *Paying the Price: The Cost of Mental Health Care in England to 2026*. 2008. King's Fund.

4. Zandi PP, Carlson MC, Plassman BL, et al. Hormone replacement therapy and incidence of Alzheimer disease in older women: the Cache County Study. *JAMA* 2002;288:2123–9.

5. Comas-Herrera A, Wittenberg R, Pickard L, Knapp M. Cognitive impairment in older people: future demand for long-term care services and the associated costs. *Int J Geriatr Psychiatry* 2007;22:1037–45.

6. Rocca WA, Bower JH, Maraganore DM, et al. Increased risk of cognitive impairment or dementia in women who underwent oophorectomy before menopause. *Neurology* 2007;69:1074–83.

7. LeBlanc ES, Janowsky J, Chan BKS, Nelson HD. Hormone replacement therapy and cognition: systematic review and meta-analysis. *JAMA* 2001;285:1489–99.

8. Maki PM, Sundermann E. Hormone therapy and cognitive function. *Hum Reprod Update* 2009;15:667–81.

9. Shumaker SA, Legault C, Rapp SR, et al. Estrogen plus progestin and the incidence of dementia and mild cognitive impairment in postmenopausal women: the Women's Health Initiative Memory Study: a randomized controlled trial. *JAMA* 2003;289:2651–62.

10. Savolainen-Peltonen H, Rahkola-Soisalo P, Hoti F, et al. Use of postmenopausal hormone therapy and risk of Alzheimer's disease in Finland: nationwide case-control study. *BMJ* 2019;364:1665.

11. Schmid NS, Taylor KI, Foldi NS, Berres M, Monsch AU. Neuropsychological signs of Alzheimer's disease 8 years prior to diagnosis. *J Alzheimer's Dis* 2013;34:537–46.

12. Gleason CE, Dowling NM, Wharton W, et al. Effects of hormone therapy on cognition and mood in recently postmenopausal women: findings from the randomized, controlled KEEPS-Cognitive and Affective Study. *PLoS Med* 2015;12(6):e1001833.

13. Henderson VW, St John JA, Hodis HN, et al. Cognitive effects of estradiol after menopause: a randomized trial of the timing hypothesis. *Neurology* 2016;87(7):699–708.

14. Maki P. Menopausal hormone therapy and cognition. *BMJ* 2019;364:1877.

15. World Health Organization. *World Health Report: Shaping the Future.* 2003. WHO.

16. Wassertheil-Smoller S, Shumaker S, Ockene J, et al. The Women's Health Initiative (WHI) – depression and cardiovascular sequelae in postmenopausal women. *Arch Intern Med* 2004;164(3):289–98.

17. Stewart DE, Boydell KM. Psychologic distress during menopause: associations across the reproductive life cycle. *Int J Psychiatr Med* 1993;23:157–62.

18. Gregory RJ, Masand PS, Yohai NH. Depression across the reproductive life cycle: correlations between events. *Prim Care Companion J Clin Psychiatry* 2000;2:127–9.

19. Payne JL, Roy PS, Murphy-Eberenz K, et al. Reproductive cycle-associated mood symptoms in women with major depression and bipolar disorder. *J Affect Disord* 2007;99:221–9.

20. Chuong CJ, Burgos DM. Medical history in women with premenstrual syndrome. *J Psychosom Obstet Gynaecol* 1995;16:21–7.

21. Morse CA, Dudley E, Guthrie J, Dennerstein L. Relationships between premenstrual complaints and perimenopausal experiences. *J Psychosom Obstet Gynaecol* 1998;19:182–91.

22. Binfa L, Castelo-Branco C, Blumel JE, et al. Influence of psycho-social factors on climacteric symptoms. *Maturitas* 2004;48:425–31.

23. Freeman EW, Sammel MD, Liu L, et al. Hormones and menopausal status as predictors of depression in women in transition to menopause. *Arch Gen Psychiat* 2004;61:62–70.

24. Aydin N, Inandi T, Karabulut N. Depression and associated factors among women within their first postnatal year in Erzurum province in eastern Turkey. *Women Health* 2005;41:1–12.

25. Bloch M, Rotenberg N, Koren D, Klein E. Risk factors associated with the development of postpartum mood disorders. *J Affect Disord* 2005;88:9–18.

26. Bloch M, Rotenberg N, Koren D, Klein E. Risk factors for early postpartum depressive symptoms. *Gen Hosp Psychiatr* 2006;28:3–8.

27. Gordon JL, Rubinow DR, Eisenlohr-Moul TA, Xia K, Schmidt PJ, Girdler SS. Efficacy of transdermal estradiol and micronized progesterone in the prevention of depressive symptoms in the menopause transition: a randomized clinical trial. *JAMA Psychiatr* 2018;75(2):149–57.

28. Schmidt PJ, Nieman L, Danaceau MA, et al. Estrogen replacement in perimenopause-related depression:

a preliminary report. *Am J Obstet Gynecol* 2000;183:414–20.

29. Soares CN, Almeida OP, Joffe H, Cohen LS. Efficacy of estradiol for the treatment of depressive disorders in perimenopausal women: a double-blind, randomized, placebo-controlled trial. *Arch Gen Psychiatr* 2001;58:529–34.

30. Studd J, Panay N. Are oestrogens useful for the treatment of depression in women? *Best Pract Res Clin Obstet Gynaecol* 2009;23:63–71.

31. Studd J. Ten reasons to be happy about hormone replacement therapy: a guide for patients. *Menopause Int* 2010;16:44–6.

32. Studd J. Why are estrogens rarely used for the treatment of depression in women? *Gynecol Endocrinol* 2007;23:63–4.

33. Studd J, Panay N. Hormones and depression in women. *Climacteric* 2004;7:338–46.

34. Studd JWW. A guide to the treatment of depression in women by estrogens. *Climacteric* 2011;14:637–42.

35. McEwen B. Estrogen actions throughout the brain. *Recent Prog Horm Res* 2002;57:357–84.

36. Kenealy BP, Kapoor A, Guerriero KA, et al. Neuroestradiol in the hypothalamus contributes to the regulation of gonadotropin releasing hormone release. *J Neurosci* 2013;33:19051–9.

37. Heldring N, Pike A, Andersson S, et al. Estrogen receptors: how do they signal and what are their targets. *Physiol Rev* 2007;87:905–31.

38. Craig MC, Cutter WJ, van Amelsvoort TAMJ, Rymer J, Whitehead M, Murphy DGM. Effects of estrogen replacement therapy on dopaminergic responsivity in postmenopausal women. *Biol Psychiatr* 2003;53:210S.

39. Craig MC, Fletcher PC, Daly EM, et al. The interactive effect of the cholinergic system and acute ovarian suppression on the brain: an fMRI study. *Horm Behav* 2009;55:41–9.

40. Davies P, Maloney AJ. Selective loss of central cholinergic neurons in Alzheimer's disease. *Lancet* 1976;2:1403.

41. Bowen DM, Smith CB, White P, Davison AN. Neurotransmitter-related enzymes and indices of hypoxia in senile dementia and other abiotrophies. *Brain* 1976;99:459–96.

42. Shytle RD, Silver AA, Lukas RJ, et al. Nicotinic acetylcholine receptors as targets for antidepressants. *Mol Psychiatr* 2002;7:525–35.

43. van Amelsvoort TAMJ, Abel KM, Robertson DMR, et al. Prolactin response to *d*-fenfluramine in postmenopausal women on and off ERT: comparison with young women. *Psychoneuroendocrinology* 2001;26:494–502.

44. Dunlop BW, Nemeroff CB. The role of dopamine in the pathophysiology of depression. *Arch Gen Psychiatr* 2007;64:327–37.

45. Backman L, Nyberg L. Dopamine and training-related working-memory improvement. *Neurosci Biobehav Rev* 2013;37:2209–19.

46. Ettigi P, Lal S, Martin JB, Friesen HC. Effects of sex, oral contraceptives, and glucose loading on apomorphine induced growth hormone secretion. *J Clin Endocrinol Metab* 1975;40:1094–8.

47. Wieck A, Hirst AD, Kumar R, Checkley SA, Campbell IC. Growth hormone secretion by human females in response to apomorphine challenge is markedly affected by menstrual cycle phase. *B J Clin Pharmacol* 1989;27:700–1.

48. Wieck A, Kumar R, Marks MN, Checkley SA. Increased sensitivity of dopamine receptors and recurrence of affective psychosis after childbirth. *Br Med J (Clin Res Ed)* 1991;303:613–16.

49. Craig M, Cutter W, Wickhham H, van Amelsvoort T, Murphy D. Effect of long-term estrogen therapy on dopaminergic responsivity in postmenopausal women. *Psychoneuroendocrinology* 2004;29:1309–16.

50. Lamar M, Craig M, Daly EM, et al. Acute tryptophan depletion promotes an anterior-to-posterior fMRI activation shift during task switching in older adults. *Hum Brain Mapp* 2014;35:712–22.

51. Halbreich U, Rojansky N, Palter S, et al. Estrogen augments serotonergic activity in postmenopausal women. *Biol Psychiatr* 1995;37:434–41.

52. Matthews KA, Kuller LH, Wing RR, Meilahn EN, Plantinga P. Prior to use of estrogen replacement therapy, are users healthier than nonusers? *Am J Epidemiol* 1996;143:971–8.

53. Resnick SM, Maki PM, Golski S, Kraut MA, Zonderman AB. Effects of estrogen replacement therapy on PET cerebral blood flow and neuropsychological performance. *Horm Behav* 1998;34:171–82.

54. Raz N, Gunning-Dixon F, Head D, et al. Aging, sexual dimorphism, and hemispheric asymmetry of the cerebral cortex: replicability of regional differences in volume. *Neurobiol Aging* 2004;25:377–96.

55. Eberling JL, Wu C, Tong-Turnbeaugh R, Jagurst J. Estrogen-and-tamoxifen-associated effects on brain structure and function. *Neuroimage* 2004;21:364–71.

56. Erickson KI, Colcombe SJ, Raz N, et al. Selective sparing of brain tissue in postmenopausal women receiving hormone replacement therapy. *Neurobiol Aging* 2005;26:1205–13.

57. Robertson DMW, Craig MC, Van Amelsvoort T, et al. Effects of estrogen replacement therapy on age-related differences in grey matter volume. *Climacteric* 2009;12:301–9.

58. Eberling JL, Wu C, Mungas D, Buoncore M, Jagurst J. Preliminary evidence that oestrogen protects against age-related hippocampal atrophy. *Neurobiol Aging* 2003;24:725–32.

59. McEwen BS. Glucocorticoids, depression, and mood disorders: structural remodeling in the brain. *Metabolism* 2005;54 Suppl 1:20–3.

60. Robertson D, Craig MC, van Amelsvoort T, et al. Effects of estrogen therapy on age-related differences in gray matter concentration. *Climacteric* 2009;12:301–9.

61. Schmidt R, Fazekas F, Reinhart B, et al. Estrogen replacement therapy in older women: a neuropsychological and brain MRI study. *J Am Geriatr Soc* 1996;44:1307–13.

62. Cook IA, Morgan ML, Dunkin JJ, et al. Estrogen replacement therapy is associated with less progression of subclinical structural brain disease in normal elderly women: a pilot study. *Int J Geriatr Psychiatry* 2002;17:610–18.

63. Raz E, Tighe H, Sato Y, et al. Preferential induction of a Th1 immune response and inhibition of specific IgE antibody formation by plasmid DNA immunization. *Proc Natl Acad Sci USA* 1996;93:5141–5.

64. Jernigan TL, Archibald SL, Fennema-Notestine C, et al. Effects of age on tissues and regions of the cerebrum and cerebellum. *Neurobiol Aging* 2001;22:581–94.

65. Sullivan EV, Marsh L, Mathalon DH, Lim KO, Pfefferbaum A. Age-related decline in MRI volumes of temporal lobe gray matter but not hippocampus. *Neurobiol Aging* 1995;16:591–606.

66. Sherwin BB, Henrya JF. Brain aging modulates the neuroprotective effects of estrogen on selective aspects of cognition in women: a critical review. *Frontiers Neuroendocrinol* 2008;29:88–113.

67. Eberling JL, Reed BR, Coleman JE, Jagust WJ. Effect of estrogen on cerebral glucose metabolism in postmenopausal women. *Neurology* 2000;55:875–7.

68. Shaywitz SE, Shaywitz BA, Pugh KR, et al. Effect of estrogen on brain activation patterns in postmenopausal women during working memory tasks. *JAMA* 1999;281:1197–202.

69. Berman KF, Schmidt PJ, Rubinow DR, et al. Modulation of cognition-specific cortical activity by gonadal steroids: a positron-emission tomography study in

women. *Proc Natl Acad Sci USA* 1997;94:8836–41.

70. Craig MC, Fletcher PC, Daly EM, et al. Gonadotropin hormone releasing hormone agonists alter prefrontal function during verbal encoding in young women. *Psychoneuroendocrinology* 2007;32:1116–27.

71. Craig MC, Fletcher PC, Daly EM, et al. Reversibility of the effects of acute ovarian hormone suppression on verbal memory and prefrontal function in pre-menopausal women. *Psychoneuroendocrinology* 2008;33:1426–31.

72. Craig MC, Brammer M, Maki PM, et al. The interactive effect of acute ovarian suppression and the cholinergic system on visuospatial working memory in young women. *Psychoneuroendocrinology* 2010;35:987–1000.

73. Jenden DJ. The metabolism of choline. *Bull Clin Sci* 1990;55:99–106.

74. Pfefferbaum A, Adalsteinsson E, Speilman D, Sullivan EV, Lim KO. *In vivo* spectroscopic quantification of the N-acetyl-moiety, creatine, and choline from large volume of brain grey and white matter: the effects of normal aging. *Magn Reson Med* 1999;41:276–84.

75. Robertson DM, van Amelsvoort T, Daly E, et al. Effects of estrogen replacement therapy on human brain aging: an in vivo 1H MRS study. *Neurology* 2001;57:2114–17.

76. Ernst T, Chang L, Cooray D, et al. The effects of tamoxifen and estrogen on brain metabolism in elderly women. *J Natl Cancer Inst* 2002;94:592–7.

77. Chang L, Ernst T, Poland RE, Jenden DJ. In vivo proton magnetic resonance spectroscopy of the normal aging human brain. *Life Sci* 1996;58:2049–56.

78. Huang W, Alexander GE, Chang L, et al. Brain metabolite concentration and dementia severity in Alzheimer's disease: a 1H MRS study. *Neurology* 2001;57:626–32.

79. Kugaya A, Epperson CN, Zoghbi S, et al. Increase in prefrontal cortex serotonin 2A receptors following estrogen treatment in postmenopausal women. *Am J Psychiatry* 2003;160:1522–4.

80. Moses EL, Drevets WC, Smith G, et al. Effects of estradiol and progesterone administration on human serotonin 2A receptor binding: a PET study. *Biol Psychiatry* 2000;48:854–60.

81. Compton J, Travis MJ, Norbury R, et al. Long-term estrogen therapy and 5-HT2A receptor binding in postmenopausal women; a single photon emission tomography (SPET) study. *Horm Behav* 2008;53:61–8.

82. Nobury R, Travis MJ, Erlandsson K, et al. Estrogen therapy and brain muscarinic receptor density in healthy females: a SPET study. *Horm Behav* 2007;51:249–57.

83. Smith YR, Minoshima S, Kuhl DE, Zubieta JK. Effects of long-term hormone therapy on cholinergic synaptic concentrations in healthy postmenopausal women. *J Clin Endocrinol Metab* 2001;86:679–84.

84. Nobury R, Travis MJ, Erlandsson K, et al. *In vivo* imaging of muscarinic receptors in the aging female brain with (R,R) [123I]-I-QNB and single photon emission tomography. *Exp Gerontol* 2005;40:137–45.

Chapter 10

Libido and Sexual Function in the Menopause

Claudine Domoney

Loss of libido is the most common sexual complaint of women, often being a final common pathway of many sexual disorders. Estimates range from 30–45 per cent depending on the population sampled, highest in the postmenopausal age group [1]. However, the degree of distress associated with loss of libido may be minimal and therefore not sexually dysfunctional. Lack of arousal and orgasmic disorders are frequently correlated with loss of libido, as are sexual pain disorders. It is important for the medical doctor to help the patient decipher the chain of events and their impact, to facilitate change and improvement. Making assumptions about a particular set of expectations is likely to lead to neglect of key factors. In psychosexual medicine, listening and observing the patient's expression of feelings can help to interpret the predominant issue(s) that may be resolved using brief psychotherapeutic intervention.

The Menopause

The menopause incorporates changes related to ageing, hormonal decline and altered social roles. Studies of the menopause and sexual relationships have reported a reduction in sexual activity with age. However, a US study of 18- to 59-year-old adults has reported sexual difficulties in 43 per cent of women and 31 per cent of men, i.e. a large proportion of the younger population [2]. An Australian longitudinal study, observing women from the age of 45 to 55, suggested that female sexual dysfunction increased from 42 to 88 per cent from the early to late menopause [3]. However, if 'distress' is included in the definition of female sexual dysfunction, this is reduced significantly [4]. As an indicator of the many factors, there is a small variation amongst European women, country by country, which indicates that the frequency of intercourse varies, but body mass index (BMI) is the only significant influencer.

However, there are well-documented increasing sexual difficulties with age: in women, these may be correlated with estrogen levels, but not consistently androgens, although testosterone levels have also not consistently been shown to reflect sexual functioning in younger women either. Predictably, women who have a sexual partner are more likely to be sexually active and to have increased satisfaction within their relationship. Cessation of sexual activity is more likely to be male-partner-driven within a relationship. A lifestyle survey from the UK, published in 2013, indicated that sexual inactivity was more common with reducing health status in both men and women, and therefore with age. One in six people reported a health condition that affected their sex life in the previous year: 24 per cent of men and 18 per cent of women had sought help or advice from a health care professional. Men report an increase in ejaculation and satisfaction problems, but less erectile dysfunction, although the wide availability of phosphodiesterase inhibitors may have changed the distribution of sexual problems in men (and the likelihood of seeking professional help). In women, sexual satisfaction rates have been increasing overall and have been linked with earlier sexual debut and more positive attitudes to female sexuality [5]. There is a greater expectation in women to continue to be sexually active and satisfied, but this is not universal. The change in social status and role of older women within their family, workplace and society in general contributes to the psychological overlay of sexual behaviour and responsivity. Individual preconceptions regarding ageing and behaviour vary hugely and overall knowledge is poor regarding the management of sexual problems in peri- and postmenopausal women. These culturally influenced factors will determine help-seeking attitudes.

Although many studies have been contradictory with respect to menopause and the cause of sexual difficulties being age or hormone related, overall when dealing with individual patients, the patient will be the 'expert' in her condition. The clinician needs to help her unravel the issues around cause and effect and determine the degree of distress.

Sexual Disorders

The *Diagnostic and Statistical Manual of Mental Disorders* (DSM) V classification now combines *desire* and *arousal disorders* as they are almost invariably linked. Isolated genital *arousal disorder* may, however, exist in postmenopausal women due to the physical changes of the menopause causing vulvo-vaginal atrophy. Over time this condition is commonly associated with reduced desire. Development of *desire disorder* may be protective from distress and dissatisfaction when preceded by dyspareunia or adverse changes in sexual responsivity.

Orgasmic disorders are a separate category, which may include a lack of or reduction in quality of sex, sometimes due to direct hormonal deficiencies or a culmination of other sexual issues. Dyspareunia and vaginismus are now also classified together, but are separate from non-coital pain disorders, which can also cause severe sexual dysfunction, for example vulvodynia and bladder pain syndrome.

The duration of the problem is an important factor in diagnosis of female sexual dysfunction. Short-term issues may be normal and a manifestation of the effects of life circumstances. Sexual difficulties may also reflect the overall psychological well-being of the individual. Of importance in the menopausal woman are the organic causes of sexual problems that may impact on psychological health. The etiological routes of anatomic, hormonal, neurologic, vascular and other abnormalities affect sexual self-esteem and functioning, given that sex is a mind and body activity.

However the academic study of sex should only inform the individual consultation – pathway-driven health care is most likely to fail where the emphasis of contributory factors is an individual response.

Sexual Response Cycle

Although the Masters and Johnson model of human sexuality [6] has been useful in explaining the sequence of phases in the human sexual response cycle, the Basson model of female sexuality [7] facilitates a clearer understanding of the drivers and difficulties specifically involved in the female sexual response cycle. A spontaneous drive to be sexually active may be less significant in a longstanding relationship than the need for emotional and physical satisfaction, and emotional and physical intimacy. A sexually neutral woman is able to be receptive to sexual stimuli in the right circumstances, and desire and arousal may occur concomitantly, rather than desire being a driver for activity. A better understanding of her emotional and relationship issues can be crucial to understanding the physical responses of a woman, particularly with the major life changes occurring at the menopause. How she perceives the changes happening to her, including her role in society, at work and within her family, all reflect her self-esteem and sexual confidence.

Management

Hormonal: Local

Estrogen deficiency has a significant impact on whole-body function for many women as detailed in this book but can be devastating for sexual function. Lack of information about the short-, intermediate- and long-term impact of the menopause can lead women and their partners to believe these are inevitable consequences of ageing. Even if the deterioration is linked to hormones, the fear of treatment may prevent any exploration of possible treatment. Yet the impact on urogenital anatomy, nerve transmission, blood flow, sleep disorders, mood, vasomotor and other symptoms may alter responsivity without the possible decline in hormonally driven sexual drive and orgasmic potential. Within the genital tract, shortening and loss of elasticity in the vagina occurs, with reduced secretions and thinning of the vaginal epithelial layers, leading to an increase in the risk of trauma and discomfort, discharge and infections, particularly in association with sexual activity. Atrophy of the tissues causes pain, dryness, lack of arousal, reduction in desire, reduced orgasm and sensitivity and increasing urinary symptoms. An alteration in vaginal pH can cause recurrent infections such as bacterial vaginosis and thrush. More covert symptoms of lack of desire and arousal, decreased orgasmic response and postcoital bleeding causing anxiety, can all lead to avoidance of sex, deterioration in a relationship and an acceptance of sexual decline. If not recognized, this becomes a repetitive cycle that is difficult to unravel or arrest. Psychologically, behavioural patterns become embedded and their initial trigger becomes less identifiable. At this point, recovery and re-engagement with a sexual partner can be troublesome.

The health care professional (HCP) consulting with a woman needs to elucidate the sequence of events and what happens when/if they try to engage with sexual activity. Local pain, increase in cystitis, postcoital bleeding, discharge or irritation should be addressed by local oestrogens or DHEA (see Chapters 18 and 19), lubricants, vaginal re-moisturizers, small antibiotic dose with intercourse, in addition to education on estrogen deficiency changes. These may be more acceptable to her than systemic HRT if she does not have generalized problematic menopause symptoms – many may feel they have 'got through' menopause without HRT and do not wish to take it now.

Hormonal: Systemic

Estrogen replacement alone has been reported to impact positively on the sexual status of women, although this may be secondary to multiple modes of action. Direct effects on sexual arousal and desire may be complementary to an improvement in sleep, mood, energy. It should be noted that local estrogens are more effective than systemic for urogenital changes and may be required in addition to systemic with no additional risk but a significant improvement in efficacy. Contraceptive concerns also need to be clarified as there is great misunderstanding of perimenopausal requirements (see Chapter 20).

Testosterone replacement therapy (see Chapter 19) is controversial, although studies have confirmed a benefit for some women with low sexual desire peri- and postmenopausally [8]. These studies have included women with bilateral oophorectomy who have a significant reduction in androgens, as postmenopausal ovaries produce at least 50 per cent of circulating androgens, and with and without estrogen replacement. Androgen levels reduce by 50 per cent in women from their twenties to their forties, yet many women feel greater satisfaction as they mature, although this may reflect more of a change in male attentiveness with age and female confidence. Transdermal estrogen therapy may be better than oral estrogen for libido as sex hormone binding globulin (SHBG) levels increase with oral therapy, leading to a reduction in free testosterone. This increase in SHBG and consequent reduction in free androgen index can also occur with other oral hormone therapy including thyroxine. Testosterone is manufactured for women in implant, gel and patch form, although licenses and availability are variable around the world. For some, testosterone may help with 'kick starting' sexual sensitivity and responsiveness, such that once a regular satisfying sexual life has been re-established, it may not be necessary, similar to the use of phosphodiesterase inhibitors in men with psychogenic erectile dysfunction. Once sexual responsiveness has been confirmed to the individual, performance anxiety may reduce and sexual encounters be less stressful, therefore more reliably pleasurable.

Non-hormonal Pharmacotherapy

The pharmaceutical holy grail of a 'cure' for female sexual dysfunction is likely to remain elusive. Flibanserin is a pharmacological treatment for *hypoactive desire disorder* causing neurotransmitter modulation [9]. It is licensed in the US for treatment of premenopausal women with a small benefit for satisfying sexual episodes but with side effects of somnolence, dizziness and nausea with an interaction with alcohol. There is some evidence of benefit for postmenopausal women. Bupropion has been used as an antidepressant with no reduction in libido compared to selective serotonin uptake inhibitors (SSRIs).

Psychosexual: Aging

The menopause is associated with specific features previously discussed that may directly contribute to sexual decline. Symptoms of mood change and lability, night sweats and flashing, sleep problems and urogenital atrophic changes can be dealt with by the use of medication, most appropriately menopausal hormone therapy (MHT). Yet the psychology of aging, particularly in the Western world, may be more pertinent. Changes in BMI and body habitus, with their impact on self-esteem, are relevant for many women. Perception of attractiveness and self-image, as a reflection of society's view of aging, may be transferred to the individual. Loss of hair and changes in skin and nails are important secondary sexual determinants for many women, particularly for those without a supportive relationship. In addition, there may be an expectation that older people should be sexually passive and discrete, but contrasted with celebrity culture of everlasting youth. Problems with teenage children and their pressures, pelvic floor dysfunction, physical illness, medication use and side effects, partner dysfunction, relationship factors and financial factors are all relevant and often coexist.

Psychosexual: Relationship

Although it may not be the role of the HCP to be a relationship counsellor, it is part of our remit to understand if this appears to be the most important factor. The couple can then be directed to the most appropriate therapist. Revelations of fear or fantasies in an atmosphere of trust and safety in the consultation room can be powerful to access and understand the psychodynamics of the relationship and her attitude to it. We should be aware of the patient's motivation for change and her defences or reluctance for this. Presenting with an overt sexual problem indicates that she is more likely to be receptive to encouragement to change her behaviours. If she has presented without her partner, accept that she may wish to 'own' and treat these problems herself – to explore the changes in her body and sexuality. If there is an obvious partner factor, they should be encouraged to seek their own help, usually separately, particularly if the woman has colluded with this to 'spare his feelings'.

We may focus on how she understands her relationship to be with her husband now, how she wishes it to be in the future, what their sexual history has been and whether there have been any other factors that have impacted on her sexuality and her ability to respond to him. Is she sad that she no longer feels sexy or wants to be sexually active, or is she accepting of the situation, or is it what she expects in middle or old age? Does she feel sexual feelings at times other than with her husband?

Psychosexual: Attitude to and Experience of Sex

When analysing loss of libido and sexual difficulties, approaching the two components of motivation and drive can be helpful. With respect to motivation, factors relating to previous experiences, relationship quality, relationship duration, previous disagreements and disputes may be important. Drive may be dependent on age, health, hormone status and mood, which all interact, depending on life events and circumstances. Asking a woman about her general sexual desire and feelings of sexuality can be important. Does she feel attractive or attracted to others? Does she have fantasies, daydreams or other desires? Does this induce a need and wish to behave sexually? Is she able or was she ever able to masturbate? With respect to her relationship: are there interpersonal conflicts such as a dysfunctional partner, miscommunications and any other family or financial problems? She may have mood changes, a history of trauma in the past, self-esteem issues or other inter- or intrapersonal conflicts. Are there any other comorbidities that coincided or overlap the onset of the sexual difficulties? Are they situational only? What is the effect of her problems and the impact on her quality of life?

How does she perceive that you might help her? Does she expect hormone management or a 'female Viagra'? Has she read about 'cures' on the Internet or been told by friends to try a product? There is clearly a strong placebo effect with medications given for sexual issues and those that are motivated to change are more likely to be thinking about sex – the lack of which may be part of the problem. Does she express feelings of pain – if she does where is that pain coming from? Pain is often expressed as physical although it can be psychological in origin. Yet this disparity is reported more commonly in younger women in comparison to older women, who often have more problems with lubrication and sexual interest.

Using the Genital Examination as a Therapeutic Tool

The genital examination is an exposure of vulnerability and attitudes to intimacy in addition to an investigation of the genitourinary tract: revelations can be made through verbal and non-verbal communication. The process of undertaking an examination may facilitate a 'moment of truth'. How she approaches getting undressed, covering herself, what she says or how she covers her genitals, how they appear, whether she has any unrecognized atrophic changes are an important part of the process of examination. Has she had any other symptoms that may have caused difficulties that she had not related to the menopause? We need to understand how the menopause is perceived and how aging is changing her. Does she have prolapse, urinary or faecal incontinence, skin changes or any other concerns about her genitals? Commenting on the observations and reflecting upon her reactions can be therapeutic: you seem to find this painful/ upsetting – has it always been like this? Her past and present issues may then be revealed.

Sex Therapy Techniques

Helping an individual understand the aetiology and impact of her sexual problems can be helpful enough alongside her presenting to an HCP to engender change. Prescribing relaxation time and acknowledging that this is an important issue, worthy of intervention, can validate her concerns. Encouraging her to discuss the consultation with her partner can be a natural way to introduce what is frequently the 'elephant in the room'.

For some women, a specific approach using the PLISSIT model may be helpful: 'Permission giving' in the form of talking or changing behaviours, 'Limited Information' regarding the areas suitable for the patient, 'Specific Suggestions' detailing exercises or regimes to help the area of sexual difficulty, and lastly 'Intensive Therapy' with deeper analysis of concerns and issues. Sensate focus is a common regime of graduated increasing re-engagement with intimacy through touch, building up to sexual intimacy. This involves 'homework' and the need for both partners to be involved. Often this may be cumbersome and awkward for those who have become resistant to their sexual feelings. As the 'patient is the expert' in her own symptoms and sexual history, it is imperative that she feels able and comfortable to engage with the reasons for her difficulties.

Summary

The interaction between the physical and psychological changes over the menopausal transition has an important impact on sexual activity and relationships. The lack of understanding of the contribution of the hormonal as opposed to those of ageing contributes to the insidious acceptance of sexual demise. Past experiences, the relationship or lack of, and treating the individual experience of menopause will impact on the ability of any woman to negotiate these changes in a sexual context. Easily accessed information, treatment and support without onward referral to counsellors will facilitate more timely interventions that prevent embedded dysfunctional adaptation that may lead to a loss of sexual functioning. The HCP involved in menopause management is the key to this.

References

1. Hayes RD, Bennett CM, Fairley CK, Dennerstein L. What can prevalence studies tell us about female sexual difficulty and dysfunction? *J Sex Med* 2006;3:589–95.

2. Laumann E, Paik A, Rosen R. Sexual dysfunction in the United States: prevalence and predictors. *JAMA* 1999;281:537–44.

3. Dennerstein L, Alexander JL, Kotz K. The menopause and sexual functioning: a review of the population-based studies. *Ann Rev Sex Res* 2003;14:64–82.

4. Dennerstein L, Guthrie JR, Hayes RD, DeRogatis LR, Lehert P. Sexual function, dysfunction, and sexual distress in a prospective, population-based sample of mid-aged, Australian-born women. *J Sex Med* 2008;5:2291–9.

5. Beckman N, Waern M, Gustafson D, Skoog I. Secular trends in self reported sexual activity and satisfaction in Swedish 70 year olds: cross sectional survey of four populations, 1971–2001. *Br Med J* 2008;337:151–4.

6. Masters WH, Johnson VE. *Human Sexual Response*. 1966. Little, Brown.

7. Basson R, Althof S, Davis S, et al. Summary of the recommendations on sexual dysfunctions in women. *J Sex Med* 2004;1:24.

8. Somboonporn W, Davis S, Seif MW, Bell R. Testosterone for peri- and postmenopausal women. *Cochrane Database Syst Rev* 2005;4: CD004509.

9. Jaspers L, Feys F, Bramer WM, Franco OH, Leusink P, Laan ET. Efficacy and safety of flibanserin for the treatment of hypoactive sexual desire disorder in women: a systematic review and meta-analysis. *JAMA Intern Med* 2016;176 (4):453–62.

Vulvo-Vaginal Atrophy (VVA)

Rossella E. Nappi

The term *vulvo-vaginal atrophy* (VVA) defines the anatomic and physiological changes in the vulvo-vaginal tissues, which are directly related to reduced circulating estrogen levels, associated with menopause and aging. Atrophic vaginitis connotes a state of inflammation or infection that may be present in some women with VVA.

VVA or atrophic vaginitis is a medical challenge because it is under-reported by women, under-recognized by health care providers (HCPs) and, therefore, under-treated. The most common symptoms associated with VVA are dryness, itching, irritation, burning and dyspareunia. These may negatively influence well-being and relationships. Urinary symptoms are also associated with VVA, and include increased frequency, urgency, dysuria, and recurrent urinary tract infections (rUTIs), as well as urinary incontinence resulting mainly from pelvic floor problems [1]. More recently, VVA has been renamed genitourinary syndrome of menopause (GSM), to highlight the many genital, sexual and urinary symptoms associated with atrophic changes of vulvo-vaginal and urological tissues, in association with estrogen deficiency, occurring at midlife and beyond. Of note, the new definition GSM includes signs and symptoms that cannot be all reversed by evidence-based endocrine therapies and may require different strategies according to their true etiology [2]. Recent surveys indicate that around 50 per cent of postmenopausal women experience vaginal discomfort attributable to VVA and symptoms are already evident during the perimenopause/early postmenopause. Longitudinal data showed that the prevalence of vaginal dryness, the most common symptom associated with VVA, ranged from about 3 per cent at premenopause to 47 per cent at 3 years postmenopause. Epidemiological findings are influenced by a range of factors, including women's age, time since menopause, frequency of sexual activity, general health, partner's availability, socio-cultural background. In addition, most of the data rely on self-reported symptoms and the severity of symptoms (from mild to severe) is rather subjective. Indeed, objective signs of VVA may be present, but women may not report symptoms because they are self-treating, feel the symptoms are not important enough, abstain from sexual activity because of no partner/a partner with health/sexual problems or are embarrassed to discuss such an intimate topic.

HCPs should be proactive in order to help their patients to disclose symptoms related to VVA and to seek adequate treatment when vaginal discomfort is clinically relevant. Women are not aware that VVA is a chronic condition with a significant impact on sexual health and quality of life and that effective and safe treatments may be available. VVA can lead to symptoms not only in response to sexual activity (reduced lubrication, pain, low desire and arousal, impaired sexual pleasure and orgasm), but also during simple activities such as walking or exercising (itching, burning, discharge, malodour, discomfort). Dyspareunia may be accompanied by postcoital bleeding and secondary vaginismus triggered by avoidance, anxiety and loss of sexual desire due to the anticipation of coital pain. A woman with VVA may also experience bleeding with minimal trauma, such as during a medical examination or whilst undertaking physical activities. That being so, it is very important to include VVA in the menopause agenda, by encouraging an open conversation on the topic of urogenital health and performing a gynaecological examination, if indicated. According to very recent guidelines on appropriate management of VVA in clinical practice, it is essential to overcome the vaginal 'taboo' in order to optimize affected women's health care [1].

VVA as a Chronic Condition

In European countries natural menopause occurs between 51 and 52 years of age and increased life expectancy means that most women will spend at least one-third of their life in the postmenopausal hypoestrogenic state. Menopause is a multidimensional phenomenon in which biological variables are modulated by intrapersonal and interpersonal factors, varying according to the socio-cultural environment and the health care system.

VVA is one of the many changes occurring at the time of the menopause transition, as a consequence of reduction of estrogen production by aging ovaries. It may occur as a consequence of other hypoestrogenic states, but this is less common. Unlike hot flushes, which usually resolve over time, VVA has a chronic/progressive course throughout the menopause transition and beyond. The areas of a woman's life most likely to be negatively impacted by VVA are sexual intimacy (64 per cent), having a loving relationship with a partner (32 per cent), overall quality of life (32 per cent), feeling healthy (21 per cent) and feeling attractive (21 per cent). The presence and severity of symptoms are variable, from mild discomfort to significant impairment, depending on age, time and type of menopause, parity and vaginal delivery, frequency of coital activity, cigarette smoking and certain medical conditions/medications. Breast cancer survivors are a special group of women that may suffer from VVA and require individualized care.

Estrogen is vital to maintain normal structure and function of the vagina and surrounding urogenital tissues. However, the science of intracrinology points to the age-related decline of circulating DHEA as an additional cause of both estrogen's and androgen's local intracellular deficiency. Estrogen receptors (both α and β), which are widely present in the vagina, vulva, muscles of the pelvic floor, endopelvic fascia, urethra and bladder trigone during reproductive life, decline with menopause and may be restored by estrogen treatment. Androgen receptors (ARs) are also well expressed at multiple levels (mucosa, submucosa, stroma, smooth muscle and vascular endothelium) and cross-talk with ERs, influencing neurovascular and neuromuscular function.

Early data show that untreated postmenopausal women with less than 50 pmol/l of estradiol suffer more from symptoms associated with VVA. The absence of estrogen stimulation contributes to the loss of mucosal elasticity by inducing fusion and hyalinization of collagen fibres and fragmentation of elastin fibres. Mucosal hydration is reduced in the dermal layer with a reduction of intracellular mucopolysaccharide and hyaluronic acid. The vagina loses its rugae, the epithelial folds that allow for dispensability, and there is a shortening and narrowing of the vaginal canal. The mucosa of the vagina, introitus, the labia minora become thin and pale and the significant reduction of vascular support induces a decrease of the volume of vaginal transudate and of other secretions. Over time, there is a progressive dominance of parabasal cells with fewer intermediate and superficial cells. This is a marker of estrogen deprivation in the vaginal squamous epithelium, which becomes friable with petechiae, ulceration and eventually bleeding after minimal trauma. With thinning of the vaginal epithelium there is a significant reduction in glycogen, which affects the population of lactobacilli and increases vaginal pH (between 5.0 and 7.5). A decrease of vaginal hydrogen peroxide supports the growth of pathogenic bacteria, including staphylococci, group B streptococci and coliforms. Similar anatomical and functional changes in the vulva as well as in the pelvic floor and within the urinary tract occur, resulting in an impairment of the pelvic floor efficiency. In particular, the vulvar introitus retracts, and hymeneal carunculae involute and lose elasticity, leading to significant entry dyspareunia. The urethral meatus appears prominent relative to the introitus and thinning of the urinary epithelium and weakening of the surrounding tissue may promote reduced urethral closure pressure, reduced sensory threshold in the bladder, and in some cases, increased risk of rUTIs [6].

In summary, VVA is a chronic condition during the postmenopausal years and it cannot regress unless adequately treated.

How to Recognize Symptoms and Signs of VVA

During menopausal consultation, women are often uncomfortable to report intimate symptoms spontaneously and they assume that problems associated with VVA are a natural part of aging. However, postmenopausal women like to be asked and very simple questions may help HCPs to 'break the ice' in order to discuss vaginal and sexual health. Unfortunately, HCPs tend not to take a proactive approach to urogenital health management in the middle- and later-life age groups, mainly because of inadequate training, constraints of time and personal attitudes and beliefs that sex is not a priority for older patients [4]. Whenever postmenopausal women report urogenital symptoms in clinical practice, an accurate pelvic examination should be performed to look for signs of VVA (Table 11.1). Dyspareunia is generally less reported later in life mainly because older women are less likely to still have a spousal or other intimate relationship and sexually related personal distress declines with age. Tissues may be easily traumatized and irritated and a gentle approach is mandatory in the most severe cases. It has been comprehensively described that the inspection should include the tissues of the vulva, vestibule, vagina and urethra, and clinical scales may be used in the attempt to quantify VVA. Organ prolapse and the muscle tone of the pelvic floor should be also noted, as well as other disorders that can cause symptoms similar to those of VVA. Although VVA is typically a clinical diagnosis, other laboratory tests may be used to support the diagnosis, such as an evaluation of vaginal pH and the vaginal maturation index (VMI), which describes the relative proportion of parabasal, intermediate and superficial vaginal epithelial cells. A more alkaline pH (>5) leads to a shift in the vaginal flora towards more coliforms and, together with the other atrophic changes, is responsible for increased susceptibility to and frequency of infections and odour, as well as traumatic bleeding associated with sexual intercourse or secondary to speculum insertion during routine gynaecological examination. Dominance of parabasal cells, calculated on

Table 11.1 Symptoms and signs associated with VVA in menopause.

Symptoms	Signs
Dryness (vaginal, vulvar, genital skin)	Decreased moisture
Decreased lubrication with sexual intercourse	Decreased elasticity
Discomfort with sexual activity	Labial resorption
Irritation/burning/itching	Pallor/erythema
Vulvo-vaginal infections	Loss of vaginal rugae
Dysuria	Tissue fragility/fissures/petechiae
Urinary frequency	Discharge
Urinary urgency	Odour/infections

Note. Supportive findings: pH > 5, increased parabasal cells on vaginal maturation index (VMI).

specimens obtained directly from the lateral upper vaginal walls, indicates hypoestrogenism and atrophy. Thus, the shift to a higher number of superficial cells is a primary end point of any treatment prescribed to relieve symptoms of VVA [1].

The potential burden of VVA should be considered not only in sexually active postmenopausal women, but also in women who abstain from sexual activity because they may suffer even more of the long-term consequence of estrogen deprivation, especially vaginal and introital stenosis, fusion of the labia minora to the labia majora, and other urogenital conditions. Special care should be devoted to women with breast cancer and other gynecological malignancies who are at very high risk of VVA and associated symptoms as a consequence of endocrine chemotherapy, surgery and/or radiation. Finally, severe VVA may be a barrier to adequately assess both cytologic and colposcopic findings to prevent cervical cancer and it is a very common reason of urgent referral to exclude endometrial cancer and other malignancies after an episode of postmenopausal bleeding.

Vaginal synechiae (adhesions) are uncommon, but can lead to occlusion of the vagina. In menstruating women this can result in haematocolpos. Adhesions prevent adequate examination and therefore significant pathology may go unrecognized [6].

Treatment Options

The therapeutic management of VVA in the menopause is multifaceted and should include non-hormonal and hormonal preparations, according to very recent guidelines [1, 3]. An open dialogue between women and their clinician is needed in order to individualize the most suitable management strategy for VVA according to the personal risk–benefit profile, women's preferences and expectations. The principles of treatment in women with a clinical diagnosis of VVA are (1) restoration of urogenital physiology and (2) alleviation of symptoms. Given the progression of VVA over time, it is mandatory to start an effective treatment as soon as the symptoms become bothersome for the woman, in order to avoid severe impairment of urogenital tissues with aging. It has been shown that more than half of affected women reported having symptoms for 3 years or longer because they did not feel comfortable discussing VVA with their HCPs. On the other hand, women who discussed VVA with HCPs were twice as likely to be current specific-treatment users.

This finding is relevant because postponing treatment unfortunately results in refractory VVA symptoms that can be amplified by psychosocial factors, such as low self-esteem and relationship problems, leading to a significant impairment of quality of life.

There is a general agreement that systemic menopausal hormone therapy (MHT) may be prescribed at the lowest effective dose, in the absence of contraindications. However, when VVA is the sole consequence of menopause, systemic MHT is not indicated and local estrogen therapy (LET) is the first-line treatment for the maintenance of urogynecological and sexual health. Moreover, around 10–25 per cent of women using systemic MHT will still experience VVA symptoms and, therefore, a combination with LET may be useful to relieve vaginal dryness, dyspareunia and other urogenital symptoms, after appropriate counselling. Low-dose vaginal estrogen (estradiol, estriol, promestriene) preparations in various formulations (creams, rings, tablets, suppositories, gels) are available with some differences among countries. They have been shown, when used as directed, to be safe and effective, without causing significant proliferation of the endometrium or increase in serum estrogen levels beyond the normal postmenopausal range. LET provides vaginal estrogen, while minimizing systemic exposure, and results in increased blood flow, increased epithelial thickness and increased secretions, as well as reduced pH. These physiological improvements lead to reversal of atrophy with a positive clinical outcome for most postmenopausal women. In older women, LET has been shown to improve urinary urge incontinence and symptoms of overactive bladder and to reduce the rUTIs. Generally, there is no need for progestogen because low-dose LET is not associated with an increased risk for endometrial hyperplasia. Given the comparable efficiency of the different low-dose, locally administered estrogen products, the best way to select the type of treatment is dependent on effectiveness and safety for the individual patient. In addition, it is important that the patient accepts and adheres to their treatment in order to fully realize the benefits, and therefore they have to like the treatment of choice. DHEA has become available very recently. It is delivered intravaginally and has shown positive effects, similar to LET, on signs and symptoms of VVA, without significantly increasing plasma levels of sex hormones. Local testosterone cream, if available, may be safely used according to a double-blind, randomized, placebo-controlled trial in postmenopausal women taking an aromatase inhibitor with VVA symptoms.

All woman may experience a beneficial effect from non-hormonal treatments, such as vaginal moisturizers and lubricants with different characteristics. Lubricants are usually used on demand to relieve vaginal dryness during intercourse and therefore do not provide a long-term solution. On the other hand, women use moisturizers on a more regular basis and these local products may induce some positive modification of genital tissues according to their composition (reduction of pH, maturation of the vaginal epithelium, improvement of natural moisture). Although over-the-counter treatments may work for women with mild symptoms, they are often inadequate for women with moderate to severe symptoms. However, non-hormonal options are primarily indicated in women wishing to avoid hormonal therapy or in high-risk individuals with a history of hormone-sensitive malignancy such as breast or endometrial cancer. In cases of severe symptoms of VVA, it may be appropriate to discuss the relative risk of using LET/DHEA/testosterone with the oncology team as well as with the patient. Whereas in women taking tamoxifen following breast cancer, there is very little concern that the use of LET may compromise the effects of tamoxifen, the situation is different in women treated with aromatase inhibitors where contraindication to LET use remains.

In general, physical therapy including pelvic floor exercises, medical devices, and other activities with the aim to learn new sexual skills are useful alone or in association with other treatments to ameliorate urogenital health. In particular, microablative fractional CO_2 laser, the non-ablative vaginal Erbium YAG laser (VEL) and energy-based devices are increasingly used to alleviate VVA/GSM symptoms with promising results and a good safety profile. It is also important to mention that regular sexual activity, when it is possible, facilitates active blood flow to the vagina and increases vaginal lubrication. Psycho-educational programs and cognitive behavioural therapy have been proved highly effective in menopause management particularly after gynaecological and breast cancers, and such techniques provide benefits both for the individual woman and also for the couple. Recent data indicate that evaluation of men's attitudes regarding VVA and the effect on their postmenopausal partners may lead to a better understanding of the impact of VVA on sexual intimacy and may help couples to address the consequences of vaginal discomfort with their HCPs.

Systemic plant-derived and herbal remedies are a very popular alternative to medical treatments, but the real effectiveness in improving VVA is not proven in well-controlled studies, even though a combination of vaginal phytoestrogens and lactobacilli has been proven to be effective in women in whom hormone therapy is contraindicated.

Finally, Ospemifene, a selective estrogen receptor modulator (SERM) with a unique estrogen-like effect in the vaginal epithelium, is the first oral treatment approved for moderate to severe dyspareunia associated with VVA and for other VVA symptoms. Randomized clinical trials have shown that Ospemifene in a dose of 60 mg can be safely used with a high rate of efficacy and without significant estrogenic or clinically relevant adverse effects reported on endometrial tissue in women with an intact uterus. Given its pharmacological characteristics, consideration should be given to the possible use of Ospemifene in breast cancer survivors who have completed their protocol of chemotherapy [5].

Conclusion

VVA is a chronic, age-dependent condition resulting mainly from estrogen (and androgen) deficiency, and may worsen without appropriate treatment leading to the vicious cycle of sexual symptoms and urogynecological consequences. Early recognition and effective treatment of VVA may enhance sexual health and quality of life of women and their partners.

Bibliography

1. Sturdee DW, Panay N, International Menopause Society Writing Group. Recommendations for the management of postmenopausal vaginal atrophy. *Climacteric* 2010;13:509–22.

2. Portman, DJ, Gass ML, Vulvovaginal Atrophy Terminology Consensus Conference Panel. Genitourinary syndrome of menopause: new terminology for vulvovaginal atrophy from the International Society for the Study of Women's Sexual Health and the North American Menopause Society. *Menopause* 2014;21:1063–8.

3. Palacios S, Castelo-Branco C, Currie H, et al. Update on management of

genitourinary syndrome of menopause: a practical guide. *Maturitas* 2015;82:308–13.

4. Simon JA, Davis SR, Althof SE, et al. Sexual well-being after menopause: an International Menopause Society white paper. *Climacteric* 2018;21:415–27.

5. Shifren JL. Genito-urinary syndrome of menopause. *Clin Obstet Gynecol* 2018;61:508–16.

6. Nappi RE, Martini E, Cucinella L, et al. Addressing vulvovaginal atrophy (vva)/ genitourinary syndrome of menopause (gsm) for healthy aging in women. *Front Endocrinol* 2019;10:561.

Chapter 12

Pelvic Floor, Urinary Problems and the Menopause

Marco Gambacciani, Eleonora Russo, Magdalena Montt Guevara and Tommaso Simoncini

The female pelvic floor undergoes a large number of adaptive changes, related to life and endocrine events. The injuries and functional modifications of female pelvic floor due to pregnancy, life events and aging are associated to several changes that may predispose to pelvic floor dysfunctions (PFD). PFD globally affects micturition, defecation and sexual activity and its incidence increases dramatically with age and menopause.

Pelvic organ prolapse (POP), female lower urinary tract symptoms (FLUTS), chronic obstructive defecation syndrome (OFD), constipation and sexual dysfunction are just a few of the many aspects of PFD. POP and FLUTS are the most common pelvic floor dysfunctions in postmenopausal women [1].

Pathophysiology

Menopause, Ageing and PFD

Symptoms and severity of PFD increase after the menopausal transition and worsen with time. The effect of ageing and menopause cannot be clearly separated in midlife women. On the other hand, the sharp decline of estrogen levels cannot be neutral in the pelvic muscular and connective tissues that are estrogen sensitive and responsive. The female genital and lower urinary tracts share a common embryological origin, arising from the urogenital sinus, and both are sensitive to the effects of the female sex steroid hormones. Estrogen receptors (ER) are present in the epithelial tissues of the bladder, trigone, urethra, vaginal mucosa and in the support structures of the utero-sacral ligaments, as well as in levator ani muscles and pubo-cervical fascia [2]. Estrogen is involved in the increase of cell maturation index of these epithelial structures. It has been shown that alterations in the ratio of estrogen to ER may be involved in the development of stress urinary incontinence [3]. Estrogens control the synthesis and metabolism of collagen in the lower genital tract and increase the amount of muscle fibres in the detrusor muscle and in the urethral muscle layer [4, 5]. Estrogens may also influence the neurologic control of micturition in the central nervous system, altering the density of sympathetic nerve fibres in the pelvis and the central and peripheral synthesis of neurotrophins, even if this set of actions is not fully understood [6]. Progesterone receptors (PR) are also expressed in the lower urinary tract, even if with less density than ER. There is evidence that progesterone has adverse effects on female urinary tract function since it is linked to an increase in the adrenergic tone, provoking a decreased tone in the ureters, bladder and urethra.

The sensitivity to sex steroid hormones of the urogenital tissues has been advocated as an explanation for the common appearance of FLUTS at menopause. Most of the urogenital dysfunctions such as urinary incontinence (UI), voiding dysfunction, recurrent urinary tract infection (UTI), dyspareunia and POP are increased by declining levels of estrogen. This observation has been recently elaborated by a panel of experts into a unifying concept called the genitourinary syndrome of menopause (GSM) [7]. GSM is defined as a collection of symptoms and signs associated with a decrease in estrogen and other sex steroids involving changes in the labia majora/minora, clitoris, vestibule/introitus, vagina, urethra and bladder. The syndrome may include but is not limited to genital symptoms of dryness, burning and irritation; sexual symptoms of lack of lubrication, discomfort or pain, and impaired function; and urinary symptoms of urgency, dysuria and recurrent urinary tract infections. Women may present with some or all of the signs and symptoms, which must be bothersome and should not be better accounted for by another diagnosis [7].

Moreover, the ageing process can induce per se several changes in the structure and function of the lower urinary and genital tract. Several physiological and pathological bladder changes that frequently occur with aging are closely related to FLUTS. With aging, the adaptive mechanisms that are able to adjust the functional bladder capacity to urine production become less evident. The bladder sensation and ability to empty the bladder seem to decrease with advancing age as a possible consequence of neuronal loss and remodelling of the bladder and urethra [8]. In women suffering from FLUTS, there is a persistent correlation between age and terminal detrusor overactivity and a reduction of the functional bladder capacity. These age-related changes have also been detected at urodynamic testing [9]. From bladder structure point of view it seems that aging is associated with several changes in bladder properties. Some studies have showed a relationship between aging, oxidative stress, inflammation and bladder dysfunctions [10, 11].

Pelvic floor laxity depends on muscle injury and progressive pelvic floor weakening during the aging process. These result from connective tissue degradation, pelvic denervation, devascularization and anatomical modifications, all determining a decline in mechanical strength and dysynergic pelvic floor function, predisposing to POP and bowel dysfunctions.

Aging can induce changes in the structure and function of the gastrointestinal tract, especially in the colon and in the anorectal region. Within the aging process, there could be a reduced rectal sensation and an increased rectal compliance, anatomical anal canal changes and anal sphincter degeneration and atrophy. These changes can impair bowel habits and evacuation mechanisms [12].

Clinical Assessment of Female Pelvic Floor

An overall assessment should include evaluations of general fitness, balance and mobility and cognitive status. If symptoms suggest a neurologic disease, a basic and pelvic neurologic examination should be performed. In midlife women, the first focus on pelvic examination should always be on overall vulvo-vaginal health.

Several signs are discoverable on pelvic examination. First the evaluation of the presence of signs of vulvo-vaginal atrophy (VVA) and of anatomical defects. Pelvic visceral support is assessed by first observing the presence or absence of a bulge at the introitus with Valsalva effort. Speculum examination is required to accurately assess support. Over the last 15 years, measures to evaluate POP were improved. There is now an internationally accepted standard for describing, quantifying and staging female pelvic support, Pelvic Organ Prolapse Quantification (POP-Q), and a number of valid, reliable and responsive symptom questionnaires and condition-specific health-related quality-of-life (HRQOL) instruments [13, 14]. The POP-Q allows a reproducible description of the support of the anterior, posterior and apical vaginal segments using precise measurements to a fixed reference point, the hymen, and established criteria for staging the various levels of pelvic organ support from good support (POP-Q stage 0 or I) to almost complete lack of support (POP-Q stage IV). Other discoverable signs include the presence of vulvar abnormalities, urethral caruncle and urethral diverticulum.

Pelvic floor muscle assessment is generally assessed by palpating levator muscle contraction and then grading it subjectively. In 2005, the Pelvic Floor Clinical Assessment Group of the International Continence Society recommended use of a simpler classification: absent, weak, normal and strong. Normal muscle tone or abnormal muscle tone in terms of hyper- or hypotonicity should be evaluated. Maximal voluntary contraction (MVC), muscle strength, local muscle endurance and muscle coordination are other important parameters. Pelvic floor muscle assessment may help determine whether a patient is a candidate for a trial of pelvic floor physiotherapy or whether she is a candidate for other treatments.

The presence of stress urinary incontinence (SUI) can be objectively documented at this time by asking the woman to cough forcibly (the 'cough stress test'). If SUI is present, where surgical intervention is being considered, it is important to ascertain the mobility of the bladder neck. Principal methods are the simple visual assessment of bladder neck descent during straining or cough or the bladder neck position evaluation by ultrasound. At the time of initial clinical assessment, it is simple to assess a postvoid residual (PVR) volume. It can be assessed either by in and out catheterization or ultrasound following a spontaneous or demand void. PVR < 100 ml is generally accepted as normal. This is a key instrument in patients with anterior vaginal wall prolapse but also in women without POP complaining of incomplete emptying or recurrent UTI. Uroflowmetry is a useful clinical adjunct to PVR measurement. It involves measurement of the voided volume, flow rate and flow pattern. As a diagnostic tool, uroflowmetry helps define the voiding function in selective patients.

Finally, a screening urinalysis should be performed to rule out infection. Urine cytology and cystoscopy are in general reserved for those patients with irritative symptoms, recurrent infections, or persistent hematuria, in order to rule out malignancy or foreign body presence in the bladder (usually a stone).

Clinical Conditions and Management

Female Lower Urinary Tract Symptoms (FLUTS)

FLUTS, such as UI, overactive bladder syndrome (OAB) and voiding dysfunctions (incomplete bladder emptying, urinary retention), are prevalent in postmenopausal and elderly women. These conditions can interfere with daily life and can lead to negative effects on HRQOL.

According to the definition of the International Continence Society (ICS), UI is the complaint of any involuntary leakage of urine. Urgency urinary incontinence (UUI) is defined as involuntary leakage of urine, accompanied or immediately preceded by urgency. SUI is the complaint of involuntary leakage on effort or exertion or sneezing or coughing. Mixed urinary incontinence (MUI) encompasses urge UI and SUI. The complaint is of involuntary leakage associated with urgency and with exertion, effort, sneezing, or coughing [15].

Prevalence and severity of UI increases with age. Current data provide very disparate prevalence estimates for UI in women. Isolated SUI accounts for approximately half of all incontinence, with most studies reporting 10–39 per cent prevalence. With few exceptions, MUI is found to be next most common, with most studies reporting 7.5–25 per cent prevalence. Isolated UUI is uncommon, with 1–7 per cent prevalence, and where recorded at all, other causes of incontinence occur with approximately 0.5–1 per cent prevalence. Prevalence rates from cross-sectional studies uniformly demonstrate an association with age [16, 17]. Annual incidence rates for broad definitions of UI ('monthly' or 'any') range from 0.9 to 18.8 per cent, while rates for weekly UI show less variation at 1.2–4.0 per cent [17]. The age distribution for incontinence of all causes reported in the EPINCONT study shows a distinct peak in slight incontinence around the time of the menopause.

Despite a number of high-quality longitudinal studies, the literature on risk factors for incontinence is very heterogeneous. Among women, age, BMI, parity and mode of delivery are associated with incontinence.

OAB is urinary urgency, with or without urgency incontinence, usually with increased daytime frequency and nocturia, if there is no proven infection or obvious pathology [15]. There is evidence that estrogen deficiency may increase the risk of developing OAB after menopause [5]. The prevalence of OAB increases with age (19.1 per cent in women between 65 and 74 years of age) [18]. OAB incidence varies between 3.7 and 8.8 per cent [19]. While age is a clear risk factor for urinary urgency and/or OAB, other risk factors have not been that well studied.

OAB and UI are terms to describe the clinical problem of urgency and incontinence from a symptomatic rather than from a urodynamic perspective [20]. Symptoms alone can help determine treatment paths and define the impact on quality of life. Urodynamic testing is performed for objective diagnosis and is often used prior to surgery. Such testing defines urodynamic stress incontinence as objective urine loss with increased intra-abdominal pressure in the absence of a detrusor contraction. This objective finding would be expected in most women complaining of SUI. Additionally, urodynamics objectively define the condition of detrusor overactivity, a bladder dysfunction with uninhibited detrusor muscle contractions (with or without urine loss) on bladder filling in the absence of infection or the obvious bladder pathology. Detrusor overactivity is most often associated with UUI and/or OAB symptoms.

Management and Treatment of Urinary Incontinence (UI)

In the management and treatment of UI different options are available, including pelvic floor muscle training (PFMT) and physical therapies, drugs, surgery and neuromodulation strategies.

Conservative Management: Behavioural Modification, Physical Therapy and PFMT

UI can successfully be managed initially at the primary care level in most patients. Referral to a specialist is usually indicated when conservative measures fail to improve symptoms. Women with all types of UI can be advised to decrease their intake of fluids, caffeine and carbonated drinks. Further behavioural modification includes timed voiding, with a goal of reducing voiding frequency to every two to three hours. Bladder training (BT) should be recommended as first-line conservative therapy for UI in women. Constipation should be managed and avoided because this contributes to UI and voiding dysfunction [21].

PFMT has a crucial role in the treatment of UI. Because PFM integrity appears to be a key factor in the continence mechanism, there is a biological rationale to support the use of PFMT in preventing and treating both SUI and UUI in women. The role of PFMT in the treatment of UUI is related to the capacity of PFM contraction to prevent the leakage during detrusor contraction as well as inhibit and suppress detrusor contraction [21].

Laser therapy has gained attention as an effective treatment for VVA and an increasing body of evidence suggests its potential in improving urinary continence and possibly pelvic support. The concept behind laser procedures to treat vulvo-vaginal conditions is to use a wavelength having high water absorption, such as the carbon dioxide (CO_2) laser and the Erbium (Er:YAG) [22, 23]. Laser treatment induces tissue remodelling, with histological evidence of the restoration of vaginal mucosa, a thickening of the epithelium, with the maturation of epithelial cells, a new formation of papillae indenting the epithelium with newly formed and extended small vessels [22, 23]. In addition, in the connective tissue underlying the epithelium, the formation of new thin fibrils and morphological features of fibroblasts supporting a renewal of the extracellular matrix with functional restoration are generated. Fractional CO_2 laser was the first used to treat vaginal atrophy. According to the concept of fractional photothermolysis, CO_2 lasers ablate a fraction of the vaginal mucosa in the treatment area. At variance, the second-generation non-ablative vaginal Er:YAG laser (VEL) induces morphological changes via a non-ablative thermal diffusion to the vaginal walls. Besides the effects of VEL on the treatment of VVA, the efficacy of VEL in SUI has been reported in observational studies, in long-term cohort studies, and confirmed in a RCT study [22–31]. VEL may provide a safe and effective alternative in women suffering from PFD, being less invasive than the current surgical gold standard for SUI, offering a possible solution for women suffering from mild-moderate SUI that are not candidates for surgery. The possible synergistic effect of VEL and PFMT is currently under investigation.

Drug Treatments and Surgical Options

Medical therapy is a usually a valid option for women with UUI and MUI. Estrogen has been used to treat incontinence over a number of years, either alone or in combination with some of these other options, and there is evidence that UI may improve with local estrogen treatment [10]. In contrast, systemic hormone replacement therapy seems to worsen UI [11]. The possible worsening of UI with systemic estrogen therapy as well as the concerns about adverse effects of systemic treatment (for example regarding breast cancer, effects on endometrium or thromboembolic diseases) makes further evaluation of local estrogen therapy in the treatment of UI of great value. The currently available evidence has to be interpreted with caution because the treatment effects are based on a relatively low number of patients and a wide range of types, dosages and durations of estrogen treatment [32]. Moreover, also in the studies regarding local estrogen treatment for urinary tract symptoms, there is a diversity in the outcomes measured (urodynamic or clinical) and populations studied. The available evidence regarding vaginal estrogen therapy in postmenopausal women with OAB symptoms (urinary urgency, frequency, nocturia, with or without UUI) is encouraging [33]. However, it is not clear if subjective improvement in OAB symptoms reflects a direct effect on lower urinary tract function or an indirect effect via reversing vaginal atrophy [34].

A positive effect of the new SERM Ospemifene administration has been reported in women suffering from mixed urinary incontinence and OAB [35]. The possible role of Ospemifene in women suffering from PFD warrants further, properly sized studies.

Drug should be initiated after conservative methods have been tried and antimuscarinic drugs, combined with local estrogens, constitute first-line medical treatment in postmenopausal women with symptoms suggestive of an OAB [36]. Antimuscarinic agents may be associated with adverse effects. The human bladder tissue, the brain, the salivary glands, the cardiovascular system and the eye contain muscarinic receptors. As a result, antimuscarinic agents are effective in treating OAB symptoms, but they may also be associated with adverse effects such as dry mouth, constipation, cognitive impairment, tachycardia and blurred vision. These side effects are not uncommon and may lead to failure of treatment due to people stopping the use of the drugs. The use of these medications is contraindicated in patients with narrow-angle glaucoma, urinary retention or gastric retention. New-generation drugs such as solifenacin and fesoterodine have been shown to be more efficacious than tolterodine [37]. A beta-3 adrenergic receptor agonist (β3-AR agonist) has been introduced as a means of medical management of OAB. It is a safe, effective and well-tolerated new class of drug. Pharmaceutical companies have developed selective β3-AR agonists targeted at urinary inconsistencies approved such as Mirabegron. Mirabegron has a particular affinity for β3 adrenoceptors and improves the storage capacity of the bladder with little effect on the contractile ability of the bladder [38]. Mirabegron can improve the symptoms of patients who have not had adequate response to antimuscarinics and its tolerability profile offers potential to improve patients' adherence with treatment for OAB [39].

In case conservative management and medical treatment are not successful after 8–12 weeks, specialized management should be considered [40]. According to the American Urology Association and European Urology Association guidelines recommendations, onabotulinumtoxin-A intravesical injection and neuromodulation are considered the third-line treatments for patients without response to medical treatment [41]. Onabotulinumtoxin-A is a neurotoxin that inhibits acetylcholine release from presynaptic neurons with decrease in acetylcholine availability in the neuromuscular junction and detrusor paralysis. The technique involves injection of onabotulinum-A in multiple sites throughout the bladder wall, whilst avoiding injecting the trigon. This technique is being increasingly used to treat severe OAB refractory to standard management both for neurogenic and idiopathic overactive bladder. The most frequent adverse effects following the administration of the toxin are urinary retention and urinary tract infection. The duration of effect of botulinum toxin type A may range from 3 to 12 months. Intravesical botulinum toxin appears to be an effective therapy for refractory OAB symptoms, but as yet little controlled trial data exist on benefits and safety compared with other interventions, or with placebo [42]. Sacral nerve stimulation can be used as an alternative to botulinum injections in patients who are dissatisfied or in whom such treatment with botulinum toxin-A treatment fails. Sacral nerve stimulation follows a test phase with temporary electrodes placed next to the S3 sacral nerve root. If sufficient symptomatic improvement is given, the definitive electrode can be placed, with a subcutaneous stimulator. Incontinence episodes and voiding frequency are both reduced while receiving sacral nerve stimulation, with a significant improvement of quality of life [43]. Percutaneous tibial nerve stimulation (PTNS) is a form of peripheral neuromodulation. PTNS uses a removable device with a fine needle, penetrating the skin at the level of the posterior tibial nerve two fingers above the malleolus medialis of the ankle. The indication of proximity to the nerve is the observation for intrinsic foot muscle contraction. The stimulus is applied for half an hour. Treatment is repeated at weekly intervals. There is strong evidence for the efficacy of PTNS on frequency and urgency UI and limited evidence for nocturia and urgency [44].

From a surgical perspective injectable bulking agents, laparoscopic suspensions (laparoscopic 'Burch' colposuspension), mid-urethral slings, pubovaginal slings and open retropubic suspensions are available strategies in treatment of SUI.

Retro pubic (RP-TVT) and trans obturator mid-urethral (TO-TVT) mid-urethral sling (MUS) are today the most popular surgical treatments for female SUI. The surgical strategy of sling stems from the 'hammock' hypothesis. This describes the urethra as being compressed against a hammock-like supportive layer to assist in the urethral closure mechanism during an increase in intra-abdominal pressure, such as during a cough. This theory originated with the work of Petros and Ulmsten, who described how alterations in connective tissue may cause laxity in the vagina and its supporting ligaments and lead to incontinence [45]. Success rates of mid-urethral slings range from 84 to 99 per cent [46]. Risks of surgical correction include bleeding, pain, infection, de novo urgency, urinary retention and failure of treatment. The long-term efficacy and safety of the procedures is still a topic of intense clinical research and several randomized controlled trials (RCTs) have been published in the last years.

Pelvic Organ Prolapse (POP)

POP is clinically defined as 'the descent of one or more of the anterior vaginal wall, posterior vaginal wall, the uterus (cervix) or the apex of the vagina (vaginal vault or cuff scar after hysterectomy)' [47]. The etiology of POP is and unique in each patient, and its thorough understanding is key to successful treatment. Risk factors include pregnancy, childbirth, obesity, congenital or acquired connective tissue abnormalities, chronic constipation, family history of POP, denervation or weakness of the pelvic floor, menopause and aging [1, 48–50].

It is estimated that nearly 50 per cent of women will develop some form of prolapse, only 10–20 per cent search medical assistance [48]. The prevalence of POP increases with age with a peak in women aged 60 to 69 [51]. POP can be identified in up to 50 per cent of women with vaginal inspection, but if POP is defined by the presence of clinically relevant symptoms, its prevalence in the general population ranges between 3–6 per cent, since mild or moderate POP is frequently asymptomatic [52].

POP-related symptoms vary based on the anatomical defect(s) or related to the degree of bladder, bowel and sexual dysfunction [47]. Patients constantly report vaginal bulge in the presence of moderate to advanced POP. The anatomic threshold for symptomatic prolapse appears to be the hymen; however, medical attention is not infrequently sought for early-stage POP [53].

Protrusion of the vagina may result in chronic discharge and/or bleeding from ulceration. Loss of support of the anterior and vaginal apex may affect bladder and urethral function. Symptoms of SUI often coexist with stage I or II of prolapse and as prolapse advances women may experience improvement in SUI but increased difficulty voiding. Common POP-related voiding dysfunctions are: hesitancy, prolonged or intermittent flow, the need to push the POP back up to aid urinary voiding and the sensation of incomplete emptying. Women with POP have also an increased risk of OAB symptoms [54].

Defecatory symptoms are more prevalent in women with POP and can occur with any posterior compartment defect, including rectocele, enterocele sigmoidocele, internal rectal prolapse or full mucosal rectal prolapse. Constipation, incomplete evacuation and obstructed defecation, are common complaints. Straining and the need to exert digital manipulation to complete evacuation are clinical hallmark of obstructed defecation syndrome (ODS).

Management and Treatment of POP

Treatment for POP should be reserved for symptomatic women. Treatment is individualized according to each patient's symptoms and their impact on her quality of life. The treatment of POP includes conservative management (lifestyle modifications and physical therapies), surgery or pessary. The choice of therapy depends also upon the patient's preference, as well as the ability to comply with conservative therapy or tolerate surgery.

First-line management of POP is conservative therapy. Conservative management is a usually a valid option for women with mild degree of prolapse and mild symptoms [21]. Lifestyle modification includes dietary modification, weight loss, reducing activities that strain the pelvic floor, treatment of constipation and ceasing smoking. While these interventions mitigate POP symptoms, whether they limit POP progression is not established.

Physical therapies improve POP symptoms and help restore pelvic floor function. These interventions include physical activity, cognitive behavioural therapy, bladder training, bowel habit training, biofeedback and electrical muscle stimulation [55]. Pelvic floor muscle training (PFMT) involves the contraction of the pelvic floor muscles to improve strength, endurance and timing of contractions to better support the pelvic organs. Several meta-analyses show that women with symptomatic mild POP treated with PFMT undergo significant improvement of prolapse symptoms and severity of POP [56]. No data are available on the efficacy of PFMT treatment in aiding POP surgery, although most experts consider it useful [57, 58].

Laser therapy is a promising option for women with mild degree of prolapse or with mild symptoms. It has been suggested that VEL can be used in the so-called vaginal relaxation syndrome (VRS), where the relaxing of the vaginal wall leads to physical and psychological problems mainly related to decreasing sexual satisfaction. There are not RCTs published to date about laser therapy for the treatment of POP. Only case series have been published mainly regarding the effects of VEL on cystocele rather than rectocele [22, 23].

Women with symptomatic prolapse who have failed conservative management are candidates for reconstructive surgery. There is no indication for repair of asymptomatic POP as an isolated procedure. It is important to identify symptoms that are attributable to each specific anatomical compartment, since this aids surgical decision-making. Several factors affect surgical planning, primarily the combination or complexity of anatomical defects and the individual risks for surgical complications. Isolated repair of anterior, apical or posterior vaginal wall prolapse is typically performed transvaginally. Abdominal surgery is more effective and safe for the management of advanced or multi-compartmental POP. Although no RCTs are available, estrogen treatment prior to surgery has been reported to ease the procedures.

Conclusion

The pelvic floor in women is a complex and highly vulnerable structure. Injuries and functional modifications of this structure due to delivery, life events, menopause and aging often lead to pelvic floor dysfunctions. Pelvic floor dysfunction determines a variable association of complaints related to the urinary, genital and low intestinal tracts. Such symptoms are extremely common in postmenopausal and aging women and can significantly impair a woman's quality of life. Pathophysiology of pelvic floor dysfunctions is unique in each patient, and their comprehensive understanding is key to successful treatment.

References

1. Tinelli A, Malvasi A, Rahimi S, Negro R, Vergara D, Martignago R, et al. Age-related pelvic floor modifications and prolapse risk factors in postmenopausal women. *Menopause* 2010;17(1):204–12.

2. Gebhart JB, Rickard DJ, Barrett TJ, Lesnick TG, Webb MJ, Podratz KC, et al. Expression of estrogen receptor isoforms alpha and beta messenger RNA in vaginal tissue of premenopausal and postmenopausal women. *Am J Obstet Gynecol* 2001;185(6):1325–30; discussion 30–1.

3. Xie Z, Shi H, Zhou C, Dong M, Hong L, Jin H. Alterations of estrogen receptor-alpha and -beta in the anterior vaginal wall of women with urinary incontinence. *Eur J Obstet Gynecol Reprod Biol* 2007;134(2):254–8.

4. Robinson D, Cardozo L. Estrogens and the lower urinary tract. *Neurol Urodyn* 2011;30 (5):754–7.

5. Robinson D, Toozs-Hobson P, Cardozo L. The effect of hormones on the lower urinary tract. *Menopause Int* 2013;19(4):155–62.

6. Zoubina EV, Mize AL, Alper RH, Smith PG. Acute and chronic estrogen supplementation decreases uterine sympathetic innervation in ovariectomized adult virgin rats. *Histol Histopathol* 2001;16(4):989–96.

7. Portman DJ, Gass ML. Genitourinary syndrome of menopause: new terminology for vulvovaginal atrophy from the International Society for the Study of Women's Sexual Health and the North American Menopause Society. *Climacteric* 2014;17(5):557–63.

8. Andersson KE, Boedtkjer DB, Forman A. The link between vascular dysfunction, bladder ischemia, and aging bladder dysfunction. *Thera Adv Urol* 2017;9 (1):11–27.

9. Camoes J, Coelho A, Castro-Diaz D, Cruz F. Lower urinary tract symptoms and aging: the impact of chronic bladder ischemia on overactive bladder syndrome. *Urol Int* 2015;95(4):373–9.

10. Tyagi P, Tyagi V, Qu X, Lin HT, Kuo HC, Chuang YC, et al. Association of inflammaging (inflammation + aging) with higher prevalence of OAB in elderly

population. *Int Urol Nephrol* 2014;46 (5):871–7.

11. Ghoniem G, Faruqui N, Elmissiry M, Mahdy A, Abdelwahab H, Oommen M, et al. Differential profile analysis of urinary cytokines in patients with overactive bladder. *Int Urogynecol J* 2011;22(8):953–61.

12. Rociu E, Stoker J, Eijkemans MJ, Lameris JS. Normal anal sphincter anatomy and age- and sex-related variations at high-spatial-resolution endoanal MR imaging. *Radiology* 2000;217 (2):395–401.

13. Digesu GA, Khullar V, Cardozo L, Robinson D, Salvatore S. P-QOL: a validated questionnaire to assess the symptoms and quality of life of women with urogenital prolapse. *Int Urogynecol J Pelvic Floor Dysfunction* 2005;16 (3):176–81; discussion 81.

14. Barber MD, Walters MD, Bump RC. Short forms of two condition-specific quality-of-life questionnaires for women with pelvic floor disorders (PFDI-20 and PFIQ-7). *Am J Obstet Gynecol* 2005;193(1):103–13.

15. Abrams P, Cardozo L, Fall M, Griffiths D, Rosier P, Ulmsten U, et al. The standardisation of terminology in lower urinary tract function: report from the standardisation sub-committee of the International Continence Society. *Urology* 2003;61(1):37–49.

16. Hunskaar S, Lose G, Sykes D, Voss S. The prevalence of urinary incontinence in women in four European countries. *BJU Int* 2004;93(3):324–30.

17. Coyne KS, Sexton CC, Kopp ZS, Luks S, Gross A, Irwin D, et al. Rationale for the study methods and design of the epidemiology of lower urinary tract symptoms (EpiLUTS) study. *BJU Int* 2009;104(3):348–51.

18. Wallace KM, Drake MJ. Overactive bladder. *F1000Res* 2015;4.

19. Irwin DE, Milsom I, Kopp Z, Abrams P, Artibani W, Herschorn S. Prevalence, severity, and symptom bother of lower urinary tract symptoms among men in the

EPIC study: impact of overactive bladder. *Eur Urol* 2009;56(1):14–20.

20. Steers WD. Pathophysiology of overactive bladder and urge urinary incontinence. *Rev Urol* 2002;4 Suppl 4:S7–s18.

21. Dumoulin C, Hunter KF, Moore K, Bradley CS, Burgio KL, Hagen S, et al. Conservative management for female urinary incontinence and pelvic organ prolapse review 2013: summary of the 5th International Consultation on Incontinence. *Neurourol Urodyn* 2016;35 (1):15–20.

22. Tadir Y, Gaspar A, Lev-Sagie A, Alexiades M, Alinsod R, Bader A, et al. Light and energy based therapeutics for genitourinary syndrome of menopause: consensus and controversies. *Lasers Surg Med* 2017;49(2):137–59.

23. Gambacciani M, Palacios S. Laser therapy for the restoration of vaginal function. *Maturitas* 2017;99:10–5.

24. Arunkalaivanan A, Kaur H, Onuma O. Laser therapy as a treatment modality for genitourinary syndrome of menopause: a critical appraisal of evidence. *Int Urogynecol J* 2017;28(5):681–5.

25. Gambacciani M, Levancini M, Russo E, Vacca L, Simoncini T, Cervigni M. Long-term effects of vaginal erbium laser in the treatment of genitourinary syndrome of menopause. *Climacteric* 2018;21 (2):148–52.

26. Gaspar A, Brandi H, Gomez V, Luque D. Efficacy of Erbium: YAG laser treatment compared to topical estriol treatment for symptoms of genitourinary syndrome of menopause. *Lasers Surg Med* 2017;49 (2):160–8.

27. Fistonic N, Fistonic I, Gustek SF, Turina IS, Marton I, Vizintin Z, et al. Minimally invasive, non-ablative Er: YAGlaser treatment of stress urinary incontinence in women–a pilot study. *Lasers Med Sci* 2016;31(4):635–43.

28. Digesu GA, Swift S. Laser treatment in urogynaecology and the myth of the scientific evidence. *Int Urogynecol J* 2017;28:1443–4.

29. Tien YW, Hsiao SM, Lee CN, Lin HH. Effects of laser procedure for female urodynamic stress incontinence on pad weight, urodynamics, and sexual function. *Int Urogynecol J* 2017;28(3):469–76.

30. Fistonic I, Fistonic N. Baseline ICIQ-UI score, body mass index, age, average birth weight, and perineometry duration as promising predictors of the short-term efficacy of Er: YAG laser treatment in stress urinary incontinent women: a prospective cohort study. *Lasers Surg Med* 2018;epub ahead of print.

31. Gaspar A, Brandi H. Non-ablative erbium YAG laser for the treatment of type III stress urinary incontinence (intrinsic sphincter deficiency). *Lasers Med Sci* 2017;32(3):685–91.

32. Cody JD, Jacobs ML, Richardson K, Moehrer B, Hextall A. Oestrogen therapy for urinary incontinence in post-menopausal women. *Cochrane Database Syst Rev* 2012;10:Cd001405.

33. Ostle Z. Vaginal oestrogen for overactive bladder in post-menopausal women. *Br J Nurs* 2015;24(11):582–5.

34. Robinson D, Cardozo L, Milsom I, Pons ME, Kirby M, Koelbl H, et al. Oestrogens and overactive bladder. *Neurourol Urodyn* 2014;33(7):1086–91.

35. Schiavi MC, D'Oria O, Aleksa N, Vena F, Prata G, Di Tucci C, et al. Usefulness of Ospemifene in the treatment of urgency in menopausal patients affected by mixed urinary incontinence underwent mid-urethral slings surgery. *Gynecol Endocrinol* 2019;35(2):155–9.

36. Baber RJ, Panay N, Fenton A. 2016 IMS Recommendations on women's midlife health and menopause hormone therapy. *Climacteric* 2016;19(2):109–50.

37. Madhuvrata P, Cody JD, Ellis G, Herbison GP, Hay-Smith EJ. Which anticholinergic drug for overactive bladder symptoms in adults. *Cochrane Database of Syst Rev* 2012;1:Cd005429.

38. Warren K, Burden H, Abrams P. Mirabegron in overactive bladder patients: efficacy review and update on drug safety. *Thera Adv Drug Saf* 2016;7(5):204–16.

39. Giarenis I, Robinson D, Cardozo L. Overactive bladder and the beta3-adrenoceptor agonists: current strategy and future prospects. *Drugs* 2015;75(15):1707–13.

40. Abrams P, Andersson KE, Birder L, Brubaker L, Cardozo L, Chapple C, et al. Fourth International Consultation on Incontinence Recommendations of the International Scientific Committee: evaluation and treatment of urinary incontinence, pelvic organ prolapse, and fecal incontinence. *Neurourol Urodyn* 2010;29(1):213–40.

41. Gormley EA, Lightner DJ, Faraday M, Vasavada SP. Diagnosis and treatment of overactive bladder (non-neurogenic) in adults: AUA/SUFU guideline amendment. *J Urol* 2015;193(5):1572–80.

42. Duthie JB, Vincent M, Herbison GP, Wilson DI, Wilson D. Botulinum toxin injections for adults with overactive bladder syndrome. *Cochrane Database Syst Rev* 2011(12):Cd005493.

43. Noblett K, Siegel S, Mangel J, Griebling TL, Sutherland SE, Bird ET, et al. Results of a prospective, multicenter study evaluating quality of life, safety, and efficacy of sacral neuromodulation at twelve months in subjects with symptoms of overactive bladder. *Neurourol Urodyn* 2016;35 (2):246–51.

44. Gaziev G, Topazio L, Iacovelli V, Asimakopoulos A, Di Santo A, De Nunzio C, et al. Percutaneous tibial nerve stimulation (PTNS) efficacy in the treatment of lower urinary tract dysfunctions: a systematic review. *BMC Urol* 2013;13:61.

45. Petros PE, Ulmsten UI. An integral theory of female urinary incontinence. Experimental and clinical considerations. *Acta Obstet Gynecol Scand Suppl* 1990;153:7–31.

46. Ogah J, Cody DJ, Rogerson L. Minimally invasive synthetic suburethral sling operations for stress urinary incontinence in women: a short version Cochrane review. *Neurourol Urodyn* 2011;30 (3):284–91.

47. Haylen BT, Maher CF, Barber MD, Camargo S, Dandolu V, Digesu A, et al. An International Urogynecological Association (IUGA)/International Continence Society (ICS) joint report on the terminology for female pelvic organ prolapse (POP). *Neurourol Urodyn* 2016;35(2):137–68.

48. Maher C, Feiner B, Baessler K, Schmid C. Surgical management of pelvic organ prolapse in women. *Cochrane Database Syst Rev* 2013(4):Cd004014.

49. Nygaard I, Barber MD, Burgio KL, Kenton K, Meikle S, Schaffer J, et al. Prevalence of symptomatic pelvic floor disorders in US women. *JAMA* 2008;300 (11):1311–6.

50. Lince SL, van Kempen LC, Vierhout ME, Kluivers KB. A systematic review of clinical studies on hereditary factors in pelvic organ prolapse. *Int Urogynecol J* 2012;23(10):1327–36.

51. Wu JM, Vaughan CP, Goode PS, Redden DT, Burgio KL, Richter HE, et al. Prevalence and trends of symptomatic pelvic floor disorders in US women. *Obstetr Gynecol* 2014;123(1):141–8.

52. Barber MD, Maher C. Epidemiology and outcome assessment of pelvic organ prolapse. *Int Urogynecol J* 2013;24 (11):1783–90.

53. Gutman RE, Ford DE, Quiroz LH, Shippey SH, Handa VL. Is there a pelvic organ prolapse threshold that predicts pelvic floor symptoms? *Am J Obstet Gynecol* 2008;199(6):683.e1–7.

54. de Boer TA, Salvatore S, Cardozo L, Chapple C, Kelleher C, van Kerrebroeck P, et al. Pelvic organ prolapse and overactive bladder. *Neurourol Urodyn* 2010;29 (1):30–9.

55. Bo K, Frawley HC, Haylen BT, Abramov Y, Almeida FG, Berghmans B, et al. An International Urogynecological Association (IUGA)/International Continence Society (ICS) joint report on the terminology for the conservative and nonpharmacological management of female pelvic floor dysfunction. *Int Urogynecol J* 2017;28(2):191–213.

56. Li C, Gong Y, Wang B. The efficacy of pelvic floor muscle training for pelvic organ prolapse: a systematic review and meta-analysis. *Int Urogynecol J* 2016;27 (7):981–92.

57. Barber MD, Brubaker L, Burgio KL, Richter HE, Nygaard I, Weidner AC, et al. Comparison of 2 transvaginal surgical approaches and perioperative behavioral therapy for apical vaginal prolapse: the OPTIMAL randomized trial. *JAMA* 2014;311(10):1023–34.

58. Hagen S, Stark D. Conservative prevention and management of pelvic organ prolapse in women. *Cochrane Database Syst Rev* 2011(12):Cd003882.

Chapter 13

The Effect of Menopause on the Musculoskeletal System

Jean Calleja-Agius and Mark P. Brincat

Menopause has an overall adverse impact on musculoskeletal health. It is associated with osteoporosis, osteoarthritis and sarcopenia [1]. Osteoporosis and related fractures, together with the consequent pain and locomotor disability, affect the quality of life and life expectancy of postmenopausal women. Poor musculoskeletal health may progress to frailty and higher incidence of falls and fractures, which further increase the associated morbidity and mortality [1]. This leads to high economic costs worldwide [1, 2].

The fact that female sex hormones play an important role in the aetiology and pathophysiology of a variety of musculoskeletal degenerative diseases and osteoporosis, is supported by the increased prevalence of these conditions in postmenopausal women [3]. For example, low back pain is commoner in postmenopausal women than age-matched men, and this is associated with the physiological changes caused by the relatively lower level of sex hormones after menopause in women [3, 4].

The pathophysiology of osteoporosis, which is characterized by progressive loss of bone tissue, is multifactorial and complex. Various cytokines, mediators and signalling pathways in combination with genetic, hormonal and environmental influences regulating the bone remodelling process are involved. The presence of osteoporosis especially in the mother and the existence of previous fractures are significant risk factors for the occurrence of osteoporosis [5]. The development and differentiation of osteoblasts and osteoclasts is tightly controlled by growth factors and cytokines synthesized in the bone marrow microenvironment in order to maintain a dynamic equilibrium between their formation, survival and function. Women with low BMD have higher levels of adipokines, and lower levels of markers of bone turnover such as PINP, PINP/CTX ratio in their circulation as compared to those with normal BMD [6]. The increase in osteoclastogenesis and impaired osteoblastogenesis, rather than the alteration in the activity of these cells, are responsible for postmenopausal osteoporosis [7].

The Role of Estrogen in Bone Turnover

Estradiol levels are significantly lower in women with low BMD of the hip and spine [6]. Estrogen regulates the secretion of cytokines involved in bone homeostasis exerting a role in bone remodelling. It inhibits the formation of locally produced pro-inflammatory cytokines and suppresses new osteoclast formation.

When there is oophorectomy, this leads to a significant increase in bone resorption. This occurs because a decline in circulating estrogen results in an increase in osteoclastogenesis and prolongation of osteoclasts' lifespan by decreasing apoptosis. However, the unlimited rise in osteoclasts number and lifespan is restrained by a compensatory increase in bone formation at each remodelling unit. Estrogen deficiency causes expansion of the pool of early mesenchymal progenitors as well as an increase in committed pluripotent precursors to the osteoblastic lineage, both enhancing the number of osteoblasts. However, lack of estrogen limits osteoblastogenesis by accelerating osteoblast apoptosis and enhancing the formation of inflammatory cytokines such as IL-7 and TNF, which inhibit the functional activity of mature osteoblasts. Thus, the overall increase in osteoblastogenesis is insufficient to compensate for osteoclastic bone resorption [8].

Decreased levels of bioavailable estradiol inhibit the activity of osteoblasts and stromal cells. This results in decreased osteoprogenitor secretion permitting more binding of RANKL to receptor activator of nuclear factor kappa-B (RANK) hence increasing osteoclastogenesis and bone resorption. In postmenopausal osteoporosis, the increase in bone resorption is brought about by a rise in paracrine production of bone resorbing cytokines. Decreased estradiol levels also increase the expression and secretion of IL-6, IL-11 and RANKL, which in turn directly activate more osteoclasts formation and activity. The secretion of these cytokines is significantly higher in bone marrow cells isolated from postmenopausal women [8, 9].

Menopausal hormone therapy (MHT) involves the administration of physiologic levels of estrogen and progestogen to replace and artificially boost the hormones which decline during menopause. MHT maintains a steady rate of bone loss in osteoporotic patients. It elevates calcium absorption and as a result of a decline in the bone resorption rate, bone balance is either maintained or becomes slightly positive. This positive bone balance is mainly pronounced in trabecular bone while bone mass is maintained in areas of the skeleton rich in cortical bone.

Estrogen is known to inhibit osteoclasts' activity. It causes a decline in erosion depth and osteoclast activation frequency by inducing apoptosis which is mediated by TGF-β and suppressing osteoclastogenesis. The decline in bone resorption is also mediated by a reduction in the formation and sensitivity of bone cells to IL-6, IL-1 and TNF-α and increase in the formation of IL-4. This causes a decrease in the differentiation of precursor cells to osteoclasts. Additionally, administering MHT to postmenopausal women causes a decline in proportion of bone marrow cell to express RANKL in lymphocytes but its concentration per cell is not altered. Hence, a decline in the osteoclasts' formation, differentiation and survival is observed. Moreover, estrogen reduces the lytic enzyme activity of osteoclasts, alters the concentration of growth factors and interferons and affects bone collagen metabolism [9].

As estrogen receptors are present on osteoblasts, estrogen supplied through MHT acts directly on such receptors to prevent bone loss. Long-term treatment with MHT administered at high doses not only decreases bone resorption but also activates bone formation by enhancing proliferation of osteoblasts resulting in a net anabolic action. This is known to result from the non-genotropic effect of estrogen on osteoblast apoptosis [9].

The indirect action of estrogen involves decreasing the responsiveness of bone to parathyroid hormone (PTH) and altering its secretion. It also elevates intestinal absorption and reduces the renal excretion of calcium.

Epidemiological studies have shown that a short-term treatment with MHT decreases the occurrence of osteoporotic fractures. It has been determined that undergoing estrogen therapy for 5 years reduces vertebral fractures by 60 per cent whilst hip fractures may decline by 50 per cent. Generally, by using estrogen treatment, bone turnover is reduced by half, decreasing postmenopausal bone loss and lowering the incidence of an osteoporotic fracture. However, once treatment with MHT is terminated, estrogen level declines and protection against osteoporosis is lost again. Most studies suggest that bone loss will progress at the same rate prior to treatment with MHT. Thus the accelerated bone loss during menopause is postponed by the duration of MHT treatment. To date, trabecular bone score, an indirect evaluation of skeletal microarchitecture, is calculated from dual-energy X-ray absorptiometry (DEXA) [10]. Several biomarkers have been studied as potential predictors of osteoporosis. One promising marker is urinary N-telopeptide U-NTX can be used early in the menopause transition to determine if a woman is about to experience significant bone loss, especially in the lumbar spine, before there is been substantial skeletal deterioration [11].

MHT has been shown to be highly effective in preventing postmenopausal osteoporosis during the first 5–10 years following the onset of menopause and treatment should be continuous and lifelong. This is because the rate of bone loss is the highest during the first 2 years of menopause. However, studies suggest that when estrogen therapy is initiated beyond the age of 60 years, BMD is either maintained or increased after 2 years of use. The increase in bone mass in such patients is a result of a decline in bone resorption more than bone formation. Women who initiate HRT at an older age, gain 5–10 per cent of bone density during the initial 2 years of therapy and then lose 0.5 per cent of bone density each year. Studies suggest that estrogen therapy initiated in the early sixties is as advantageous as continuous treatment that began immediately after menopause. When MHT is discontinued, 2 per cent of bone density is lost each year for 5 years and 1 per cent each year thereafter [7].

Progestogens (either natural progesterone, or a progestin, which is a synthetic analogue) decrease the rate of bone resorption as they reduce urinary calcium excretion. Administration of progestogen in combination with estrogen not only decreases the rate of bone loss but it has been proven to promote bone formation by enhancing osteoblasts' activity via suppression of glucocorticoid action. A number of studies have shown the positive effect of progesterone on bone proliferation and inhibition of bone resorption. Administration of estrogen and progestogen alone may have distinct yet complementary roles in the maintenance of bone architecture.

Intervertebral Discs

Each intervertebral disc is composed of high collagen content and glycosaminoglycans. Intervertebral discs are responsible for 20 per cent of the spinal column height and allow flexion and extension of the back, and also act as 'shock absorbers' of the spinal column. This may have an important role on osteoporotic compression fractures. With the ageing process, there is a change in collagen type, with a more profound difference with increasing years since menopause. The collagen types I, III and VI predominate at the expense of collagen types II, IV and IX. There is also a significant decrease in glycosaminoglycans and elastin in the aged intervertebral disc.

The lumbar intervertebral disc height as measured by DEXA bone densitometry has been shown to be significantly higher in the premenopausal group and hormone-treated group, compared to the untreated postmenopausal women. The premenopausal women and hormone-treated women had disc heights of 2.01 ± 0.09 cm and 2.15 ± 0.08 cm, respectively, the latter results being significantly higher than the untreated postmenopausal group (height of three lumbar discs 1.82 ± 0.06 cm) and the osteoporotic fracture group (1.58 ± 0.1 cm) ($p < 0.0001$) [12]. This association between menopause and disc degeneration in the lumbar spine has further been confirmed using a magnetic resonance imaging-based eight-level grading system, and has been shown to occur in the first 15 years after the menopause [13, 14].

This does strongly suggest that estrogen deficiency might be a risk factor of disc degeneration of the lumbar spine. This may lead to loss of the shock-absorbing properties of the intervertebral discs and an altered discoid shape, influencing the occurrence of osteoporotic vertebral body fractures. Hormone-treated and premenopausal women have thicker intervertebral discs than untreated postmenopausal women. Alterations in the extracellular matrix in the intervertebral discs appear to be intimately related to the menopausal process. Loss of disc height may predate osteoporotic fracture [12].

Postmenopausal women show accelerated disc degeneration due to relative estrogen deficiency, resulting in narrower intervertebral disc space in women than age-matched men, increased prevalence of spondylolisthesis, and increased prevalence of facet joint osteoarthritis [4]. Postmenopausal women also show higher osteoporosis-related spine fracture rate, particularly at the thoracic-lumbar junction site [4].

In rat models ovariectomy induces oxidative stress, autophagy and intervertebral disc degeneration. The level of autophagy of the intervertebral disc, which is negatively correlated with oxidative stress, can be reduced by estrogen replacement therapy through modulating the redox balance and downregulating the autophagy level [15].

Similarly, menopause has also been associated with cartilage degeneration of the knee joint. After menopause, cartilage showed progressive severe degeneration that occurred in the first 25 years after the menopause, suggesting estrogen deficiency might be a risk factor of cartilage degeneration of the knee joint. Further studies are needed to investigate whether age or menopause plays a more important role in the progression of cartilage degeneration in the knee joint [16].

Considering MHT's consistent efficacy reported with menopause-associated osteoarthritis and osteoporosis, an in-depth understanding of the role of the gonadal hormones in low back pain modulation warrants further study. MHT initiated at early postmenopausal phase may be protective for recurring low back pain. If this is the case, further cost–benefit analysis should be performed for optimal MHT regimen in cases of women with high risk of recurring severe low back pain [4].

Muscle

Sarcopenia includes age-related muscle wasting as well as loss of muscle function. It is a relatively newly recognized condition and is known to be accelerated by estrogen deficiency [1]. In menopause, there is a decline in muscle mass and strength when serum estrogen declines. Estrogen improves muscle strength. The underlying mechanism involves estrogen receptors to improve muscle quality rather than quantity. MHT attenuates exercise-induced skeletal muscle damage in postmenopausal women. Postmenopausal women not using hormonal therapy experience greater muscle damage. MHT modifies skeletal muscle composition and function. It gives better mobility, greater muscle power, prevents muscle weakness and thus prevents mobility limitation [17].

Many elderly postmenopausal women experience physical disabilities and loss of independence related to sarcopenia, which reduces life quality and is associated with substantial financial costs. There is inverse correlation between dominant hand grip strength (measured with a digital dynamometer) and age, and earlier age at menopause was associated with an increased dynapenia risk [18].

Thus, in order to maintain the integrity of the musculoskeletal system, the main recommendations are to do regular physical exercise, maintain protein intake and in the postmenopause, consider estrogen replacement. Resistance training and dietary optimization can counteract or at least decelerate the degenerative ageing process, but lack of estrogen in postmenopausal women may reduce their sensitivity to these anabolic stimuli and accelerate muscle loss.

Tendons and ligaments are also affected by sex hormones, but the effect seems to differ between endogenous and exogenous female hormones and seems to depend on the age, and as a result influence the biomechanical properties of the ligaments and tendons differentially. Since it seems to play a significant role with regard to skeletal muscle protein turnover, estrogen/hormonal replacement therapy may counteract the degenerative changes in skeletal muscle [19]. Women differ from men with regard to muscle and tendon, most likely because of sex differences in estrogen. Experimental findings support the hypothesis that estrogen has an anabolic effect on muscle primarily by lowering the protein turnover and enhancing sensitivity to resistance training. Furthermore, estrogen may reduce the stiffness of tendons, an effect that may be modified by physical training [20].

In response to acute estrogen treatment, FOXO3 activation (dephosphorylation) and MuRF1 protein expression were shown to decrease in early postmenopausal women but increase in late postmenopausal women ($p < 0.05$). Preliminary studies suggest the effects of estrogen treatment on skeletal muscle protein breakdown markers are dependent on time since menopause [21].

Nevertheless, there is a need for greater insight into the direct and indirect mechanistic effects of female hormones before any evidence-based recommendations regarding type, dose, duration and timing of hormone replacement therapy can be provided.

Treatment and Alternatives

As long as their benefits and risks are assessed on an individual basis, and each patient is aware of the risks, older women with continuing symptoms should not be denied MHT. In fact, the key recommendation of most societies, including the British Menopause Society, is that all women should be able to access advice on how they can optimize their menopause transition and beyond, with particular reference to lifestyle and diet and an opportunity to discuss the pros and cons of complementary therapies and HRT [22]. A global consensus statement on menopausal MHT concludes that it is effective and appropriate for the prevention of osteoporosis-related fractures in at-risk women before age 60 years or within 10 years after menopause [23].

Effective prophylactic strategies are needed for the suppression of age-related muscle wasting and bone loss after menopause. The effect of exercise is now taking a more central role in the prevention and as an adjuvant treatment for postmenopausal-related musculoskeletal degeneration. Higher volumes of exercise, especially impact exercise, lead to a smaller decline in total bone mineral density, which may remain following intervention completion [24]. Aerobic dance intervention was also shown to result in a lower incidence of bone fracture through increasing BMD and decreasing fall risk for postmenopausal women [25]. In ovariectomized rats, interval running significantly inhibited the expression of inflammatory molecules, and improved antioxidant activity via down-regulation of mitogen-activated protein kinases (MAPKs) in the ageing-induced ovariectomized rats skeletal muscle. When compared with continuous running, interval running improved muscle mass and growth in these rats by promoting muscle growth-related factors including MyoD, myogenin, phospho-mechanistic target of rapamycin (p-mTOR), sirtuins (SIRTs), and bone morphogenic proteins (BMPs). This also effectively reversed bone loss via the down-regulation of bone resorption and osteoclast formation in receptor activator of nuclear factor κB ligand (RANKL)-treated bone marrow macrophages (BMMs). There was also an increased expression of SIRT1 and 6, which promoted osteogenic differentiation and bone formation via modulating the BMP signalling pathway compared with continuous training [26].

The use of calcium with or without vitamin D supplements is associated with less BMD loss of the lumbar spine and femoral neck, especially in premenopausal women [27].

Selective estrogen receptor modulators (SERMs), such as raloxifene, now have a more central role in the prevention and management of postmenopausal osteoporosis. SERMs act through estrogen receptors and are agonists for bone and antagonists for breast and uterine tissue. Bisphosphonates are also widely used. Zoledronic acid infusion combined with percutaneous kyphoplasty could provide more benefits in the treatment of T12 or L1 osteoporotic vertebral compression fracture [28]. Also there are newer drugs which act by interplaying with cytokines [29] (Table 13.1).

Obesity in Postmenopausal Women

Obesity is a current epidemic which is also effecting postmenopausal women. Trabecular bone score, an indirect evaluation of skeletal microarchitecture, calculated from DEXA in postmenopausal women is negatively correlated with age and BMI, and positively with BMD and BMD to BMI ratio [30]. Severe obesity may weaken the impact of menopause on bone mass and turnover. Also, soft tissue body composition appears to poorly influence bone density in these women [31]. Sarcopenia and obesity (sarcobesity) have adverse outcomes as they lead to morbidity due to increased incidence of lifestyle diseases like diabetes mellitus, hypertension [1].

Conclusion

The ideal prevention of postmenopausal bone loss is a healthy active lifestyle ideally while maintaining premenopausal estrogen status. Health care providers and policy makers need to focus on menopause-related musculoskeletal disorders and by including prevention in national programs, health resources will be utilized more cost-effectively.

Table 13.1 Current pharmacological agents indicated for the treatment of postmenopausal osteoporosis

Conventional pharmacological treatment	
Menopause Hormone Therapy (MHT)	• Increases calcium absorption • Decreases the erosion depth and osteoclast activation frequency by inducing apoptosis and suppressing osteoclastogenesis • Decreases the responsiveness of bone to PTH and altering its secretion • Promotes calcium intestinal absorption • Decreases the renal excretion of calcium • Long-term treatment with HRT administered at high doses stimulates proliferation of osteoblasts hence promoting bone formation
Bisphosphonates	• Decreases the activity of osteoclasts • Stimulates osteoclasts' apoptosis • Decreases the formation of oxygen free radicals produced by polymorphonuclear cells which are known to promote inflammation • Decreases pro-inflammatory cytokines and adhesion molecules • Promotes proliferation of T-lymphocytes
Strontium ranelate	• Dual action; anti-resorptive and anabolic actions • Inhibits the osteoclasts' recruitment and augments osteoblasts' proliferation and differentiation • Decreases both hip and vertebral fractures
Teriparatide	• Recombinant synthetic form of the natural human hormone • Daily subcutaneous injection enhances bone formation by activating osteoblasts and increase BMD • Enhances calcium intestinal absorption as well as calcium reabsorption from the kidney fractures • Decreases significantly vertebral (by 65%) and non-vertebral fractures (by 35%) excluding hip fractures • Mainly used in severe osteoporotic patients with a high fracture risk
Calcitonin	• Peptide hormone synthesized by the thyroid gland • Can be administered via subcutaneous, intramuscular or nasal routes • Nasal spray calcitonin effective in decreasing vertebral fractures in postmenopausal osteoporotic women but no effect on non-vertebral fractures • Administer calcium and vitamin D supplementation concurrently as calcitonin decreases blood calcium levels • Indicated mainly for osteoporotic women who are beyond their fifth year of menopause
Calcitriol	• Active vitamin D metabolite used to treat low calcium levels in postmenopausal women • Aids in calcium intestinal absorption

Table 13.1 (cont.)

Conventional pharmacological treatment	
	• Reduces the rate of vertebral fractures whereas it has no effect on hip fractures
Selective estrogen receptor modulators	• Non-steroidal compounds with tissue-specific activity; oestrogenic effects in certain tissues and anti-oestrogenic effects in others
	Raloxifene: • Anti-resorptive agent administered either to young postmenopausal osteoporotic women or those having low bone mass • Prevents and decreases osteoporosis-related vertebral fractures by 30–50% and increases BMD at the hip and the spine by 0.5% to 1.0%, respectively • Decreases the risk of breast cancer in osteoporotic women and is also cardioprotective • Vasomotor symptoms and thromboembolic events placed raloxifene as a second-line agent in patients who have developed intolerance to previous osteoporotic treatment
	Bazedoxifene: • Elevates BMD • Reduces the bone turnover markers • Decreases the occurrence of vertebral fractures in postmenopausal women • As opposed to other SERMs, bazedoxifene has an antagonistic activity on the uterus and the breast
Tibolone	• Synthetic steroid known as selective tissue estrogenic activity regulator (STEAR) • Exerts tissue-specific actions by enzymatic conversion of steroid into three bioactive metabolites • Suppresses bone turnover by decreasing osteoclasts' activity • Bone loss is prevented at the lumbar spine and proximal femur while it can increase BMD in the phalanges and the hip • Low dose of tibolone also decreases the occurrence of vertebral and non-vertebral fractures in elderly postmenopausal women
Vitamin D/ calcium	• Postmenopausal women have the highest calcium requirements • Adequate amount of dietary or supplemental calcium and vitamin D to postmenopausal women serves as a baseline treatment of postmenopausal osteoporosis • Dietary calcium intake without estrogen therapy retards but not entirely prevents postmenopausal bone loss • Concomitant intake of vitamin D with calcium enhances calcium absorption from the gastrointestinal tract

Table 13.1 (cont.)

Conventional pharmacological treatment
• Calcium supplementation may lower the rate of bone loss following 2 years of treatment; however, during the initial 5 years of menopause, it exerts little effect on bone loss as it can be attributed to the decline in estrogen synthesis • Calcium supplementation regarded as an adjunct to other treatment regimens unless sufficient dietary intake is ensured • Vitamin D may decrease the risk of hip and non-vertebral fractures in ambulatory elderly patients only if an oral supplementation of 700–800 IU is administered each day • Vitamin D/calcium supplementation increase BMD and decrease the risk of fracture. The latter is negated by some recent randomized controlled clinical trials

References

1. Khadilkar SS. Musculoskeletal disorders and menopause. *J Obstet Gynaecol India* 2019 Apr;69(2):99–103.

2. Lello S, Sorge R, Surico N, OMERO Study Group. Osteoporosis's Menopausal Epidemiological Risk Observation (OMERO) study. *Gynecol Endocrinol* 2015;31(12):992–8.

3. Wang YX, Wang JQ, Kaplar Z. Increased low back pain prevalence in females than in males after menopause age: evidences based on synthetic literature review. *Quant Imaging Med Surg* 2016 Apr;6(2):199–206.

4. Wang YXJ. Menopause as a potential cause for higher prevalence of low back pain in women than in age-matched men. *J Orthop Translat* 2016 Jun;14(8):1–4.

5. Bijelic R, Milicevic S, Balaban J. The influence of non-preventable risk factors on the development of osteoporosis in postmenopausal women. *Mater Sociomed* 2019 Mar;31(1):62–5.

6. Azizieh FY, Shehab D, Al Jarallah K, Mojiminiyi O, Gupta R, Raghupathy R. Circulatory pattern of cytokines, adipokines and bone markers in postmenopausal women with low BMD. *J Inflamm Res* 2019 Apr 26;12:99–108.

7. Calleja-Agius J, Brincat M. The effect of menopause on the skin and other connective tissues. *Gynecol Endocrinol* 2012 Apr;28(4):273–7.

8. Rachner TD, Khosla S, Lorenz C, Hofbauer LC. Osteoporosis: now and the future. *Lancet* 2011;377:1276–87.

9. Salari P, Abdollahi M. A comprehensive review of the shared roles of inflammatory cytokines in osteoporosis and cardiovascular diseases as two common old people problem – actions toward development of new drugs. *Int J Pharmacol* 2011;7(5):552–67.

10. Brincat M, Calleja-Agius J, Vujovic S, Erel T, Gambacciani M, Lambrinoudaki I, et al. EMAS position statement: bone densitometry screening for osteoporosis. *Maturitas* 2011 Jan;68(1):98–101.

11. Shieh A, Greendale GA, Cauley JA, Karvonen-Gutierrez C, Lo J, Karlamangla AS. Urinary N-telopeptide as predictor of onset of menopause-related bone loss in pre- and perimenopausal women. *JBMR Plus* 2018 Dec 30;3(4): e10116.

12. Muscat BY, Brincat MP, Galea R, Calleja N. Low intervertebral disc height in postmenopausal women with osteoporotic vertebral fractures compared to hormone-treated and untreated postmenopausal women and

premenopausal women without fractures. *Climacteric* 2007 Aug;10(4):314–9.

13. Lou C, Chen HL, Feng XZ, Xiang GH, Zhu SP, Tian NF, Jin YL, Fang MQ, Wang C, Xu HZ. Menopause is associated with lumbar disc degeneration: a review of 4230 intervertebral discs. *Climacteric* 2014 Dec;17(6):700–4.

14. Lou C, Chen H, Mei L, Yu W, Zhu K, Liu F, Chen Z, Xiang G, Chen M, Weng Q, He D. Association between menopause and lumbar disc degeneration: an MRI study of 1,566 women and 1,382 men. *Menopause* 2017 Oct;24(10):1136–44.

15. Jin LY, Lv ZD, Wang K, Qian L, Song XX, Li XF, Shen HX. Estradiol alleviates intervertebral disc degeneration through modulating the antioxidant enzymes and inhibiting autophagy in the model of menopause rats. *Oxid Med Cell Longev* 2018 Dec 23;2018:7890291.

16. Lou C, Xiang G, Weng Q, Chen Z, Chen D, Wang Q, Zhang D, Zhou B, He D, Chen H. Menopause is associated with articular cartilage degeneration: a clinical study of knee joint in 860 women. *Menopause* 2016 Nov;23 (11):1239–46.

17. Dieli-Conwright CM, Spektor TM, Rice JC, Sattler FR, Schroeder ET. Hormone replacement therapy and messenger RNA expression of estrogen receptor coregulators after exercise in postmenopausal women. *Med Sci Sports Exerc* 2010;42(3):422–9.

18. Garcia-Alfaro P, Garcia S, Rodríguez I, Tresserra F, Pérez-López FR. Factors related to muscle strength in postmenopausal women aged younger than 65 years with normal vitamin D status. *Climacteric* 2019 Aug;22 (4):390–4.

19. Hansen M. Female hormones: do they influence muscle and tendon protein metabolism? *Proc Nutr Soc* 2018 Feb;77 (1):32–41.

20. Hansen M, Kjaer M. Influence of sex and estrogen on musculotendinous protein turnover at rest and after exercise. *Exerc Sport Sci Rev* 2014 Oct;42(4):183–92.

21. Park YM, Keller AC, Runchey SS, Miller BF, Kohrt WM, Van Pelt RE, Kang C, Jankowski CM, Moreau KL. Acute estradiol treatment reduces skeletal muscle protein breakdown markers in early- but not late-postmenopausal women. *Steroids* 2019 Jun;146:43–9.

22. Panay N, Hamoda H, Arya R, Savvas M, British Menopause Society and Women's Health Concern. The 2013 British Menopause Society and Women's Health Concern recommendations on hormone replacement therapy. *Menopause Int* 2013 Jun;19(2):59–68.

23. de Villiers TJ, Gass ML, Haines CJ, Hall JE, Lobo RA, Pierroz DD, Rees M. Global consensus statement on menopausal hormone therapy. *Climacteric* 2013 Apr;16(2):203–4.

24. Gonzalo-Encabo P, McNeil J, Boyne DJ, Courneya KS, Friedenreich CM. Dose-response effects of exercise on bone mineral density and content in post-menopausal women. *Scand J Med Sci Sports* 2019 Apr 29;29:1121–9.

25. Yu PA, Hsu WH, Hsu WB, Kuo LT, Lin ZR, Shen WJ, Hsu RW. The effects of high impact exercise intervention on bone mineral density, physical fitness, and quality of life in postmenopausal women with osteopenia: a retrospective cohort study. *Medicine (Baltimore)* 2019 Mar;98(11): e14898.

26. Kim JS, Jeon J, An JJ, Yi HK. Interval running training improves age-related skeletal muscle wasting and bone loss: experiments with ovariectomized rats. *Exp Physiol* 2019 May;104(5):691–703.

27. Bailey R, Wallace T, Weaver C, Zou P. Premenopausal calcium with or without vitamin d supplementation: a critical window of opportunity for preventing bone loss across menopause transition (P18-049-19). *Climacteric* 2019 Aug;22 (4):390–4.

28. Zhang J, Zhang T, Xu X, Cai Q, Zhao D. Zoledronic acid combined with percutaneous kyphoplasty in the treatment of osteoporotic compression fracture in a single T12 or L1 vertebral body in postmenopausal women. *Osteoporos Int* 2019 Apr 11;30:1475–80.

29. Tan X, Wen F, Yang W, Xie JY, Ding LL, Mo YX. Comparative efficacy and safety of pharmacological interventions for osteoporosis in postmenopausal women: a network meta-analysis (Chongqing, China). *Menopause* 2019 Apr 21;26:929–39.

30. Torgutalp ŞŞ, Babayeva N, Kara ÖS, Özkan Ö, Dönmez G, Korkusuz F. Trabecular bone score of postmenopausal women is positively correlated with bone mineral density and negatively correlated with age and body mass index. *Menopause* 2019 Oct;26:1166–70.

31. Crivelli M, Chain A, Bezerra F. Association between body composition and bone density in morbidly obese women according to menopausal status (P01–023–19). *Curr Dev Nutr* 2019 Jun 13;3(Suppl 1):pii: nzz028.P01-023-19.

Hormonal Management of Osteoporosis during the Menopause

Panagiotis G. Anagnostis and John C. Stevenson

Bone Pathophysiology

Therapies for osteoporosis have been traditionally based on our understanding of bone cell activities. Bone tissue is constantly being removed and replaced (bone turnover) by osteoclasts, which resorb bone, and osteoblasts, which lay down new bone. Bone turnover is essential for the maintenance of a healthy skeleton by removing or repairing the microscopic damage that results from everyday physical activity. These processes of resorption and formation are linked or 'coupled' so that bone turnover proceeds in an orderly fashion.

When these processes become imbalanced or uncoupled, resorption can exceed formation and bone loss then occurs leading to an increased risk of fractures [1–4]. Traditionally, drugs which reduce osteoclastic activity have been the mainstay of treatment. Thus, agents such as estrogens and bisphosphonates have been widely used with considerable success. Agents that act directly on osteoblasts to increase bone formation are few, with parathyroid hormone (PTH) and PTH-related peptide (PTHrP) analogues being the main ones. However, more recent understanding of bone biology has led to the recognition of cell signalling systems that regulate both osteoclasts and osteoblasts. New therapies are being developed which target these cell signals. Receptor activator of nuclear factor kappa-B ligand (RANKL) plays a key role in the differentiation, activation and survival of osteoclasts. RANKL, which is produced by preosteoblasts and osteoblasts, is a member of the tumour necrosis factor super-family and plays a pivotal role in osteoclastogenesis. Another member of this system is osteoprotegerin (OPG), a soluble receptor for RANKL produced by osteoblasts, which acts in the opposite way by inhibiting RANKL-induced bone resorption.

Antibodies to RANKL have been developed and act as powerful inhibitors of bone resorption [1–4]. A major signalling pathway to the osteoblasts is the Wnt low-density lipoprotein receptor-related proteins (LRP) pathway, which stimulates differentiation of preosteoblasts into mature bone-forming osteoblasts. This signalling pathway has two natural inhibitors, sclerostin and Dickkopf-1 (Dkk-1), and these have become targets for the development of antibodies blocking their actions and hence enhancing the stimulatory signals of Wnt-LRP. Finally, an understanding of the mechanisms by which osteoclasts resorb bone has led to the development of inhibitors of proteases secreted by osteoclasts, thereby inhibiting their resorptive actions without influencing their cell activity or numbers. This potentially avoids a concomitant reduction of osteoblastic activity via the coupling mechanisms, which is normally seen with agents that reduce osteoclastic cell activity [5].

Therapeutic Options

Osteoporosis is a term used to describe a condition of bone microarchitecture deterioration and subsequent predisposition to fractures. It constitutes a major health problem, affecting millions of people worldwide and is associated with increased morbidity and mortality. The hallmark of osteoporosis diagnosis is low bone mineral density (BMD), usually assessed by dual-energy X-ray absorptiometry (DXA). Although women with the lowest BMD have the highest risk of fracture, the majority of fractures occur in women with osteopenia rather than osteoporosis, highlighting the importance of assessing fracture risk on an individual basis. The decision for treatment should thus be based both on BMD measurement and individual fracture risk profile. Medical history and clinical examination (in order to exclude causes of secondary osteoporosis and estimate fracture risk), taking into account the patient's age, lifestyle habits (exercise, smoking, alcohol) and specific medications associated with bone loss, should always precede DXA assessment [1,2].

General Management

Anti-fall strategies and nutritional measures, including a balanced diet with adequate calcium and vitamin D, should precede any major therapeutic intervention. Interventions which aim at modifying several risk factors associated with falls, such as decreased visual acuity, medications affecting balance, and home environment obstacles such as slippery floors, insufficient lighting and the installation of handrails, are recommended. Furthermore, avoidance of smoking, excessive alcohol and caffeine intake are also helpful in maintaining bone mass.

To gain the best available benefit with anti-osteoporosis medications, optimal calcium and vitamin D intake must be assured. Assessing 25-hydroxy-vitamin D [25(OH)D] levels prior to commencing any major anti-osteoporosis treatment may be prudent if there is suspected deficiency because optimizing vitamin D status may significantly increase the anti-fracture efficacy of osteoporosis treatment [1]. In general, doses >800 IU/day are more effective than lower doses. In patients with severe vitamin D deficiency (<25 nmol/l or <10 ng/ml) high loading doses, i.e. 300 000 IU, may be considered, which correspond to weekly doses of 50 000 IU for 6 weeks, followed by maintenance doses of 800–2000 IU/day. Specific considerations are recommended for special patient groups, such as pregnant or lactating women, obese women, those with malabsorption disorders or receiving corticosteroid or anti-convulsant medication. Regarding obesity, there is an inverse association between 25(OH)D concentrations and BMI or waist circumference, although the exact mechanisms have not been fully elucidated. The decreased bioavailability of vitamin D metabolites in adipose tissue and the reduced sun exposure due to a sedentary lifestyle are the most plausible explanations.

In general, the evidence for anti-fracture efficacy of vitamin D supplementation is weak [1]. However, this seems to be the case when vitamin D is co-administered with calcium. Indeed, calcium, either as monotherapy (dietary or supplement) or in combination with vitamin D, seems to modestly reduce hip and non-vertebral fracture risk, especially in older individuals. Compliance is always a key factor determining anti-fracture efficacy [1].

Major Pharmacological Interventions

Menopause Hormone Therapy (MHT) and Tibolone

The findings from the Women's Health Initiative (WHI) trial, which was designed to assess the prevention of common chronic diseases in women, such as cardiovascular disease, cancer and osteoporosis, showed a beneficial effect of estrogen on bones. In particular both estrogen [conjugated equine estrogen (CEE), at a daily dose of 0.625 mg] plus progestin (medroxyprogesterone acetate 2.5 mg/day) and CEE alone were efficient in reducing the risk of vertebral and hip fractures by 35 per cent and 33 per cent, respectively, in comparison with placebo. Mean BMD in lumbar spine and total hip and femoral neck increased by a mean of 7.6 per cent and 4.5 per cent, respectively, after 3 years of treatment, compared with 1.5 per cent and −0.3 per cent in the placebo group.

However, there was a small increased risk of venous thromboembolism (VTE) [1,4]. An increased risk of stroke in those initiating therapy at older ages was not seen in those initiating therapy below age 60 years. Breast cancer incidence was significantly reduced with cumulative follow-up of the estrogen-alone users. Moreover, breast cancer incidence was not significantly increased with combination therapy after adjustment for confounding variables, a finding confirmed in a more recent smaller but longer-duration randomized MHT trial. For those initiating estrogen-alone MHT below the age of 60, a reduction in coronary heart disease became evident during long-term follow-up. Although not currently recommended by regulatory authorities, we believe that the use of MHT for the sole treatment of osteoporosis should be considered as first-line therapy in postmenopausal women. The risks of VTE and stroke may be minimized or even prevented by the use of appropriately low doses of estrogen on initiating therapy or by the use of non-oral administration.

MHT is an effective, safe and cheap therapy for osteoporosis prevention [1,4]. The bone-preserving effect of estrogen is dose dependent and lower-than-standard doses are effective in older women. Higher doses may be necessary in young women who have premature ovarian insufficiency or have undergone a menopause induced by surgery, radiation or chemotherapy. However, rapid bone loss at pretreatment rates usually occurs after MHT discontinuation, although a recent study showed preservation of benefit at the level of bone microarchitecture.

Tibolone is a synthetic steroid, with a mixed estrogenic, progestogenic and androgenic profile, used as an alternative to estrogen for relief of menopausal symptoms [1,4]. Clinical trials have shown that tibolone 2.5 mg/day can prevent bone loss in both spine and proximal femur. In comparative studies, tibolone seems to be as effective as MHT regimens regarding its effect on BMD. Data show a significant reduction in vertebral and non-vertebral fracture risk by 45 per cent and 26 per cent, respectively. No adequate data exist with respect to its effect on hip fracture prevention. Tibolone has some adverse metabolic effects on lipid metabolism and insulin resistance. It may also increase the risk of stroke and its effect on breast cancer risk is unclear.

Selective Estrogen Receptor Modulators

Selective estrogen receptor modulators (SERMs) [1,4] exert estrogenic and anti-estrogenic properties, depending on the target tissue(see Chapter 24). In terms of bone, SERMs inhibit osteoclast-mediated bone resorption. Two members of this family are currently available for the treatment of postmenopausal osteoporosis, these being raloxifene and bazedoxifene. Raloxifene has estrogen agonist effects on bone and lipid metabolism and estrogen antagonist effects on uterine and breast tissue. Raloxifene administered at 60 mg daily has been associated with a significant reduction in the incidence of new vertebral fractures by 61 per cent in women without prevalent vertebral fractures and by 37 per cent in those with prevalent vertebral fractures. However, it has not shown any significant effect with respect to the risk of non-vertebral fractures. Raloxifene has also been approved for the prevention of invasive breast cancer. The most common side effects include increased risk of deep vein thrombosis (DVT), hot flashes, leg cramps and endometrial hyperplasia.

The other representative [1,4] of this drug category, bazedoxifene, is effective in reducing vertebral fracture risk in postmenopausal women with osteoporosis (by 42 per cent, compared with placebo) and that of non-vertebral fractures in high-risk populations (50 per cent and 44 per cent compared with placebo and raloxifene, respectively). Its effect on the endometrium is neutral. Other SERMs which have not been approved for osteoporosis treatment are tamoxifen and toremifene (used for prevention and treatment of breast cancer), ospemifene (approved for treatment of dyspareunia from menopausal vaginal atrophy) and lasofoxifene. A new promising formulation is the tissue-selective estrogen complex (TSEC), a pairing of CEE with bazedoxifene, which allows both relief of vasomotor symptoms and prevention of bone loss without any stimulatory effect on the breast or the endometrium.

Bisphosphonates

Bisphosphonates [1,4] are synthetic analogues of pyrophosphate, in which the oxygen atom has been substituted by a carbon atom. Their different action is dependent on the variable R2 side chain, bound to the carbon atom and in particular the nitrogen compound. The main representatives of this category used for the treatment of osteoporosis are alendronate, ibandronate (with their nitrogen found in the straight alkyl chain), risedronate and zoledronate (with their nitrogen being part of a cyclized aromatic ring). Their main action is inhibition of bone resorption, by inhibition of farnesyl pyrophosphate synthase, a key enzyme in the mevalonic acid pathway, which blocks specific signalling molecules (GTPases) involved in major osteoclastic functions, such as maintenance of the cytoskeleton and formation of ruffled borders. Because of the coupling of bone resorption to bone formation, the inhibition of resorption by these agents is associated with a reduction in bone formation, but the former effect is initially greater than the latter, leading to a refilling of the remodelling space and a subsequent increase in mineralization density. Consequently, they are associated with a reduction in fracture risk due both to a decrease in bone remodelling and to an increase in bone mass.

Both oral (weekly administered alendronate and risedonate or monthly ibandronate) and intravenous (i.v.) bisphosphonates (ibandronate administered every 3 months and zoledronate administered annually) have been associated with significant reductions in vertebral fractures (40–70 per cent) and non-vertebral fractures (30–40 per cent) [1,4]. Hip fracture efficacy has been shown for alendronate, risedronate and zoledronate (40–50 per cent). Greater antifracture efficacy has been seen with the latter in terms of vertebral, non-vertebral and hip fractures, although direct head-to-head comparisons between bisphosphonates do not exist with regard to fracture risk. It is of note that the anti-resorptive effect of zoledronate may persist for at least 5 years after a single injection, as demonstrated by a sustained reduction in bone turnover markers and increase in BMD. Extension trials show maintained benefit with 5 years of oral bisphosphonates (alendronate) and 6 years with zoledronate in patients at high fracture risk, such as those with femoral neck T-score less than −2.5 or with prevalent vertebral fractures. In cases at low fracture risk, a 'drug holiday' may be considered, in particular after 5 years with alendronate and 3 years with zoledronate or risedronate therapy. In these cases, BMD seems to be generally preserved above pretreatment values. Continuous monitoring at regular intervals, depending mainly on acquisition of BMD at the time of bisphosphonate withdrawal, and re-initiation of therapy if fracture risk increases, is recommended.

The overall benefits of bisphosphonate therapy generally outweigh its risks [3]. Some concerns with oral bisphosphonates are symptoms from the upper gastrointestinal tract, such as esophagitis, esophageal ulcer and bleeding, although these have been minimized with less frequent dosing. There is conflicting evidence concerning an association with increased risk of esophageal cancer. An acute phase reaction (characterized by fever, headache, myalgia, arthralgia, malaise) may occur in 18 per cent of patients with in 24–36 hours after zoledronate infusion, lasting up to 3 days. This reaction can be significantly reduced with acetaminophen and with subsequent infusions. In the HORIZON trial, the pivotal trial of zoledronate, there was an increased risk of serious atrial fibrillation (1.3 per cent vs 0.5 per cent with placebo), but the overall incidence of atrial fibrillation did not differ between the two groups. This risk has also been observed in some studies of oral bisphosphonates.

The two major concerns with bisphosphonate use are the risk of atypical subtrochanteric and diaphyseal femur fractures (AFF), and osteonecrosis of the jaw (ONJ) [1]. The absolute risk for AFF is very low (around 5 cases per 10 000 person-years), taking also into account that these fractures constitute <1 per cent of all hip and femoral fractures. It is increased in cases of prolonged bisphosphonate use (>5 years) and use of other concomitant drugs, such as glucocorticoids. With regard to ONJ, this is mostly seen in patients with underlying malignancies treated with high doses of i.v. bisphosphonates (4 mg zoledronic acid/3–4 weeks), with a reported risk of 1–10 per cent. ONJ is associated with prolonged suppression of bone turnover and its risk is mainly increased in patients undergoing tooth extractions, and in those with other comorbidities. The absolute risk of ONJ when bisphosphonates are administered for osteoporosis is extremely low (1 case per 100 000 person-years). The prevalence of ONJ with oral bisphosphonates was found to be one case in 250 000, in a German registry of osteoporotic patients treated with oral bisphosphonates. However, higher prevalence has been reported in studies by oral and maxillofacial surgeons, varying from 1 in 1000 to 1 in 100 000. It has been speculated that a 'drug holiday' may reduce the risk of ONJ and AFF, although evidence for the effectiveness of this policy is still lacking. Only one prospective study has shown a 71 per cent reduction in AFF risk per year since bisphosphonate discontinuation.

Finally, it should be remembered that bisphosphonates have a prolonged skeletal retention time, perhaps around 12–15 years for alendronate and probably considerably longer for the more potent bisphosphonates [1,4]. The very long-term consequences of this skeletal retention are not known, and hence caution should be taken when considering their use in younger patients. In 80-year-old osteoporotics, unknown clinical consequences some 20 years later are unlikely to be considered important, but this may not be true for those aged around 60 years. A very recent study also showed anti-fracture efficacy with zoledronate after four infusions (at 18 months apart) in older patients with osteopenia.

Parathyroid Hormone (PTH) and PTH-Related Peptide (PTHrP) Analogues

Although continuous endogenous production of PTH (i.e. in primary hyperparathyroidism) exerts detrimental effects on bone, intermittent PTH administration leads to an increase in bone mass due to increased number and activity of osteoblasts [1]. Recombinant PTH, consisting of the 1–34 N-terminal fragment of natural PTH molecule (which is the active one) (PTH(1–34) or teriparatide) or the intact PTH molecule (amino acids 1–84) have both been used for the treatment of osteoporosis. They stimulate bone formation and increase BMD to a greater extent than other agents, such as bisphosphonates, both in lumbar spine and femoral neck. Teriparatide appears also to improve bone microarchitecture (trabecular connectivity) at both trabecular and cortical skeletal sites, which further contributes to the reduction in fracture risk and cannot be detected by DXA. Teriparatide treatment has been associated with a significant reduction in the incidence of both vertebral and non-vertebral fractures by 70 per cent and 38 per cent, respectively. In a recent comparative study, teriparatide was more effective in reducing vertebral and clinical fracture risk than risedronate. It is recommended for patients at very high risk for fracture, such as those with T-score less than or equal to −3.5, or severe or multiple vertebral fractures, failure with anti-resorptive agents or with established glucocorticoid-induced osteoporosis for the reduction of vertebral and non-vertebral fractures. Moreover, a recent meta-analysis showed a 56 per cent relative risk reduction in hip fractures in comparison with placebo. Teriparatide is administered by subcutaneous injections, at a daily dose of 20 µg, for up to 2 years.

The most common adverse events are of minor concern and include hypersensitivity reactions, nausea, pain in the limbs, headache and dizziness [1,2,4]. Hypercalcemia or hypercalciuria may occur, but are usually transient and of minor significance. Hypercortisolism has been reported. The risk of osteosarcoma reported in rats has not been confirmed in human clinical studies. Contraindications to teriparatide and PTH administration are states of abnormally increased bone turnover (such as hyperparathyroidism and Paget's disease), elevated alkaline phosphatase, prior radiation therapy of the skeleton and renal impairment. The high cost of teriparatide further limits its use.

PTHrP is a 34 amino acid polypeptide, which also binds to PTH type 1 receptor (PTH1 R), as PTH [1,4]. It increases bone resorption and renal tubular calcium reabsorption. It also regulates chondrocyte differentiation and osteoblast function. Knockout models have shown that selective deletion of *PTHrP* gene leads to decreased bone formation and low bone mass, whereas *PTHrP* loss of function results in skeletal deformities, such as in Blomstrand's chondrodysplasia. Abaloparatide is a synthetic analogue, sharing the first 22 amino acid sequence with PTHrP, differing in amino acids 23–34. In comparison with teriparatide, it exerts a higher affinity for the RG and a lower affinity for the R0 conformation of the PTH1 R, which provides a greater osteoanabolic effect. Abaloparatide shows comparable vertebral and non-vertebral anti-fracture efficacy with teriparatide (86 per cent and 43 per cent relative risk reduction, respectively). However, the reduction in the risk of major osteoporotic fractures (including those of the upper arm, wrist, hip or clinical spine) was greater with abaloparatide and the risk of hypercalcaemia was lower. Abaloparatide has been recently approved by the FDA for the treatment of postmenopausal women with osteoporosis at very high risk of fracture, as with teriparatide. Of note, both regimens should be followed by an anti-resorptive agent to maintain BMD gain [5].

Strontium Ranelate

Strontium ranelate consists of two atoms of stable strontium combined with ranelic acid, acting as carrier. It is postulated to have a dual osteoanabolic and anticatabolic effect, although it has not been convincingly demonstrated in humans Although its action is not fully elucidated, strontium increases preosteoblast replication and osteoblast differentiation (via expression of Runx2 gene), collagen type I synthesis and bone matrix mineralization. The latter effect is mediated probably through a calcium-sensing receptor (CaR)-dependent mechanism, since strontium is a divalent cation which closely resembles calcium in its atomic and ionic properties and, thus, could act as an agonist for the CaR. Strontium also inhibits osteoclast differentiation and activity via an increase in OPG and a decrease in RANKL.

Therapy with strontium ranelate (administered daily as 2 g sachets) has been associated with a 41 per cent, 16 per cent and 19 per cent reduction in the risk of vertebral, total and major non-vertebral fractures, respectively, after 3 years of treatment [1,4]. In patients older than 74 years and with T-score less than or equal to -2.4, strontium ranelate has been also associated with a 36 per cent reduction in the risk of hip fractures. The anti-fracture efficacy of strontium ranelate seems to be independent of the level of fracture risk. Extension studies show continuous increases in BMD for >10 years of treatment. Renal impairment is a contraindication to treatment. Most common adverse events include nausea and diarrhea. Rare and serious adverse events are increased incidence in venous thromboembolism, eosinophilia and systemic symptoms syndrome, which may prove fatal. Recent serious concerns about a potential association with increased cardiovascular disease (CVD) risk have severely limited its use for the treatment of osteoporosis [1,4].

Denosumab

Denosumab, a human monoclonal antibody, which acts in a similar way to OPG, exerting high affinity to RANKL, is approved for the treatment of postmenopausal osteoporosis. Given by subcutaneous injections of 60 mg every 6 months, it is a powerful anti-resorptive agent and reduces incidence of vertebral, non-vertebral and hip fractures by 68 per cent, 20 per cent and 40 per cent, respectively, after 3 years of treatment. Recent data support that extending its administration to 10 years is safe and associated with a continuous increase in BMD and a decrease in fracture risk. Interestingly, a plateau in non-vertebral anti-fracture efficacy is observed after completion of 10 years of continuous denosumab use and achievement of total hip T-scores between -2 and -1.5, independently of age and prevalent vertebral fractures.

Denosumab is particularly indicated for the treatment of postmenopausal women with high fracture probability, defined as those with a history of osteoporotic fracture or multiple risk factors for fracture or those who have inadequate response or are intolerant to other therapies [1–3]. It has a quite favourable safety profile. However, due to the fact that RANKL is also involved in other functions of the immune system, it has been associated with an increased risk of infections, such as cellulitis and urinary tract infections.

Rare adverse effects that have been reported include increased muscle pain, increased cholesterol, hypocalcemia, ONJ and AFF. Renal impairment is not a contraindication to treatment.

In contrast to bisphosphonates, BMD declines after discontinuation of treatment (although it remains higher than baseline) and bone turnover markers increase above baseline within 3–6 months posttreatment [3]. In several cases reports have been recently published showing an increased risk of 'rebound' vertebral fractures after denosumab withdrawal, potentially attributed to increased osteoclastogenesis. Thus, denosumab should always be followed by an anti-resorptive agent (i.e. bisphosphonates) in order to maintain its BMD gain, although data from randomized controlled trials are lacking [3].

Novel Therapies under Development

Further insights to bone metabolism have significantly contributed to a more targeted drug development. Novel therapies are already tested in phase 3 trials, such as cathepsin K inhibitors and sclerostin antibodies. The first category is a truly 'anti-resorptive' agent, which inhibits a key osteoclast enzyme, cathepsin K, involved in bone matrix resorption. Because it does not affect osteoclast activity but only function, it does not influence the coupling of osteoclast and osteoblast activities and the latter does not decrease. Odanacatib, the first representative, has already been developed. Early studies have shown a significant dose-response increase in spine and hip BMD (7.9 per cent and 5.8 per cent, respectively, after treatment with 50 mg/weekly for 3 years), along with a significant reduction in bone resorption and a minimal effect on bone formation markers. However, concerns about an increased risk in CVD events have currently suspended its further promotion.

Sclerostin, which is produced by osteocytes, reduces bone formation and has been considered as an attractive target for treating osteoporosis [5]. Romosozumab, the first humanized anti-sclerostin antibody, has already been developed and tested in a phase II multicentre study. The greatest gain in BMD was noticed in lumbar spine and it was shown with a 210 mg subcutaneous dose every 3 months (+11.3 per cent), an effect that was significantly greater than the one observed with alendronate or teriparatide. Romosozumab also increased total hip and femoral neck BMD by 4.1 per cent and 3.7 per cent, respectively. It was associated with significant dose-dependent increases in bone formation markers and, in contrast with teriparatide, there is no compensatory increase in bone resorption. Phase III trials have shown a significant vertebral, non-vertebral, hip and clinical fracture risk reduction with romosozumab compared with placebo or alendronate. It has been recently approved by the FDA for the treatment of postmenopausal women at high fracture risk, administered at monthly doses of 210 mg for 12 months. This regimen should be followed by an anti-resorptive therapy, such as alendronate, to maintain or even enhance its therapeutic effect. Of note, romosozumab should be avoided in patients at very high CVD risk, such as those a history of heart attack or stroke within the previous year.

Antibodies against dickkopf-1 (Dkk) [5] are also under development. Combination therapies have also been tested recently. In patients at high risk for fracture, co-administration of teriparatide with denosumab seems to be highly effective both in lumbar spine and hip to a greater extent than either medication alone and than what has been reported with any current therapy. Thus, it may appear to be an attractive treatment option in these patients [5].

Conclusions and Recommendations

Osteoporosis treatment should be commenced and selected on an individual basis. Optimal nutritional and lifestyle measures, and exclusion and potential treatment of secondary causes of osteoporosis, should always precede any major pharmaceutical intervention. It must be noted that although *T*-scores are commonly used in clinical practice for monitoring purposes, the change in BMD does not always reflect the change in fracture risk, which seems to be multifactorial. Treatment failure, after exclusion of causes of secondary osteoporosis and suboptimal adherence, is considered in cases of (1) ≥ 2 incident fragility fractures; (2) one incident fracture and elevated bone turnover markers or a significant decrease in BMD or both; and (3) both no significant decrease in bone turnover markers and a significant decrease in BMD. Three general rules are proposed in cases of inadequate response to therapy: a weaker anti-resorptive may be replaced by a more potent drug of the same class; an oral drug may be replaced by an injectable agent; a strong antiresorptive drug may be substituted by an anabolic agent.

A patient who has sustained two low-trauma fractures and possibly vertebral fractures has a significantly increased the risk of a new fracture. A BMD scan should be performed by DXA and treatment should be offered in the case of osteopenia. Plain radiographs of the spine, or DXA vertebral fracture risk assessment (VFA) when available, will provide further information on fracture prevalence. A low-dose HRT preparation or possibly a bisphosphonate appears to be a reasonable initial approach, depending on other menopausal risk factors and patient preference. Clinical reassessment in a year's time and BMD re-evaluation in 2 years to assess efficacy of treatment seems appropriate management.

Bibliography

1. Eastell R, Rosen CJ, Black DM, Cheung AM, Murad MH, Shoback D. Pharmacological management of osteoporosis in postmenopausal women: an endocrine society clinical practice guideline. *J Clin Endocrinol Metab* 2019;104:1595–622.

2. Diez-Perez A, Adachi JD, Agnusdei D, et al., IOF CSA Inadequate Responders Working Group. Treatment failure in osteoporosis. *Osteoporos Int* 2012;23:2769–74.

3. Anagnostis P, Paschou SA, Mintziori G, et al. Drug holidays from bisphosphonates and denosumab in postmenopausal osteoporosis: EMAS position statement. *Maturitas* 2017;101:23–30.

4. Gerval MO, Stevenson JC. Treatment of osteoporosis. In: Studd J, Tan SL, Chervenak FA, eds. *Current Progress in Obstetrics and Gynaecology*. 2014. Tree Life Media pp. 379–93.

5. Anagnostis P, Gkekas NK, Potoupnis M, Kenanidis E, Tsiridis E, Goulis DG. New therapeutic targets for osteoporosis. *Maturitas* 2019;120:1–6.

Cardiovascular Disease and the Menopause

Marta Caretto, Andrea Giannini, Tommaso Simoncini and Andrea R. Genazzani

The age of the natural menopause among women in developed countries is between 50 and 52 years [1, 2], whereas in the less developed countries, it is 3–4 years earlier [3]. Deprivation of sex steroid hormones is an important consequence of normal aging and gonadal failure that potentially increases vulnerability to disease in hormone-responsive tissues, including the brain, bone and the cardiovascular system. After menopause, several chronic diseases may emerge, usually by the sixth decade, and these include obesity and metabolic disease, CVD, osteoporosis and arthritis, dementia and cognitive decline, cancer [4]. Obesity is a growing worldwide problem which exacerbates several chronic diseases. In menopausal women, the incidence of insulin resistance and diabetes has risen exponentially: this translates into an increased risk of CVD and death. If estrogen deprivation leads to altered fat distribution, MHT appears to decrease the incidence of diabetes and also improves diabetes control as indicated by assessment of glycosylated haemoglobin concentrations [5]. CVD is the most common cause of death in women over the age of 50 years. The overall prevalence of coronary heart disease (CHD) is estimated to be 5.1 per cent in women compared with 7.9 per cent in men, and the lifetime risk of developing CHD after 40 years of age is 32 per cent in women and 49 per cent in men; in addition, the incidence of CHD in women lags behind men by 10 years for CHD overall and by 20 years for myocardial infarction (MI) and sudden death. Prior studies have investigated the relationship between menopause and CVD [6]; however, the results have been inconsistent, and the direct causal relationship between menopause and increased cardiovascular risk is still being debated [7]. Major primary prevention measures are smoking cessation, weight loss, blood pressure reduction, regular aerobic exercise and diabetes and lipid control. Primary prevention strategies which are effective in men (use of aspirin and statins) do not afford a protective effect for coronary disease, cardiovascular mortality or all-cause mortality in women [4]. MHT has the potential for improving the cardiovascular risk profile through its beneficial effects on vascular function, lipid levels and glucose metabolism.

Cardiovascular Risk

Estrogen deficiency associated with the menopausal transition leads to many distressing symptoms, including vasomotor symptoms, sexual disorders and, in the long term, hormonal depletion results in changes in the risk of metabolic syndrome and increases in diabetes and cardiovascular disease. All these symptoms negatively impact on quality of life. Attention should focus on the estrogens' fundamental functions on cardiovascular system and metabolic balance.

Estrogens and Cardiovascular Risk

Estrogens and the other sex hormones regulate fundamental cardiovascular functions including blood pressure, blood flow, vasodilatation and vasoconstriction, vascular inflammation and remodelling, atherosclerosis [8]. These actions of endogenous estrogens on the cardiovascular system can be mediated directly on the vessels or indirectly through the modulation of cardiovascular risk factors. Estrogen exerts pleiotropic functions on the cardiovascular system through both genomic and non-genomic effects [9, 10]. Traditionally, estrogen receptors (ERs) work via the regulation of transcriptional processes, involving nuclear translocation and binding on specific response elements, thus leading to regulation of target gene expression (ERE). The non-transcriptional mechanisms of signal transduction, called 'non-genomic' effects, are independent by gene transcription or protein synthesis and involve steroid-induced modulation of cytoplasmic or of cell membrane-bound regulatory proteins. Relevant biological actions of steroids have been associated with this signalling in different tissues. Ubiquitary regulatory cascades such as mitogen-activated protein kinases (MAPK), the phosphatidylinositol 3-OH kinase (PI3 K) and tyrosine kinases are modulated through non-transcriptional mechanisms by steroid hormones. Furthermore, steroid hormone receptors' modulation of cell membrane-associated molecules such as ion channels and G-protein-coupled receptors has been shown in diverse tissues. The vascular wall is a site where non-genomic steroid hormones' actions are particularly prominent. For instance, estrogens and glucocorticoids trigger rapid vasodilatation due to rapid induction of nitric oxide (NO) synthesis in endothelial cells via the estrogen receptor-dependent activation of MAPK and PI3 K, leading to relevant pathophysiological consequences, in vitro and in vivo. Estrogen triggers rapid vasodilatation, exerts anti-inflammatory effects, regulates vascular cell growth and migration, leading to a protective action on vessels [11]. Recent advancements in the characterization of the molecular basis of estrogen's actions help us to understand the biological functions of estrogen and would be beneficial in elucidating current controversies on estrogen's clinical efficacy in the cardiovascular system [12–14].

Endothelium represents an elective cellular target for estrogens. It is well established that estrogen improves vascular function, maintaining and repairing endothelium, reduces atherosclerosis. ERs are expressed in endothelial cells and have an athero-protective effect. Through the recruitment of ERs, estradiol increases endothelial NO and prostacyclin synthesis, thus slowing early atheroma formation. Estradiol also decreases synthesis of pro-inflammatory cytokines by circulating or resident immune cells. In addition, estradiol facilitates endothelial vascular healing and neoangiogenesis. Emerging evidence suggests that protective effects exerted by estrogens on endothelium include multiple cellular mechanisms. Estrogen has been demonstrated to activate calcium-dependent potassium channels and induce a rapid increase in NO release [15]. These non-genomic effects of estrogens on NO production are paralleled by their genomic actions exerted by activation of endothelial NO synthase (eNOS) through a receptor-mediated system [16]. Estrogen has antioxidant and anti-inflammatory properties, acting through multiple effects. Among

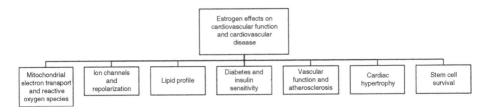

Figure 15.1 Estrogen effects and cardiovascular system.

them, estrogen may upregulate prostacyclin synthase and the expression of vascular endothelial growth factor. Conversely, it inhibits endothelin-1 release, and modulates adhesion-molecule and tumour necrosis factor α (TNF-α) expression and endothelial cell apoptosis [17, 18]. Moreover, estrogen can act by upregulating superoxide dismutase in the vascular district, which contributes to increased superoxide ion clearance [19]. Estrogen may also influence the redox balance through modulation of mitochondrial enzyme activity: these antioxidant effects are a main mechanism by which hormones protect women during their fertile life. In fact, oxidative stress is generally higher in men compared to premenopausal women. After menopause, when hormonal levels markedly fall, the risk of cardiovascular events rapidly rise in women, in parallel to a rapid increase of oxidative stress biomarker levels [20].

ERα is important in reducing endothelial dysfunction after ischemia and reperfusion [21]. The overall protection afforded by estrogen is likely mediated by effects on both myocytes and endothelial cells, and possibly other tissues such as inflammatory cells and endothelial progenitor cells (EPCs). Estrogen promotes EPCs' survival and plays an important role in cardiac repair by bone marrow–derived endothelial progenitor cells after infarction [22]. Estrogen increases survival of cardiomyocytes after myocardial infarction, and females have increased activity of the antiapoptotic kinase Akt, which may contribute to the protection observed in females. The inflammatory response and inflammatory cytokines are also regulated by estrogen [23], and this could influence the ischemia-reperfusion injury and remodelling. EPCs repair endothelial structure and enhance activity of eNOS, restoring the functional status of the endothelium. Contrary to mature endothelial cells which have limited regenerative capacity, EPCs home in the endothelial injury and ischemia sites proliferating and integrating into the endothelium. In addition, they produce vascular growth factors [24]. EPCs are higher in fertile women than men; their numbers fall after menopause. It seems that EPCs are a better predictive factor for vascular health than conventional risk factors, such as lipid profile, hypertension and diabetes [25] (Figure 15.1).

Diabetes, Lipid Profile and Obesity

Cardiovascular risk has been associated with insulin resistance and diabetes in different clinical trials [26]. Estrogen seems to contribute to glucose homeostasis through increased glucose transport into the cell, whereas lack of estrogens has been associated with a progressive decrease in glucose-stimulated insulin secretion and insulin sensitivity as well as an increase in insulin resistance [27]. After menopause, women begin to gain weight and their body fat is redistributed from a gynecoid to an android pattern. The increases in body mass index (BMI) and proportion of visceral fat are strongly correlated with the development of hypertension, insulin resistance and a number of metabolic risk factors for CVD. Menopause is associated with an increase in triglycerides (TGs), total cholesterol (TC) and low-density lipoprotein cholesterol (LDL-C) and lipoprotein (a) [Lp(a)]. Levels of high-density lipoprotein cholesterol (HDL-C) gradually fall after the menopause, although concentration remains always significantly higher in women with respect to men; this finding is considered a protective factor for female subjects.

Perimenopausal Hypertension in Cardiovascular Risk

In addition to factors comprising the metabolic syndrome and type 2 diabetes, several molecular mechanisms play a role in hypertension occurring in women at the time of the menopause [28]. Oxidative stress, endothelin levels, sympathetic nervous system activity and plasma renin activity are increased. The resultant endothelial dysfunction leads to changes in vasomotor tone, arterial stiffness, arterial remodelling and inflammation, which contribute to atherosclerosis and target-organ damage. The renin–angiotensin-aldosterone system (RAAS) plays a central role in regulating sodium balance, fluid volume and blood pressure. Chronic long-term inhibition of the RAAS using angiotensin-converting enzyme-inhibitors or angiotensin receptor blockers, as well as lowering blood pressure, may prevent most of the deleterious effects due to aging within the cardiovascular system. Aldosterone, independent of angiotensin II, has also been implicated in cardiovascular disease [29]. Blockade of the aldosterone receptor prevents sodium and water retention, with the control of blood pressure, and may prevent vascular injury and fibrosis, arrhythmias and cardiac fibrosis. It has also been shown that one synthetic progestin, drospirenone, is an aldosterone receptor antagonist with antimineralocorticoid activity [30]. When combined with estradiol as a MHT for use in the perimenopausal woman, it has been shown to have antihypertensive activity [31]. This blood pressure-lowering action of drospirenone has also been shown in women with diabetes. Drospirenone, however, has no effect on blood pressure in normotensive women [29].

Management of Cardiovascular Risk Factors in Women

Screening for CVD at regular intervals after menopause is extremely important. This includes measurement of blood pressure, lipids and perhaps inflammatory markers, BMI and ascertainment of lifestyle factors such as activity level and smoking status. In addition, a family history of heart disease and stroke is important. Risk assessment tools allow the calculation of a 10-year risk of myocardial infarction based on gender and race for individuals aged 40–79 years [29]. The main risk calculators used are the Framingham model [32] and a new one from the American Heart Association [33]. The latter is also used as part of the algorithm to decide about initiating statin therapy. The main components of these risk models are age, sex, race, total cholesterol, HDL cholesterol, systolic blood pressure, treatment for high blood pressure, diabetes and smoking status. Interventions to reduce the risk of CVD after menopause include smoking cessation, weight control through diet and exercise, aggressive treatment of elevated blood pressure, and therapies directed at elevated cholesterol and thrombosis risks. The American Heart Association has outlined diet and lifestyle recommendations to reduce CVD, resulting in better population health. The prevailing belief is that statins reduce

CHD events and all-cause mortality under primary and secondary prevention conditions in women and men. However, careful examination and meta-analyses of randomized controlled trial (RCT) data do not provide clear evidence that statins reduce CHD events or all-cause mortality in women under primary prevention conditions. The sex-specific effects are similar for aspirin. In meta-analyses of primary CHD prevention trials, aspirin significantly reduced myocardial infarction (MI) by approximately 32 per cent, with a null effect on stroke in men, whereas in women, aspirin had a null effect on MI but significantly reduced ischemic stroke by approximately 17 per cent [34]. The primary CHD prevention trials and sex-specific meta-analyses of primary prevention trials shows no evidence that aspirin therapy relative to placebo reduces CHD events or all-cause mortality in women.

The Role of Hormone Replacement Therapy

MHT has been subject of discussion and debate. In the early 1990s, the effects of MHT were thought to be beneficial because of a reduction of 30–50 per cent in risk of cardiovascular disease and osteoporosis. These effects were confirmed by a large number of observational studies, thus in 1992 the American College of Physicians published guidelines strongly advising a preventative use of MHT [35]. In those years an escalation in the use of MHT was registered across the world. However, in the late 1990s, the protective role and the safety of MHT was questioned. RCTs overturned the previous hypothesis about the advantage of MHT showing evidence of no cardiovascular benefit from MHT, rather indeed a negative effect on women's health: the Women's Health Initiative (WHI) trial had a great impact on it. Over 16 000 menopausal women between the ages of 50 and 79 (mean age 63 years) were enrolled. After a mean of 5.2 years of follow-up the study was stopped because of increased risk of cancer and adverse effects on cardiovascular system. The principal findings from the WHI were associated with a substantial decline in MHT use by postmenopausal women. Nevertheless, more recent subgroup analyses suggested that the lack of benefit or increase in CVR observed in the WHI resulted from the harmful effect of MHT in older women further from menopause [36]. It is clear that the characteristics of women selected for RCTs were different from those of women studied from the general population or from which the estrogen cardioprotective hypothesis was generated. There is strong evidence that estrogen therapy may be cardioprotective if started around the time of menopause (often referred to as the 'window of opportunity' or 'timing' hypothesis). These hypotheses could have biological basis: around the time of menopause, women still have healthy arteries, allowing a 'window' for MHT to produce cardiovascular benefit [37]. However, with aging, arteries become less responsive to the beneficial effects of estrogens. Indeed, menopause is associated with endothelial dysfunction, decreased NO-dependent relaxation and intimal thickening; moreover, age-related changes in ER-amount, distribution or affinity may also contribute to cardiovascular risk. It is well established that estrogen may have different and controversial effects on the atherosclerotic process depending on its stage. In more than 15 years of follow-up of women in the WHI, the cumulative data in the 50- to 59-year-old age group showed a reduction of CHD [38]. Meta-analyses of RCTs, including data from the WHI, have shown a significant reduction in CHD as well as mortality in women treated with estrogen under the age of 60. In the most recent Cochrane analysis, women using MHT within 10 years of menopause had a reduction of all-cause mortality of 0.70 (95 per cent CI 0.52–0.95) and of cardiovascular mortality of 0.52 (95 per cent CI 0.29–0.96) [39].

Not only the timing, but also the role of the type, dose and route of MHT should be analysed. These hypotheses have encouraged different recent prospective trials using MHT with CHD as the endpoint: the Kronos Early Estrogen Prevention Study (KEEPS) [40], the Early versus Late Intervention Trial with Estradiol (ELITE) [41]. KEEPS is a randomized clinical, double-blinded, placebo-controlled trial to test the hypothesis that initiation of MHT (oral conjugated equine estrogens [CEE 0.45 mg] or transdermal estradiol (0.05 mg) with oral micronized progesterone (MP) for 12 days of each month) in healthy, recently postmenopausal women (n = 727) would reduce the progression of atherosclerosis as measured by changes in carotid artery intima-media thickness (CIMT). KEEPS was designed to understand the effects of timely menopausal MHT on cardiovascular health. KEEPS did not show a difference between CEE 0.45 mg, transdermal estradiol 0.05 mg and placebo in terms of carotid artery intima-media thickness and coronary calcium. After 4 years, the MHT did not affect the rate of increase in CIMT and there was a trend for reduced accumulation of coronary artery calcium with CEE [42]. The ELITE trial studied the effects of oral estradiol 1 mg and placebo in two groups of women, one <6 years from menopause and the other >10 years from menopause, and showed that initiation of MHT in elderly women (<60 years old) or those who are more than 10 years postmenopause may be associated with increased risk for coronary events [41]. Venous thromboembolism (VTE) and stroke could increase with initiation of oral MHT in the older age groups, but concomitant use of statins may mitigate the risk of VTE events following initiation of MHT in women over age 60. In a study published in the *British Medical Journal*, Schierbeck and colleagues report the long-term follow-up of a cohort of postmenopausal women originally enrolled in the Danish Osteoporosis Prevention Study (DOPS). The study enrolled 1006 patients aged 45–58 who were recently menopausal or had perimenopausal symptoms between 1990 and 1993 and they prospectively received standard doses of estradiol and norethisterone in an open-label fashion, or no treatment for 10 years, and had 16 years of follow-up [43]. The main result is that women receiving MHT had a significantly lower incidence of CHD without an increased risk of stroke, VTE or breast cancer. There are at least two main differences between these studies and the WHI trial: the age of the women enrolled and the characteristic of therapy. In fact, additional variables also may alter the cardiovascular effects of MHT, including the choice of progestin. The WHI trial employed just one route of administration (oral), one formulation of estrogen (CEE, 0.625 mg), and only one progestogen (medroxyprogesterone acetate [MPA], 2.5 mg). Synthetic MPA is vasoconstrictive, whereas natural progesterone has vaso-relaxation effects and a neutral or slightly salutary effect on blood pressure. The KEEP trial, for example, studied healthy postmenopausal women aged 42–58 years who received oral CEE 0.45 mg/day or transdermal estradiol patch 50 mg/week, each with cyclic oral MP 200 mg for 12 days/month, and it found no effect on CIMT progression. MPA is associated with higher risk of CVD as compared to estrogen-only therapies. In contrast to most synthetic progestins, progesterone causes little or no reduction in HDL cholesterol levels and has compared favourably in its effects on LDL cholesterol, low-density lipoprotein phospholipids and very low-density lipoprotein triglycerides. Oral micronized progesterone has been demonstrated to provide endometrial protection from estrogen stimulation and to protect against endometrial hyperplasia and carcinoma, it may be used in lieu of synthetic progestins [44].

Nevertheless, after nearly 20 years the never-ending contradiction between studies showing the 'benefit of MHT' and guidelines stating that 'MHT should not be used to prevent chronic disorders' still exists.

In conclusion, CHD events and all-cause mortality benefits occur when MHT is initiated in younger women (<60 years old) in close proximity to menopause (<10 years since menopause) and a null and possible adverse effect occurs when initiated in older women (≥60 years old) remote from menopause (>20 years since menopause). The cumulative MHT randomized trial data initiated in younger women contrast to lipid-lowering and aspirin therapy in the primary prevention of CHD and, most importantly, in the reduction of all-cause mortality in women under primary prevention conditions. As with men, hypertension in women is the single most important treatable risk factor for stroke. With reduction of blood pressure, the risk of stroke is reduced by between 30 and 40 per cent, MI risk is reduced by 20–25 per cent and heart failure is reduced by 50 per cent. The use of statins therapy in women in the primary prevention of stroke is less clear than that in men. According to recent cross-sectional studies, there is no convincing evidence that rises in BP will occur in otherwise normotensive menopausal women due to MHT containing estrogens, or that BP will increase further due to MHT in menopausal hypertensive women. Moreover, MHT is not contraindicated in women with hypertension, and women with hypertension may be prescribed MHT as long as BP levels can be controlled by antihypertensive medication [45].

The most recent Position Statement of the North American Menopause Society on MHT published in 2017 [46] clarifies the existing data and provides easy recommendations for menopause management, suggesting that 'for healthy, and chronologically young perimenopausal women within 10 years of the onset of menopause, the lower dose regimens of MHT (estrogen alone or with a progestogen) offers benefits that outweigh risks, with fewer CVD events in younger versus older women' (Figure 15.2).

In the management of the perimenopausal woman, the cardiologist and gynaecologist should work together to assess and control cardiovascular risk and to minimize vasomotor symptoms. For the primary prevention of cardiovascular disease, the gynaecologist should advise patients about the importance of lifestyle modification, and cardiovascular risk factors should be aggressively managed [29].

Conclusions

Evidence has clearly established a link between the menopause and increased cardiovascular risk. Estrogen deficiency, which is responsible for the vasomotor and urogenital symptoms and osteoporosis in menopausal women, is also responsible for changes in metabolism and physiology to a more android pattern. The European Society of Hypertension–European Society of Cardiology guidelines recommended increasing physical activity, stopping smoking, maintaining moderate alcohol consumption: the first interventions are lifestyle changes, such as changes in diet, and can also have a favourable effect on dyslipidaemia. Many women will require pharmacological intervention with the use of antihypertensives to reduce blood pressure and statins to improve LDL cholesterol profiles, but statins have only a moderate beneficial effect on HDL cholesterol. According to the most recent guidelines of Menopause International Society, personal and familial risk of CVD, stroke and VTE should be

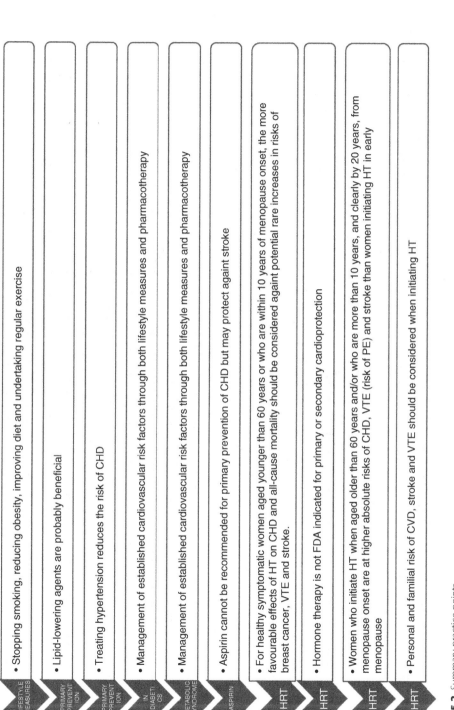

LIFESTYLE MEASURES
- Stopping smoking, reducing obesity, improving diet and undertaking regular exercise

PRIMARY PREVENTION
- Lipid-lowering agents are probably beneficial

PRIMARY PREVENTION
- Treating hypertension reduces the risk of CHD

IN DIABETICS
- Management of established cardiovascular risk factors through both lifestyle measures and pharmacotherapy

METABOLIC SYNDROME
- Management of established cardiovascular risk factors through both lifestyle measures and pharmacotherapy

ASPIRIN
- Aspirin cannot be recommended for primary prevention of CHD but may protect against stroke

HRT
- For healthy symptomatic women aged younger than 60 years or who are within 10 years of menopause onset, the more favourable effects of HT on CHD and all-cause mortality should be considered against potential rare increases in risks of breast cancer, VTE and stroke.

HRT
- Hormone therapy is not FDA indicated for primary or secondary cardioprotection

HRT
- Women who initiate HT when aged older than 60 years and/or who are more than 10 years, and clearly by 20 years, from menopause onset are at higher absolute risks of CHD, VTE (risk of PE) and stroke than women initiating HT in early menopause

HRT
- Personal and familial risk of CVD, stroke and VTE should be considered when initiating HT

Figure 15.2 Summary practice points.

considered before starting MHT. For healthy symptomatic women aged younger than 60 years or who are within 10 years of menopause onset, the more favourable effects of MHT on CHD and all-cause mortality should be considered against potential rare increases in risks of breast cancer, VTE and stroke. However, FDA doesn't indicate MHT for primary or secondary cardioprotection. Women who initiate MHT when aged older than 60 years and/ or who are more than 10 years, and clearly by 20 years, from menopause onset are at higher absolute risks of CHD, VTE and stroke than women initiating MHT in early menopause.

References

1. Gold EB, Bromberger J, Crawford S, et al. Factors associated with age at natural menopause in a multiethnic sample of midlife women. *Am J Epidemiol* 2001;153:865–74.

2. Dratva J, Gomez RF, Schindler C. Is age at menopause increasing across Europe? Results on age at menopause and determinants from two population-based studies. *Menopause* 2009;16:385–94.

3. Kriplani A, Banerjee K. An overview of age of onset of menopause in northern India. *Maturitas* 2005;52:199–204.

4. Lobo RA, Davis SR, De Villiers TJ, Gompel A, Henderson VW, Hodis HN, et al. Prevention of diseases after menopause. *Climacteric* 2014;17:1–17.

5. Manson JE, Chlebowski RT, Stefanick ML, et al. Menopausal hormone therapy and health outcomes during the intervention and extended poststopping phases of the Women's Health Initiative randomized trials. *JAMA* 2013;310:1353–68.

6. Wellons M, Ouyang P, Schreiner PJ, Herrington DM, Vaidya D. Early menopause predicts future coronary heart disease and stroke: the Multi-Ethnic Study of Atherosclerosis. *Menopause* 2012;19:1081–7.

7. Tom SE, Cooper R, Wallace RB, Guralnik JM. Type and timing of menopause and later life mortality among women in the Iowa Established Populations for the Epidemiological Study of the Elderly (EPESE) cohort. *J Womens Health (Larchmt)* 2012;21:10–11.

8. Mendelsohn ME, Karas RH. The protective effects of estrogen on the cardiovascular system. *N Engl J Med* 1999;340 (23):1801–11.

9. Fu XD, Simoncini T. Non-genomic sex steroid actions in the vascular system. *Semin Reprod Med* 2007;25(3):178–86.

10. Simoncini T, Genazzani AR. Non-genomic actions of sex steroid hormones. *Eur J Endocrinol* 2003;148(3):281–92.

11. Simoncini T, Mannella P, Fornari L, Caruso A, Varone G, Genazzani AR. Genomic and non-genomic effects of estrogens on endothelial cells. *Steroids* 2004;69(8–9):537–42.

12. Saito T, Ciobotaru A, Bopassa JC, Toro L, Stefani E, Eghbali M. Estrogen contributes to gender differences in mouse ventricular repolarization. *Circ Res* 2009;105:343–52.

13. Lagranha CJ, Deschamps A, Aponte A, Steenbergen C, Murphy E. Sex differences in the phosphorylation of mitochondrial proteins result in reduced production of reactive oxygen species and cardioprotection in females. *Circ Res* 2010;106:1681–91.

14. Razmara A, Duckles SP, Krause DN, Procaccio V. Estrogen suppresses brain mitochondrial oxidative stress in female and male rats. *Brain Res* 2007;1176:71–81.

15. Sader MA, Celermajer DS. Endothelial function, vascular reactivity and gender differences in the cardiovascular system. *Cardiovasc Res* 2002;53:597–604.

16. Simoncini T, Hafezi-Moghadam A, Brazil DP, Ley K, Chin WW, Liao JK. Interaction of oestrogen receptor with the regulatory subunit of phosphatidylinositol-3-OH kinase. *Nature* 2000;407:538–41.

17. Nathan L, Pervin S, Singh R, Rosenfeld M, Chaudhuri G. Estradiol inhibits leukocyte adhesion and transendothelial migration in rabbits in vivo: possible mechanisms for

gender differences in atherosclerosis. *Circ Res* 1999;85:377–85.

18. Simoncini T, Garibaldi S, Fu XD, Pisaneschi S, Begliuomini S, Baldacci C, Lenzi E, Goglia L, Giretti MS, Genazzani AR. Effects of phytoestrogens derived from red clover on atherogenic adhesion molecules in human endothelial cells. *Menopause* 2008;15:542–50.

19. Strehlow K, Rotter S, Wassmann S, Adam O, Grohe C, Laufs K, Böhm M, Nickenig G. Modulation of antioxidant enzyme expression and function by estrogen. *Circ Res* 2003;93:170–7.

20. Signorelli SS, Neri S, Sciacchitano S, Pino LD, Costa MP, Pennisi G, Ierna D, Caschetto S. Duration of menopause and behavior of malondialdehyde, lipids, lipoproteins and carotid wall artery intima-media thickness. *Maturitas* 2001;39:39–42.

21. Favre J, Gao J, Henry JP, Remy-Jouet I, Fourquaux I, Billon-Gales A, Thuillez C, Arnal JF, Lenfant F, Richard V. Endothelial estrogen receptor {alpha} plays an essential role in the coronary and myocardial protective effects of estradiol in ischemia/reperfusion. *Arterioscler Thromb Vasc Biol* 2010;30:2562–7.

22. Hamada H, Kim MK, Iwakura A, Ii M, Thorne T, Qin G, et al. Estrogen receptors alpha and beta mediate contribution of bone marrow–derived endothelial progenitor cells to functional recovery after myocardial infarction. *Circulation* 2006;114:2261–70.

23. Corcoran MP, Meydani M, Lichtenstein AH, Schaefer EJ, Dillard A, Lamon-Fava S. Sex hormone modulation of proinflammatory cytokine and C-reactive protein expression in macrophages from older men and postmenopausal women. *J Endocrinol* 2010;206:217–24.

24. Mayr M, Niederseer D, Niebauer J. From bench to bedside: what physicians need to know about endothelial progenitor cells. *Am J Med* 2011;124:489.

25. Strehlow K, Werner N, Berweiler J, Link A, Dirnagl U, Priller J, Laufs K, Ghaeni L, Milosevic M, Böhm M, Nickenig G. Estrogen increases bone marrow–derived endothelial progenitor cell production and diminishes neointima formation. *Circulation* 2003;107:3059–65.

26. Hu G, Tuomilehto J, Silventoinen K, Barengo N, Jousilahti P. Joint effects of physical activity, body mass index, waist circumference and waist-to-hip ratio with the risk of cardiovascular disease among middle-aged Finnish men and women. *Eur Heart J* 2004;25:2212–9.

27. Steinberg HO, Paradisi G, Cronin J, Crowde K, Hempfling A, Hook G, Baron AD. Type II diabetes abrogates sex differences in endothelial function in premenopausal women. *Circulation* 2000;101:2040–6.

28. Reckelhoff JF, Fortepiani LA. Novel mechanisms responsible for postmenopausal hypertension. *Hypertension* 2004;43:918–23.

29. Collins P, Rosano G, Casey C, Daly C, Gambacciani M, Hadji P, Kaaja R, Mikkola T, et al. Management of cardiovascular risk in the peri-menopausal woman: a consensus statement of European cardiologists and gynaecologists. *Eur Heart J* 2007;28:2028–40.

30. Krattenmacher R. Drospirenone: pharmacology and pharmacokinetics of a unique progestogen. *Contraception* 2000;62:29–38.

31. Archer DF, Thorneycroft IH, Foegh M, Hanes V, Glant MD, Bitterman P, Kempson RL. Long-term safety of drospirenone-estradiol for hormone therapy: a randomized, double-blind, multicenter trial. *Menopause* 2005;12:716–27.

32. Lerner DJ, Kannel WB. Patterns of coronary heart disease morbidity and mortality in the sexes: a 26-year follow-up of the Framingham population. *Am Heart J* 1986;111:383–90.

33. Grundy SM, Brewer HB Jr, Cleeman JI, Smith SC Jr, Lenfant C. Definition of metabolic syndrome: Report of the National Heart, Lung, and BloodInstitute/

American Heart Association conference on scientific issues related to definition. *Circulation* 2004;109:433–8.

34. Hodis HN, Mack WJ. The timing hypothesis: a paradigm shift in the primary prevention of coronary heart disease in women: part 1, comparison of therapeutic efficacy. *J Am Geriatr Soc* 2013 June;61(6):1005–10.

35. Guidelines for counseling postmenopausal women about preventive hormone therapy. *Ann Intern Med* 1992;117(12):1038–41.

36. Ghazal S, Pal L. Perspective on hormone therapy 10 years after the WHI. *Maturitas* 2013;76(3):208–12.

37. Hodis HN, Mack WJ. A 'window of opportunity': the reduction of coronary heart disease and total mortality with menopausal therapies is age- and time-dependent. *Brain Res* 2011;1379:244–52.

38. Baber RJ, Panay N, Fenton A, IMS Writing Group. 2016 IMS recommendations on women's midlife health and menopause hormone therapy. *Climacteric* 2016;19 (2):109–50.

39. Boardman HM, Hartley L, Eisinga A, et al. Hormone therapy for preventing cardiovascular disease in post-menopausal women. *Cochrane Database Syst Rev* 2015;3:CD002229.

40. Miller VM, Naftolin F, Asthana S, Black DM, Brinton EA, Budoff MJ, et al. The Kronos Early Estrogen Prevention Study (KEEPS): what have we learned? *Menopause* 2019 Sep;26:1071–84.

41. Hodis HN, Mack HJ, Henderson WV, Shoupe D, Budoff MJ, et al. Vascular effects of early versus late postmenopausal treatment with estradiol. *N Engl J Med* 2016;374:1221–31.

42. Harman SM, Black DM, Naftolin F, et al. Arterial imaging outcomes and cardiovascular risk factors in recently menopausal women: a randomized trial. *Ann Intern Med* 2014;161:249–60.

43. Schierbeck LL, Rejnmark L, Tofteng CL, et al. Effect of hormone replacement therapy on cardiovascular events in recently postmenopausal women: randomized trial. *BMJ* 2012;345:e6409.

44. Hormone therapy and heart disease. *Obstet Gynecol* 2013;121:1407–10.

45. Williams B, Mancia G, Spiering W, Rosei EA, Azizi M, Burnier M, et al. ESC/ESH guidelines for the management of arterial hypertension. *Eur Heart J* 2018;39 (33):3021–104.

46. The 2017 hormone therapy position statement of the North American Menopause Society. *Menopause* 2017;24 (7):728–75.

Gynecological Pathology in the Menopause (Excluding Cancers)

John Eden

The forties are a time of irregular and sometimes heavy menstrual loss due to fluctuating levels of sex hormones. Some months are characterized by low estrogen secretion and anovulation and others by extremely high levels of estradiol (E2). In a 20-year-old woman, E2 usually peaks at 500–1000 pmol/L. In contrast, some perimenopausal women may have cycles where E2 levels peak at around 5000 pmol/L. These high levels of estrogen are often not followed by ovulation and so progesterone is either not secreted at all, or levels are too low to counter these high-estrogen months. As we will see shortly, many gynecologic pathologies are driven by these unbalanced sex hormone levels.

The perimenopause is also a time when gynecologic pathology is common. By age 40 years, around one in three women will have at least one fibroid; adenomyosis and endometriosis are also common. All three of these conditions are driven by sex hormones and are cured by menopause. Prior to the advent of the levonorgestrel-containing intrauterine system (LNG-IUS) and endoscopic surgery, as many as one in three women had an abdominal or vaginal hysterectomy for painful, heavy periods associated with fibroids, adenomyosis and/or endometriosis.

Abnormal uterine bleeding is very common at this stage of life. Apart from the conditions already mentioned, the endometrium is often the target of pathology as well. Polyps are common and can cause pain and bleeding. Potentially more sinister, endometrial hyperplasia can be a precursor to endometrial carcinoma. In contrast to younger women, where the vast majority of ovarian cysts are benign and transient, in this age group, persistent, premalignant cysts are common.

In this chapter, we will examine the pathophysiology of those gynecologic conditions that can cause significant distress for the woman who is approaching her menopause. First, the pathophysiology of these pathologies will be considered and then second, the various clinical presentations.

Pathology

Fibroids

Fibroids are benign fibromuscular tumours arising from the myometrium. Some are very slow growing, but occasionally they can grow rapidly. Malignant transformation into a sarcoma is possible but exceedingly rare (around 1/1000). The site of the fibroid is critically important. Those that are intramural or growing subserosally (under the uterine serosa) are less likely to result in menorrhagia than those inside the uterine cavity (intracavity) or under the endometrium (submucus).

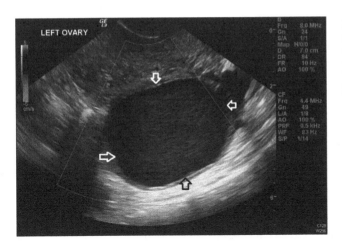

Figure 16.1 An ultrasound scan of an ovarian endometrioma. Note the homogenous appearance of the ovarian mass. Picture courtesy of Dr Yasmin Tan, Women's Health and Research Centre of Australia.

Beneath the endometrium is a rich plexus of blood vessels. Thus, a fibroid that is growing towards the uterine cavity will 'push' these vessels ahead of it. Hysteroscopic examination of such a submucus fibroid typically shows large vessels coursing over the benign tumour. When these vessels bleed, haemorrhage can be quite vigorous. Submucus fibroids can become pedunculated over time and so crampy pain is common. Occasionally pain can be severe, especially if the uterus attempts to pass a pedunculated fibroid through the cervix.

Fibroids probably arise from a somatic myometrial stem cell. They usually have estrogen receptors (ERs) and progesterone receptors (PRs). After menopause, with the loss of sex steroid drive, fibroids typically shrink, although some will become calcified.

Adenomyosis

Adenomyosis is defined by the presence of endometrial tissue within the uterine wall. It is probably due to the basalis layer of the endometrium growing into the myometrium. It usually affects the posterior wall of the uterus more than the anterior. Typically, the uterus is diffusely enlarged, although it is possible for adenomyosis to resemble a fibroid, producing a localized tumour (Figure 16.1). Adenomyosis usually hyperexpresses ER. It is often associated with fibroids, polyps and endometrial hyperplasia [1].

Endometriosis

This is an estrogen-dependent inflammatory disease that affects around 10 per cent of reproductive-aged women. It is typified by the presence of endometrial-like tissue found outside the endometrial cavity, often associated with bleeding and inflammation (leading to scarring). The inflammation can irritate nerve fibres causing severe pain, as well as damaging adjacent structures such as the fallopian tubes (leading to blockage) or bowel (leading to pain and rectal bleeding). Infertility may result from the factors already mentioned or by adverse effects on uterine receptivity, sperm function or even the embryo itself. There may be a link with ovarian cancer.

Blood levels of CA-125 can be elevated in cases of endometriosis, but the only sure method of diagnosis is visual, usually by laparoscopy. The lesions are typically black or red but can be clear and are often seen on the pelvic peritoneum, especially the Pouch of Douglas, on the ovaries, bladder, bowel and uterine serosa. It can form (chocolate-) cysts within the ovary. There does appear to be a link between endometriosis and other autoimmune conditions [2].

The etiology of endometriosis still remains elusive. One theory speculates that endometrial cells implant on the peritoneum because of retrograde menstruation. Another theory suggests that the disease is the result of celomic metaplasia. It can be inherited in a polygenic way and it often runs in families. Endometriosis usually hyperexpresses ER; whereas PR is usually downregulated and within the lesions, aromatase is hyperexpressed also. Prostaglandins are produced in high amounts by the endometriotic tissue and so contribute to the pain and inflammation.

Simple Ovarian Cysts

These are benign tumours, greater than 4–5 cm in diameter with a simple thin capsule and no internal solid features. As in younger patients, if they are ovulation-type cysts, they typically resolve in a couple of months. Cystadenomas are increasingly common as women age and are seen in this age group. Most are of a serous or mucinous type. They do not resolve spontaneously, but rather increase in size over time and can become malignant.

Most serous tumours are predominantly cystic and less solid. Inside the cystic component are papillary structures and grossly, they can resemble ovarian cancer but without invasion or atypia. Microscopically, there are small uni- or multilocular cysts lined by a single layer of tall, columnar, ciliated cells resembling normal tubal epithelium, or cuboidal non-ciliated cells resembling ovarian surface epithelium. In a third of cases they are bilateral. Autoimplants may occur on the ovarian surface that appear identical to non-invasive desmoplastic (serous epithelium with or without Psammoma bodies within abundant fibrous or granulation-like tissue) changes that can occur outside the ovary (e.g. on the fallopian tube).

Mucinous cystadenomas can grow very large and mimic fibroids or even pregnancy from localized pressure in the pelvis or abdomen. The epithelium is usually tall and columnar with basal nuclei and abundant intracellular mucin. Stroma may be fibrous. Calcifications and microscopic cyst rupture may be present. Around 5 per cent are bilateral. If the tumour ruptures (spontaneously or at surgery), spill into the peritoneal cavity can result in pseudomyxoma peritonei (a gelatinous type of ascites).

Solid or Complex Ovarian Cysts

Solid or complex ovarian cysts are fluid-filled structures with a diameter greater than 4–5 cm which also contain some internal solid tissue (Figure 16.2). A corpus luteum can appear as a complex ovarian cyst but will resolve over time. The differential diagnosis of a growing complex cyst includes a dermoid (teratoma; containing skin, neuronal tissue, teeth, hair, etc.), ovarian cancer or an endometrioma (an ovarian cyst of endometriosis; a so-called chocolate cyst) [3].

The lesion size, mobility, and presence of internal septation or solid areas (with assessment of the degree of vascularity within the solid areas), bilaterality and the presence of ascites are all important features in determining the malignant potential of a lesion.

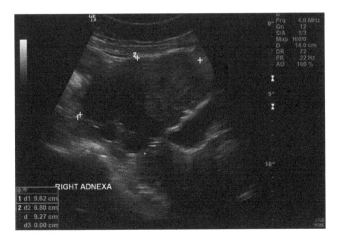

Figure 16.2 A complex ovarian mass as seen on ultrasound. Fluid shows up as 'black' on ultrasound. This mass has both cystic and solid features. Picture courtesy of Dr Yasmin Tan, Women's Health and Research Centre of Australia.

Endometrial Hyperplasia

This condition is characterized by proliferation and thickening of the endometrium. It is typically due to a prolonged, unopposed estrogen effect, which of course commonly occurs during the perimenopausal years. It is also linked to age over 40 years, tamoxifen usage and postmenopausal bleeding. It may progress to a variety of degrees of atypia (mild, moderate or severe). In its simplest form, endometrial hyperplasia is microscopically characterized by mild stratification of the endometrium with round glands, perhaps with some cystic dilatation; mitotic figures are occasional and vessel uniform in distribution.

As the disease progresses to complex endometrial hyperplasia (with varying degrees of atypia), the microscopic features become more intricate. This may include rounding of nuclei and nucleoli formation, epithelial stratification, an increase in mitosis rate, cytomegaly and pleomorphism. Endometrial hyperplasia (with or without atypia) may progress to endometrial carcinoma and can often be reversed by moderately high doses of progestins. This usually presents with abnormal uterine bleeding, as will be discussed later.

Endometrial Polyps

These are benign lesions that arise from the endometrium on a stalk fed by, often, a single blood vessel (Figure 16.3). They can range from a few millimetres to centimetres in size. They often present as abnormal uterine bleeding and are rarely premalignant (unlike bowel polyps).

Clinical Scenarios and Diagnostic Options

Pelvic Pain

Acute sudden and severe pelvic pain suggests either torsion or rupture of an ovarian cyst or perhaps rarely, in the setting of a perimenopausal woman, an ectopic pregnancy. Often the patient presents to the emergency ward and is in so much pain that she may be difficult to examine adequately.

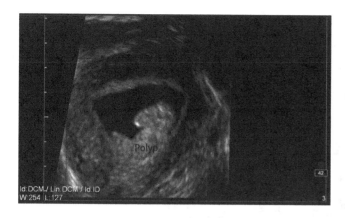

Figure 16.3 An endometrial polyp as seen on a sonohysterogram. Saline is instilled via the cervix to better define the uterine cavity. Picture courtesy of Dr Yasmin Tan, Women's Health and Research Centre of Australia.

Most of the time, pelvic pain is more chronic and often relates to the cycle. Patients with fibroids and/or adenomyosis may describe the pain as a dull ache, or feeling 'bloated'. Pressure symptoms from the bladder or rectum may be present. Endometriosis often produces pain that is more sharp and crampy and relates to the menses. Premenstrual spotting or staining and pain with intercourse are also often present with endometriosis. Gynecologic pain is often also referred down the legs and around to the back.

Clinical examination might reveal a large, firm irregular mass arising out of the pelvis (fibroids or ovarian cancer). The presence of ascites would make the diagnosis of ovarian cancer much more likely. If endometriosis is present, often painful nodules can be palpated vaginally (in the Pouch of Douglas, behind the uterus) and in severe cases, the uterus might be fixed in position and non-mobile. Sometimes endometriotic nodules on the rectum can be palpated too.

Blood testing may demonstrate iron deficiency and anaemia. Tumour markers such as CA-125 can be elevated in cases of endometriosis as well as some ovarian cancers.

Abdominal and transvaginal ultrasound is the single most useful test. In expert hands, high-quality ultrasound can usually easily diagnose fibroids and describe their location; adenomyosis is often, but not always, picked up on ultrasound. In contrast, most patients with endometriosis have a normal scan, unless an endometrioma is present.

Abnormal Uterine Bleeding

The perimenopausal phase is a time when irregular menstrual loss is common and it may be challenging for the clinician to decide which patient needs investigation. A variety of types of abnormal uterine bleeding (AUB) are described [4]. Heavy menstrual bleeding (HMB) or menorrhagia is usually defined as more than 80 ml of measured blood per menses (at least for research purposes). However, in clinical practice, few clinicians will actually measure menstrual loss. Typically, menorrhagia is associated with the passage of menstrual clots and flooding. Prolonged menstruation is usually defined as bleeding for more than 8 days. Intermenstrual bleeding is also considered abnormal. The causes of AUB are typically benign but malignancy (endometrial, cervical) should always be considered. In most series of AUB around 70 per cent will have a benign cause, 15 per cent a malignancy and 15 per cent a premalignant lesion.

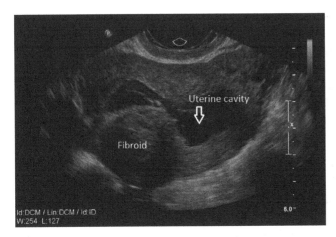

Figure 16.4 Sonohysterogram. Note that a fibroid is protruding into the uterine cavity. Picture courtesy of Dr Yasmin Tan, Women's Health and Research Centre of Australia.

Postmenopausal bleeding, defined as bleeding after 12 months of amenorrhea, always requires uterine assessment. The cervix should be visualized and cytology performed. Systematic reviews have shown that transvaginal (TV) ultrasound is a very good first test and if the endometrial thickness (ET) is 4 mm or less, then significant endometrial pathology is unlikely. Endometrial thickness greater than 4 mm (5 mm or more) or repeated episodes of postmenopausal bleeding (even if the ET is 4 mm or less) is an indication for a sonohysterogram (SHG) or (usually) hysteroscopy, and biopsy.

A SHG involves the instillation of saline into the uterine cavity (Figure 16.4). It is an accurate test and cheaper than hysteroscopy. A SHG misses around 7 per cent of intracavity lesions, usually a small polyp. The workup aims to document the cause of the bleeding, exclude malignancy and precisely locate any pathology such as fibroids.

Hysteroscopy can be performed under local or general anaesthetic and involves inspecting the endocervical canal and uterine cavity using either CO_2 or saline (or another solution). Targeted biopsies can be performed and polypoid lesions resected.

For most episodes of AUB, the minimum workup is a TV scan, cervical smear (if due) and an endometrial biopsy. Sexually transmitted infections (STIs) such as chlamydia can present with irregular vaginal bleeding and should always be considered in the differential diagnosis. A sensitive PCR-based test is available and can be performed on a swab, urine or liquid cytology. Endometrial biopsy may be performed using a Pipelle in the consulting room, or at the time of hysteroscopy.

Pelvic Mass

Sometimes patients may present with a large mass arising out of the pelvis. Pressure symptoms on the bowel or bladder are common too. Ultrasound again is extremely helpful at clarifying the type of mass. If ovarian cancer is suspected then tumour markers should be ordered.

Management

In the recent past hysterectomy with or without removal of the ovaries was often performed to cure these gynecologic pathologies. Over the last 20 years, many more medical options have become available, along with endoscopic approaches, so that far fewer hysterectomies are now performed.

Fibroids

Depending on the patient's symptoms, fibroids can be managed expectantly, medically, radiologically or surgically. For many patients with few or no symptoms, it is reasonable to simply monitor the fibroids using ultrasound, anticipating that the menopause will cure the disease. The patient with heavy menstrual bleeding has many choices. If she is healthy, normotensive and a non-smoker then a low-estrogen contraceptive pill may be adequate to control her heavy periods. Tranexamic acid (1 g three to four times a day) can be taken during menses and often markedly reduces blood loss. Another approach can be to suppress menstruation completely using a moderate dose of a progestin (e.g. norethisterone 5 mg daily, medroxyprogesterone acetate [MPA] 30–50 mg or by injection 150 mg three monthly, Depo Provera). If there are no intracavity fibroids, a LNG-IUS has around an 80 per cent success rate in reducing the degree of blood loss. A novel approach recently described is the use of ulipristal acetate (Esmya, PreLem SA) administered orally at 5 mg/day for several weeks, thus shrinking the fibroids and enabling the insertion of a LNG-IUS [5]. There have been reports of abnormal function associated with this drug and so it may be prudent to measure monthly liver function tests whilst the patients takes ulipristal.

Gonadotropin-releasing hormone (GnRH) agonists used for 3–6 months can effectively shrink fibroids, but are not a useful long-term option because of the risk of osteoporosis (and in some cases, severe hot flashes). Furthermore, the fibroids often regrow after stopping the hormone. Uterine artery embolization (UAE) involves an angiogram performed via the femoral artery. The uterine arteries are identified and then microspheres are injected to embolize the distal branches that supply the fibroids. Most patients will get a very good result but around 20 per cent will still need a surgical option. Systematic reviews have shown that around 3 per cent will develop severe pain and fever (occasionally requiring emergency hysterectomy), 1.5 per cent will expel the fibroid, 1.5 per cent will suffer a uterine infection and 0.3 per cent will have a groin complication from the angiogram [6].

Removal of the fibroids, or myomectomy, is usually performed where fertility preservation is requested. The patient may opt for an endometrial ablation, which often controls heavy menstrual loss in this setting. Any submucus fibroids should be resected first. Finally, she may opt for a hysterectomy, which could be performed abdominally or endoscopically (depending on the size of the uterus). A large uterus can sometimes be shrunk with a 3-month course of GnRH agonist so that a subtotal hysterectomy can be performed endoscopically. The body of the uterus can be morcellated (minced) to facilitate removal through a small port. Rarely a malignant fibroid may be morcellated and so this risk needs to be discussed with a patient who is considering endoscopic removal of a fibroid.

Adenomyosis

A minority of patients with adenomyosis have no symptoms. Most will have heavy painful bleeding. Some have continual pelvic pain and some have painful sexual intercourse. Over 90 per cent of cases occur in multiparous women. Tamoxifen appears to be a definite risk factor for this disease. It can reactivate adenomyosis in menopausal women. In one study more than half of women on tamoxifen had evidence of adenomyosis. Also, the majority of women with adenomyosis have other uterine pathologies such as fibroids, polyps or endometrial hyperplasia.

Pain may respond to anti-inflammatories. GnRH agonists, danazol, LNG-IUS and high-dose systemic progestins have all been used to treat adenomyosis with varying success. Superficial disease may respond to endometrial ablation, but if the disease has penetrated deeply into the myometrium, then an ablation can result in severe pelvic pain. The only definitive cure for this problem is hysterectomy, which may be performed endoscopically, abdominally or vaginally.

Endometriosis

Since endometriosis can only be definitively diagnosed by laparoscopy it follows that most will also be treated surgically. Lesions can be excised or vaporized using laser or diathermy. Ovarian endometriomas need to have the capsule removed, otherwise the disease will recur. However, there are also many effective medical options. Endometriotic lesions hyperexpress ER, prostaglandins and aromatase, and so treatments that suppress the menstrual cycle, ER and aromatase can be effective. As such, anti-inflammatories often relieve the pain and combined oral contraceptives (COCs), moderate doses of progestins, aromatase inhibitors and GnRH agonists can be useful. Patients who wish to delay child-bearing can have a LNG-IUS fitted at the time of endoscopic surgery.

A minority of patients with endometriosis and other painful pelvic conditions will develop neuralgias, often involving the pudendal nerve or its branches. This type of pain is often described as 'burning', 'tingling', like 'electricity' or 'sharp' and can be severe and disabling. Commonly, the pelvic floor becomes involved in this pain syndrome and goes into a state of chronic contraction (pelvic floor myalgia) causing more pain and dyspareunia. The neuralgic component sometimes responds to nerve modulators such as low-dose amitriptyline, gabapentin or pregabalin. Pelvic floor myalgia requires skilled physiotherapy (pelvic floor relaxation and/or dilators) and sometimes responds to Botox (infiltrated into the pelvic floor muscles under an anesthetic).

Ovarian Cysts

Small ovarian cysts found on ultrasound (size <5 cm) are followed up with a repeat scan in 2 months or so and many will resolve. If still present, or are larger on the repeat scan, then surgery will be required (usually endoscopic). Ovarian cysts with solid features are always viewed as potentially more sinister. However, a corpus luteum often has solid features, and will resolve in 2 months. A high CA-125 level does not inevitably indicate cancer, as it can be raised in the presence of endometriosis. Thus a solid ovarian lesion could be an endometrioma, a dermoid or ovarian cancer. A persistent ovarian cyst with solid (and vascular) features will always need to be removed.

Endometrial Hyperplasia

Simple endometrial hyperplasia usually responds to progestins given orally or by the endometrial route using the LNG-IUS. The risk of progression to carcinoma is low (around 2–3 per cent). In contrast, if atypia is present on the biopsy, then the risk of malignant progression is much higher (8–30 per cent). In one systematic review simple hyperplasia responded equally well to oral progestin or the LNG-IUS (89 per cent vs 96 per cent) [8]. However, the LNG-IUS was superior to oral progestin when the hyperplasia was complex (92 per cent vs 66 per cent) or when atypia was present (90 per cent vs 69 per cent). Patient compliance is also higher with the LNG-IUS over oral therapy.

Conclusions

The time leading up to the menopause is commonly associated with a number of sex hormone-responsive gynecologic pathologies. These typically present clinically with pelvic pain and/or AUB. When menopause finally occurs, these conditions such as fibroids, endometriosis and adenomyosis go into remission. Premalignant conditions such as endometrial hyperplasia with/without atypia are common after 40 years of age and usually present with AUB (including postmenopausal bleeding).

In the recent past, most of these pathologies were treated by hysterectomy (and often bilateral removal of tubes and ovaries). With the advent of improved medical options, in particular the LNG-IUS, the hysterectomy rate has fallen from around 30 per cent to 3 per cent now [7]. Radiologic options are now also available for those with symptomatic fibroids. Finally, the rise of endogynecology and operations such as endometrial ablation has now made many gynecologic techniques day (or overnight) procedures.

References

1. Bergeron C, Amant F, Ferenczy A. Pathology and pathophysiology of adenomyosis. *Best Prac Res Clin Obstet Gynaecol* 2006;20:511–21.

2. Bulun SE. Endometriosis. *N Eng J Med* 2009;360:268–79.

3. McCluggage WG. Ovarian borderline tumours: a review with emphasis on controversial areas. *Diag Histopath* 2011;17:178–91.

4. Munro MG, Critchley HOD, Fraser IS. The FIGO classification of causes of abnormal uterine bleeding in the reproductive years. *Fert Ster* 2011;95:2204–8.

5. Briggs P. The management of heavy menstrual bleeding associated with uterine fibroids using Ulipristal acetate, 5 mg daily (Esmya®, Preglem) followed by the introduction of a Levonorgestrel – Intrauterine System (LNG-IUS, Mirena®, Bayer). *Giorn Ital Ostet Ginecol* 2013;35:150–2.

6. Martin J, Bhanot S. Complications and reinterventions in uterine artery embolization for symptomatic uterine fibroids: a literature review and meta-analysis. *Cardiovasc Intervent Radiol* 2013;36:395–402.

7. Heliövaara-Peippo S, Hurskainen R, Teperi R, et al. Quality of life and costs of levonorgestrel-releasing intrauterine system or hysterectomy in the treatments of menorrhagia: a 10 year randomized controlled trial. *Am J Obstet Gynecol* 2013;209:535e1–e14.

Nutrition and Weight Gain in the Menopause

Nigel Denby

Eating well and keeping active remain the cornerstone of a healthy menopause, regardless of menopausal hormone therapy (MHT) status. During a consultation, it can be all too easy to gloss over lifestyle aspects of menopause care assuming the patient knows what a healthy diet and lifestyle is. There remains both lay and health professional confusion about the evidence-based approach to nutrition. Poor science and celebrity 'anecdote' flood consumer and social media with misinformation about what a healthy diet and lifestyle should look like.

For the purpose of this chapter the focus is on the practical elements of diet and lifestyle which are relevant to the majority of women. My focus will also be on the methods you can use to encourage and motivate a woman to make changes and put these into practice.

In my experience, the menopause is a window of opportunity in a woman's life. Now, she may have the motivation, time and mindset to make positive changes to her diet and activity levels. As health professionals, our role is to help her understand exactly what she'd benefit from changing and to help her make an effective, personalized plan of action.

Throughout the chapter, I have referenced several Food Fact Sheets produced by the British Dietetic Association [1].

Weight Management and Menopause: The Big Issue

The women who come to my clinic complain more about weight gain than any other aspect of their menopause – they tell me its 'unexplainable, persistent and all sits around the abdomen and upper body'. Usually they feel miserable and out of control. Their self-esteem, confidence and general outlook on life can all be significantly affected by their excess weight. Often, they're convinced their weight gain has occurred since commencing hormone therapy.

Rarely does a woman tell me she's worried about her bone health or her increased risk of cardiovascular disease. Fortunately, the dietary strategies to help manage her weight concerns will also improve her bone density and help manage her CVD risk.

The 2018 All Party Parliamentary Group on Obesity found that only 26 per cent of people with obesity reported being treated with dignity and respect by health care professionals.

In my experience, the greatest skill required to give good menopause dietary advice is listening and understanding. If you understand what is motivating the woman, and can support her in the way that's right for her, the technicalities of a good diet and lifestyle are easy.

Tip: It is important to ask for permission to discuss the woman's weight. This can often be achieved by simply asking what issues surrounding her menopause bother her the most. If weight gain is mentioned, simply ask 'are you happy if we talk about your weight?'

Menopause Diet and Lifestyle: Facts and Trends

- **Weight gain** at the menopause affects around 50 per cent of women. It is due to a fall in metabolic rate by around 10 per cent, and equates to an average weight gain of 1.5 kg/year and as hormone levels change the additional weight tends to be deposited centrally leading to increased risk of metabolic disorders such as diabetes and cardiovascular disease [2].
- **HRT does not cause weight gain:** The evidence is just not there to support this theory.
- **Bone health:** Bone loss is escalated during the menopause and continues for up to 10 years after [3]. The daily recommended amount of calcium intake for women of menopause age is 700 mg, but the National Osteoporosis Society suggest that those with or at risk of osteoporosis should have 1000–1200 mg/day. Weight-bearing exercise, possible Vitamin D supplementation and weight training may all help too.
- The risk of **breast cancer** can be reduced by some simple dietary measures such as avoiding excess weight gain, eating more brassica vegetables [4], upping fibre intake, especially soluble fibre, and replacing some meat with oily fish. Keeping to dietary fat recommendations and obtaining enough Vitamin D are all relevant.
- **Less active:** Regular aerobic exercise can reduce the severity and frequency of vasomotor symptoms, and if exercise is combined with diet for weight loss there may be a 30 per cent reduction in symptom severity for every 5 kg lost [5, 6]. Both aerobic and resistance exercise are an essential part of managing menopause weight gain.
- **Lipids and blood pressure:** Total cholesterol tends to rise but levels of HDL cholesterol tend to fall after menopause. This is exacerbated if accompanied by weight gain, especially centrally deposited fat and a sedentary lifestyle. Blood pressure may increase too so with the fall in cardioprotective estrogen women's risk of heart disease equals that of men.
- Strategies to lower LDL cholesterol and raise HDL cholesterol include keeping a healthy weight, reducing saturated fat intake (replacing with polyunsaturated and monounsaturated fats), keeping physically active, eating more soluble fibre and adopting a more Mediterranean diet [7]. Eating more soya-based foods may also help [8].
- **Caffeine and alcohol drinks** can exacerbate hot flushes and are often but not always high in empty calories – stick to DoH guidelines.

Menopause: Weight Gain, Body Composition and Fat Deposition

Weight gain is a common complaint among about half of women during the menopause. The transition to menopause is associated with changes in body composition and body shape, and increasing weight and BMI.

Evidence from the SWAN study and The Healthy Women's Study suggest that on average, women gain around 1.5 kg weight per year during their forties, fifties and sixties. Much of this weight gathers around the upper body and abdomen. As estrogen levels decrease, visceral fat deposition increases from 5 to 8 per cent total body fat premenopause, to 10–15 per cent total body fat postmenopause. To add to the problem, lean muscle mass and metabolic rate reduces. Most of the evidence supports changes in BMI and weight gain with ageing and changes in body composition with reproductive hormone changes [9].

Treatment and Advice: Where to Start

If you are fortunate to work amongst a multidisciplinary team including dietitians, exercise specialists and psychologists they can provide this advice and support for women. However, if it falls to you to support your patient, this section will help you focus more on the lifestyle modifications needed.

Eat Less and Move More

High-quality studies evaluating the effectiveness of interventions targeting body weight and composition changes in women during the menopause are needed. Evidence from one high-quality study indicates that women who followed a year-long plan of calorie restriction and increased exercise improved their body weight and reduced central adiposity. Reductions in waist circumference and body fat were also maintained for over 4 years [10, 11].

Dietary Change

The fundamental elements of any effective weight loss plan require a daily calorie deficit of around 500 Kcals or 3500 calories per week and a regular increase of both aerobic and resistance exercise [12]. How the calorie deficit is achieved is best assessed by determining where the majority of excess calories are coming from in the woman's diet.

Potential high-calorie contributors include

- Snacks and grazing
- Alcohol
- Large portions

The most practical and accurate way to gain an understanding of woman's dietary habits is a 3-day food and activity diary. This should be completed by the woman prior to the consultation. The diary should also be accompanied by guidance supporting accurate completion. Mobile phone applications such as My fitness Pal and Nutricheck are also easy to use, accurate and inexpensive (www.myfitnesspal.com/; www.nutracheck.co.uk/CaloriesIn/).

It can be useful to quantify regular excess calories in the context of a cumulative, weekly proportion of a woman's daily recommended calorie allowance, e.g. 'Your wine intake over the week equates to more than an entire day's worth of calories (Table 17.1). Is that something you think you could reduce?'

Agreeing on 2–3 dietary changes to achieve a total saving of 3500 calories over a week is a good and effective starting point. The weight loss plan is based on adjusting the woman's existing diet – not a prescriptive, 'one-diet-fits-all' approach.

Table 17.1 Calories contained within popular snacks/drinks

Excess calories	Per item	Typical daily intake	Equivalent in daily calorie allowance 1800 Kcals
175 ml glass of wine	159 cals	2 glasses per night × 7 days	2226 = 1.2 days' worth of calories
34.5 g bag of crisps	180 cals	1 bag × 5 days	900 = 0.5 days' worth of calories
36 g peanuts	216 cals	1 × 5 days	1080 = 0.6 days' worth of calories
Garlic bread slice	204 cals	3 slices × 2 days	1224 = 0.7 days' worth of calories
Twix	142 cals	1 × 5 days	710 = 0.4 days' worth of calories
Mayonnaise 36 g	246 cals	1 × 5 days	1230 = 0.7 days' worth of calories

Note. Calorie values: www.nhs.uk/live-well/healthy-weight/calorie-checker/; www.drinkaware.co.uk/understand-your-drinking/unit-calculator

TIP: It can also be helpful to put individual daily dietary changes into a check list to formalize the personal plan of action the woman is agreeing to undertake.
The diet plan has four changes for the woman to focus on

- Reduce wine to one glass per night (1113 calories saved)
- Cut out crisps at lunchtime (900 calories saved)
- Cut out mayonnaise (1230 calories saved)
- Only have garlic bread 1 day/week (612 calories saved)
- Total calories saved 3855

Other Calorie-Saving Considerations

Portion Sizes

It is well documented that large portion sizes can often be a contributory factory for people who are overweight. It's difficult to visualize portion sizes in a clinical setting; however, it can be useful to ask a patient if their main meal of the day would 'fit into their cupped hands' (a rough guide to the amount of food you need to satiate hunger). If the woman thinks her meal is larger than that, suggest using a smaller plate or taking a modest first helping and then assessing if she wants more after the first helping has been eaten. She should allow around 5–10 min after completing her first helping before going back for more. These are helpful, effective ways to reduce portion sizes.

Snacks

There is confusion about whether snacking is a helpful part of a healthy eating plan. Three modest-sized meals plus two small snacks per day can be perfectly healthy and in

Table 17.2 Suggested snacks that have low calorie content

Snack	Calorie value < 100
Slice of malt loaf	
Small pot of low-fat fromage frais	
2 tablespoons fresh fruit salad	
1 tablespoon low-fat hummus and crudités	
Large rice cracker with low-fat cheese spread or peanut butter	
1 crumpet with a low-fat spread	
Scotch pancake	
	Calorie value < 150
Around 20 almonds	
100 g edamame beans	
15 Pringles	
3 Jaffa cakes	
Baby Bel light or Laughing Cow cheese light with a Ryvita	
25 g baked ready salted crisps	

some instances helps prevent unconscious grazing. The reality is that it's usually more important to establish what someone is snacking on and why – rather than changing whether they do or don't snack at all.

Skipping meals and avoiding whole food groups, specifically carbohydrates, have both been identified as behaviours which tend to increase snacking. If someone is snacking and grazing unconsciously they will be more inclined to choose foods which satisfy hunger quickly – these foods are high in fat and sugar, such as confectionery, crisps and biscuits.

A planned snack mid-morning or mid-afternoon should provide around 100–150 calories (Table 17. 2). It's useful to suggest women keep snacks with them when they are away from the home.

Getting More Active

To increase physical activity levels, the food and activity diary will provide some information on baseline activity levels, for example walking to and from work, taking a lunchtime walk or using the stairs.

Most smartphones have a built-in 'health app' which counts daily steps and this can also be very helpful. Many women are unaware of the importance of daily physical activity levels in maintaining muscle mass.

European guidelines recommend >150 min of endurance exercise training at moderate to vigorous intensity. Brisk walking appears to be as effective as vigorous exercise in women, and women tend to be familiar with the guide to take 10 000 steps per day, which equates to around 9 km walking each day or around 90 min brisk walking each day [13].

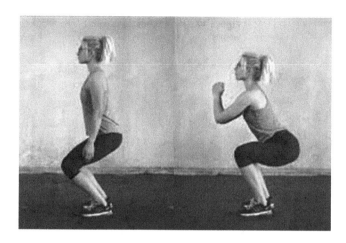

Figure 17.1 How to perform squats.

In order to effect change in muscle mass the important thing is to achieve consistent, daily increase from the woman's baseline activity level.

Tip: If the baseline is well below 10 000 steps per day, agree a realistic increase which can be built up over time. Consistency and regularity of physical activity is the most effective way to increase muscle mass when combined with regular resistance exercise.

- I will walk 7000 steps per day

Resistance Exercise

Resistance exercise should be regular (ideally daily), moderate and within the capability of the woman. The is not about 'pumping iron' once or twice a week, it's about gently challenging the major muscle groups to reach a natural fatigue.

Ideal resistance exercise for building muscle mass: Start with 10 repetitions of squats (Figure 17.1), bicep curls (Figure 17.2), box press-ups (Figure 17.3) and abdominal curls (Figure 17.4).

- I will set aside 10 min/day to do my resistance exercises

A weight loss of between 0.5 lbs/week and 2 lbs/week is ideal, safe most likely to be maintained.

It's useful to take bust, waist and hip measurements as well as keeping a track of weight. The dietary changes accompanied with resistance and aerobic exercise are aimed to help a woman lose fat and gain muscle mass – she may change shape before significant weight loss is shown on the scales.

Other Weight Management Advice for Menopause

Carbohydrates

Carbohydrates are never far from controversy when it comes to weight loss. It's vital that menopausal women include carbohydrates in their diet while trying to manage their weight, especially if they are increasing their activity and exercise levels. Exercising without sufficient carbohydrate intake will result in muscle loss not muscle gain and will of course be counterproductive.

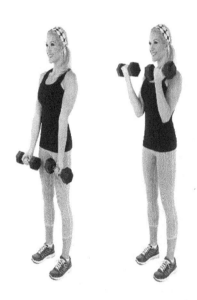

Figure 17.2 Bicep curls using light 1–2 kg hand weight.

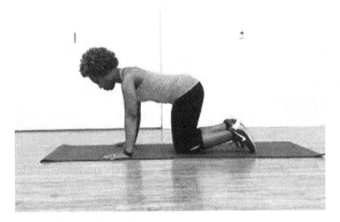

Figure 17.3 Box press-ups.

Slow Carbs, Not No Carbs

Complex carbohydrates like bread, potatoes, rice, pasta and grains are digested at different rates, which affect blood glucose levels. The glycaemic index (GI) is a ranking of how quickly carbohydrate-containing foods are converted into blood glucose. High GI foods are converted quickly while low-GI foods convert slowly into blood glucose (Table 17.3). There is some evidence to suggest that slower rises and falls in blood glucose levels may help appetite control so choosing low-GI foods can be a useful way to reassure 'carb-phobic' women to include carbohydrates at meal times.

Table 17.3 Types of carbohydrate-containing foods with low GI value

Carbohydrate food	Lower-GI choice
Bread	Multigrain, granary, rye, seeded, whole grain, oat, pitta and chapatti
Potatoes	New potatoes in skin, sweet potato, yam
Pasta	All pasta, cooked until al dente, and noodles
Rice	Basmati, long grain and brown rice
Other grains	Bulgur wheat, barley, couscous, quinoa
Breakfast cereals	Porridge, muesli, most oat- and bran-based cereals

Note. Include low-glycaemic carbohydrates with meals and snacks.

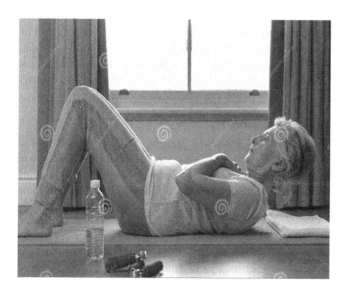

Figure 17.4 Abdominal curls.

Fruit and Vegetables

Adult UK fruit and vegetable intakes remain below the recommended five a day, with most adults achieving around 3 × 80 g servings of fruit and vegetables each day. As well as being good sources of antioxidant vitamins and minerals and dietary fibre most fruit and vegetables are also low in fat and calories. For women who are reducing other aspects of the dietary intake it's useful to encourage more consumption of fruit and vegetables to help manage hunger and satiety.

Protein

When looking at the food and activity diary try to assess how varied the protein sources are. If a woman eats meat see if there is a mixture of red meat, fish, poultry and eggs eaten. Make sure you stress the value of varying protein foods in order to reach dietary requirements for iron, omega-3 fatty acids, etc.

- 2–3 × 120 g servings of lean red meat per week is sufficient to provide a good supply of iron. Eggs are another good source of iron for women who eat little red meat – aim for six eggs per week.
- 1–2 × 125 g servings of oily fish – salmon, trout, sardines, mackerel (not tuna) – per week meets recommendations for omega-3 intake.
- Have your five a day.
- Mix and vary protein sources at meal times.

What About Popular Diets?

Weight loss diets which are popular in the media are often endorsed by celebrities and may have little scientific background. The majority consist of various regimens and rules to differentiate themselves from other diets. The reality is that if a diet limits calories, it will work. As long as the diet doesn't recommend excluding a whole food group, recommend calorie intakes below 1300 per day or suggest woman need to take dietary or herbal supplements it's probably safe enough.

So, if a woman is keen to follow an intermittent fasting diet, a low-glycaemic diet or a home delivery calorie-counted diet, ask what is appealing about the diet to the woman. If her reasoning sounds sensible, then support her. Alternatively, if she wants to follow a popular diet because a celebrity or her friend has done well on it, it doesn't necessarily translate that she will do equally well. She may be better following your suggestions.

Commercial Weight Loss Groups and Organizations

Commercial slimming groups such as www.weightwatchers.com, www .slimmingworld.co.uk, www.rosemaryconley.com and online resources like www .rosemaryconley.com and www.dietchef.co.uk can also be helpful. They all offer different styles of support and eating plans and just like every aspect of weight management their appeal will be very individual.

Find a Dietitian

NHS dietetic departments are increasingly unable to support people for simple weight management but there are an increasing number of registered dietitians working independently who will be able to support women on an individual basis.

www.bda.uk.com/improvinghealth/yourhealth/find_a_dietitian_near_me

Other Dietary Concerns with Menopause

Bone Health

The original 2008 ROGG guidelines for the prevention and treatment of osteoporosis were reviewed in 2017, where it was concluded that the original lifestyle advice should be continued. The provision of adequate calcium and vitamin D through diet or supplementation also forms the basis of the British Menopause Society's guidance for the non-pharmacological intervention for the management of osteoporosis [14, 15].

A daily calcium intake of between 700 and 1200 mg should be advised, where possible achieved through dietary intake, but with use of supplements if necessary.

- In postmenopausal women at increased risk of fracture a daily dose of 800 IU cholecalciferol should be advised.

Table 17.4 Calcium content of foods

Calcium source	Calcium provided
Milk, all types, 1/3 pint (200 ml)	240 mg
Cheese, cheddar type, matchbox size 30 mg	240 mg
Yoghurt, any, 150 g	240 mg
Calcium-enriched soya/oat alternative milk, 200 ml	240 mg
Sardines with bones, 1/2 tin, 60 g	240 mg
Lesser calcium sources	
Tofu/soya bean curd, 60 g	180 mg
Spinach, steamed, 120 g	180 mg
White bread, two large slices	120 mg
Baked beans, small tin, 220 g	120 mg
Broccoli, boiled, two florets	60 mg
Brazil nuts or almonds, 30 g	60 mg

- In postmenopausal women receiving bone protective therapy for osteoporosis, calcium supplementation should be given if the dietary intake is below 700 mg/day, and vitamin D supplementation considered in those at risk of or with evidence of vitamin D insufficiency.
- Regular weight-bearing exercise should be advised, tailored according to the needs and abilities of the individual woman.

Table 17.4 will help you assess if a woman's diet is providing enough calcium when checking her food and activity diary.

Look Out for Dairy-Free Diets

It is becoming increasingly popular to follow dairy-free diets. These can make it much more difficult for a woman to reach her daily calcium requirements. If a woman is choosing to follow a dairy-free diet it's important to advise her to check if her soya, almond, oat or rice milk alternative is calcium enriched.

If you feel a woman is going to struggle to meet her calcium requirements from diet alone a supplement providing 400–600 mg calcium and 5–10 µg vitamin D should be recommended.

Public Health England recommended in 2016 that all adults and children in the UK should consider taking a 10 µg daily supplement of vitamin D during the autumn and winter. Vitamin D-rich foods are limited but include oily fish, liver, eggs and milk and meat (summer months only). Margarine is fortified with vitamin D in the UK – butter and spreadable butter are not fortified.

Alcohol intakes above 14 units per week are associated with increased risks of osteoporosis.

- Ensure adequate calcium and vitamin D intakes

Diet and CVD Risk

By far the most effective action a woman can take to reduce her risk of postmenopausal cardiovascular disease is to maintain a healthy weight. Much evidence has focused on the distribution of fat with a more apple shape representing a higher cardiac risk than a pear shape. Thus a waist circumference of 76.2 cm (30 in) or more was associated with more than a two-fold higher risk of CHD [16].

Lower rates of coronary heart disease have also been attributed to the Mediterranean diet. The INTERHEART case control study showed that a diet containing fruit and vegetables and regular alcohol consumption was associated with a reduced risk of myocardial infarction.

Practical Mediterranean diet advice

- Switch from saturated to unsaturated fats by cutting down on fatty meats, using low-saturate oils like olive, sunflower and rape seed oils and spreads. Choose low-fat dairy foods and drinks. Grill rather than fry foods.
- Include at least two main meals a week based on fish and pulses, e.g. beans and lentils.
- Eat at least 4–5 portions of unsalted nuts, seeds and legumes each week.
- Reduce intake of sugars from sweetened beverages, cakes and confectionery.
- Reduce salt intake by cutting back on processed foods – particularly ready meals, ready-made sauces and soups. Cook from scratch as often as possible.
- Have at least two servings of fish each week – make one of them an oily fish like salmon, sardine, trout or mackerel (tuna, fresh or canned, does not count as an oily fish).
- Have a minimum of five fruit and vegetables per day.
- Swap to higher-fibre and whole-grain breads, cereals and grains – brown rice, oats, couscous, quinoa and rye are all excellent sources of fibre.
- Enjoy safe intakes of alcohol – no more than two to three units per day.

What About Plant Estrogens?

Soya beans are the main dietary source of isoflavones. A large glass (250 ml) of soya drink will provide around 25 mg isoflavone. Choosing whole soya foods and drinks is important as some processing methods can remove up to 90 per cent of the isoflavone in products like isolated soya protein, which is often used in supplements and isoflavone-enriched foods.

There is now general consensus that the controversy around the potential negative side effects of consuming soya was fuelled by findings from laboratory and animal studies using pure isoflavones or high doses which would not be consumed in a normal diet. Comprehensive reviews by the European Food Safety Authority, World Cancer Research Fund and the World Health Organization all conclude that soya as part of a healthy balanced diet is safe.

Consuming 40 mg of isoflavones daily, equivalent to 2 × 250 ml glasses of soya milk or 100 mg soya mince daily, could reduce hot flush frequency by 20 per cent and severity by up to 26 per cent. It's worth making women aware that it can take 2–3 months for the potential benefits of plant oestrogens to be seen.

They seem to work better for some women than others, which may be linked to the integrity of their gut microbiome. Women who choose to include soya isoflavones as part of their menopause management could consider taking a good-quality probiotic.

There appears to be a greater effect for women who consume soya throughout the day rather than in one large dose.

Soya isoflavones only have an 'active' effect on some estrogen receptors, so the concept that soya might provide relief from all menopausal symptoms is greatly overstated.

- If considering including more soya foods in the diet, stick to whole soya foods rather than enriched foods or supplements.

Microbiome

A review comparing the changes identified in the vaginal microbiota of menopausal women outlines alterations in the microbiome associated with specific menopausal symptoms. The review goes on to define how hormone replacement therapy impacts the vaginal microbiome and menopausal symptoms; it concludes by considering the potential of probiotics to reinstate vaginal homeostasis following menopause [17].

Lactobacillus species is particularly relevant to maintaining vaginal homeostasis. The vaginal microbiome structure in postmenopausal women changes with decreasing levels of circulating estrogen. This alteration in the microbiome is associated with changes in the vaginal epithelium that can lead to vaginal symptoms associated with menopause such as vulvo/vaginal atrophy and vaginal dryness. Hormone replacement therapy directly influences the dominance of Lactobacillus in the microbiota and can resolve vaginal symptoms.

Alternatively, both oral and vaginal probiotics hold great promise and initial studies complement the findings of previous research efforts concerning menopause and the vaginal microbiome; however, additional trials are required to determine the efficacy of probiotics alone to modulate or restore vaginal homeostasis.

- It may be useful to include a good-quality oral probiotic supplement.

References

1. www.bda.uk.com/foodfacts/home

2. www.menopause.org/for-women/menopause-take-time-to-think-about-it/consumers/2018/01/23/midlife-weight-gain-sound-familiar-you-re-not-alone

3. North American Menopause Society. Position statement of osteoporosis in postmenopausal women. *Menopause* 2010;17(1):25–54.

4. Fowke JH, Longcope C, Herbert JR. Brassican vegetable consumption shifts oestrogen metabolism in healthy postmenopausal women. *Cancer Epidemiol Biomarkers Prev* 2000;9(8):773–9.

5. Huang AJ, Subak LL, Wing R, West DS, Hernandez AL, Macer J, Grady D. An intensive behavioural weight loss intervention and hot flushes in women. *Arch Intern Med* 2010;170(13):1161–71.

6. Bailey TG, Cable NT, Aziz N, Atkinson G, Cuthbertson DJ, Low DA, Jones H. Exercise training reduces the acute physiological severity of post-menopausal hot flushes. *J Physiol* 2015;594:657–67.

7. Llaneza P, Gonzalez C, Fernandez-Inarrea J, Alonso A, Diaz-Fernandez MJ, Arnott I, Ferrer-Barriendos J. Soy isoflavone, Mediterranean diet and physical exercise in postmenopausal women with insulin resistance. *Menopause* 2010;17(2):372–8.

8. Ma DI, Taku K, Zhang Y, Jia M, Wang Y, Wang P. Serum lipid-improving effect of soybean β-conglycin in hyperlipidaemic menopausal women. The National Institute for Health AARP Diet and Health Study. *Am J Clin Nutr* 2013;90(3):664–71.

9.   Karvonen-Gutierrez C, Kim C. Association of mid-life changes in body size, body composition and obesity status in the Menopausal Transition. *Healthcare (Basel)* 2016 Sep;4(3):42.

10. Simkin_Silverman LR, Wing RR, Boraz MA, Kuller LH. Lifestyle intervention can prevent weight gain during menopause: results from a 5 year randomized clinical trial. *Ann Behav Med* 2003;26(3):212–20.

11. Jull J, et al. Lifestyle interventions targeting body weight changes during the menopause transition: a systematic review. *J Obese* 2014;2014:824310.

12. Piepoli MF, Hoes AW, Agewall S, et al. European guidelines on cardiovascular disease prevention in clinical practice: the Sixth Joint Task Force of the European Society of Cardiology and Other Societies on Cardiovascular Disease Prevention in Clinical Practice (constituted by representatives of 10 societies and by invited experts): developed with the special contribution of the European Association for Cardiovascular Prevention and Rehabilitation (EACPR). *Eur J Prev Cardiol* 2016;23:NP1–NP96.

13. Manson JE, Greenland P, LaCroix AZ, et al. Walking compared with vigorous exercise for the prevention of cardiovascular events in women. *N Engl J Med* 2002;347:716–25.

14. www.ncbi.nlm.nih.gov/pmc/articles/ PMC5397452/

15. https://thebms.org.uk/members/full-consensus-statements/prevention-and-treatment-of-osteoporosis-in-women/

16. https://thebms.org.uk/members/full-consensus-statements/primary-prevention-of-coronary-heart-disease-in-women/

17. Muhleisen A, Herbst-Kralovetz M. Menopasue and the vaginal microbiome. *Maturitas* 2016;91:42–50.

Chapter 18

The Use of Estrogens and Progestogens in Menopausal Hormone Therapy

Kugajeevan Vigneswaran and Haitham Hamoda

In November 1929, clinicians first attempted to develop an 'ovary stimulating hormone' extracted from the human placenta for the treatment of symptoms resulting from the menopause. The team at Montreal General Hospital named it 'Emmenin' and it had to be purified from the urine of pregnant women to be administered orally. It was later discovered that pregnant mares' urine could provide an abundant supply of a compound with high estrogenic activity. This conjugated equine estrogen (CEE) was commercially produced as Premarin and made available as an oral estrogenic agent in 1939.

Premarin still remains commercially available, but since then various other estrogenic compounds have been developed for the management of menopausal symptoms. These include the synthetic estradiol ethynyl estradiol, estradiol, and the synthetic estrogen in Tibolone.

Estradiol is plant derived and has a similar biochemical structure to estradiol released by the human ovary. Estradiol has gradually become the more commonly used estrogen in current MHT preparations with studies showing a more favourable benefit–risk profile with its use over CEE especially when estradiol is administered transdermally. Estradiol is available in oral, transdermal, vaginal preparations as well as subcutaneous implants.

In the late 1970s, the link between unopposed estrogen exposure and endometrial hyperplasia was highlighted and subsequently the use of cyclic or continuous progestogen alongside estrogen became the standard therapy for women with an intact uterus.

The results from the Women's Health Initiative study (WHI) concluded that the expected benefits of menopausal hormone therapy (MHT) may be outweighed by the risks of breast cancer and stroke. This caused great concern amongst both clinicians and patients alike and has had a negative impact on the uptake and use of MHT that has continued to this day.

This chapter outlines the use of oestrogens and progestogens in MHT.

Estrogen Physiology

The term *natural* has been used to describe estrogen sourced from plants or animals, but also to describe preparations that have the same chemical structure to human estrogens. The latter consist of estrone (coded E1), 17β-estradiol (E2) and estriol (E3).

17β-estradiol is the most potent naturally occurring estrogen; with estrone (the main estrogen produced in the body after the menopause) being half as active and estriol (main estrogen released during pregnancy) even less active than estrone. Estradiol is available in oral and transdermal delivery systems and as subcutaneous implants for systemic use, as well as preparations for local vaginal administration.

For MHT, 17β-estradiol is commonly administered at oral doses of 0.5–2.0 mg/day, transdermal doses of 25–100 µg/day when administered through transdermal patches or estradiol gel preparations (one to four measures a day) [4]. Bioavailability will differ between women but as a rough estimate 1 mg of oral 17β-estradiol is equivalent to two measures (each measure delivering 0.6 mg) of estradiol gel and 50 µg/day delivered through a patch.

Routes of Administration of Estrogens

Oral Administration

Both estrone and estriol cannot be absorbed through the gastrointestinal tract. Estradiol once ingested orally undergoes rapid conversion to estrone within the intestinal tract. This is further metabolized and conjugated in the liver, via the first-pass liver effect, resulting in glucuronidation of up to 30 per cent of the initial oral dose.

Oral estrogens can be micronized to enhance oral bioavailability and prevent degradation. Micronization describes the process of breaking down the product into very small particles, thereby increasing surface area and speed of absorption. Despite this step, due to first-pass metabolism, approximately only 5 per cent of the oral dose of estradiol becomes available as unchanged estradiol in the circulation and therefore able to exert an estrogenic effect.

Esterification of estradiol aims to improve absorption and bioavailability after oral administration. Following absorption, the esters are cleaved, resulting in the release of endogenous estradiol.

The route of administration of estrogen therapy (ET) impacts upon the risk profile of the medication due to the first-pass liver metabolism associated with oral administration of estradiol. Transdermal ET avoids the first-pass effect through the liver and does not alter coagulation factors and has been shown to have a neutral effect on liver pro-inflammatory markers. Evidence from large observational studies and meta-analyses has shown that transdermal administration of estradiol is unlikely to increase the risk of venous thromboembolism (VTE) above that in non-users of MHT and is associated with a lower risk compared with oral administration of estradiol. This is particularly relevant for women with an increased background risk of VTE including those with raised BMI and increased genetic risk [1]. The latter is discussed in further detail later in this chapter.

Smoking has been shown to increase estrogen clearance from the liver. Consequently, serum concentrations of estrone and estradiol have been found to be lower in smokers when compared to non-smokers following oral administration of estrogen. This difference, however, is not noted with transdermal therapy.

Transdermal Administration

Transdermal estradiol delivery systems currently used in practice include patch and gel preparations. Patches contain estradiol dissolved onto an adhesive matrix. Depending on the system, these patches have to be changed once or twice a week.

Estradiol gel preparations are commonly applied to the skin daily. Absorption occurs within minutes and serum concentrations reach a steady state within a few days.

Vaginal Estrogens

ET is one of the most effective interventions used to manage the symptoms of vaginal atrophy and urogenital ageing [2]. Estrogen increases mucosal proliferation, thus increasing blood supply to the urogenital tissues, and improves vaginal lubrication. ET also restores an acidic tissue pH by increasing lactobacilli dominance within the vaginal flora.

It has been shown that approximately 25–40 per cent of women receiving systemic ET without topical vaginal estrogen replacement continue to experience symptoms related to estrogen deficiency and this is often significantly improved by the addition of topical vaginal estrogens.

Meta-analysis data have shown that ET, in particular vaginal ET, is highly effective in improving symptoms of vaginal atrophy, through the reversal of cytomorphologic changes typically seen with the menopause. Vaginal estrogen has also been shown to have a beneficial effect in managing urinary urge incontinence symptoms as well as for the prevention of recurrent urinary tract infections in postmenopausal women.

Vaginal estrogen delivery preparations include micronized estradiol tablet (Vagifem 10), Estriol cream (Ovestin 0.1 per cent or Gynest 0.01 per cent) and low-dose estradiol-releasing rings made from a silicone elastomer that require replacing every 3 months. All are considered equally effective. In addition, vaginal estrogen preparations are associated with minimal systemic absorption and long-term data with vaginal therapy has shown no adverse effect on endometrial proliferation in follow-up studies ranging from 6 to 24 months with no increase in the risk of endometrial hyperplasia compared with controls. There is therefore no need for concomitant progestogen therapy nor endometrial surveillance in asymptomatic women receiving vaginal estrogen therapy.

When the vaginal mucosa is at its most atrophic, greatest permeability occurs and as the mucosa matures permeability decreases. It is therefore common practice to start administering vaginal estrogens more frequently, initially often given daily for the first 2–3 weeks then continued in maintenance dose commonly given two to three times a week, which can be continued long term.

Vaginal estrogen therapy may be considered in women with a history of hormone-sensitive malignancy particularly those with estrogen receptor negative tumours and in women not receiving aromatase inhibitors after considering the advantages and disadvantages of each case with the patient. This should be weighed up carefully in collaboration with the woman's oncology team and menopause specialist. This is discussed in further detail elsewhere in this book.

Vaginal moisturizers and lubricants used alone or in conjunction with estrogen therapy may also be considered for the management of vaginal dryness and dyspareunia.

Progestogens

Unopposed systemic ET has been shown to increase the risk of endometrial hyperplasia and endometrial cancer in women with an intact uterus. To counteract this risk, progestogens are used in conjunction with systemic ET. Studies have shown that the protective effect of progestogens used within combined MHT regimens is both dose and duration dependent. There is, therefore, a need to ensure that progestogens administered within both sequential and continuous combined MHT regimens are given in adequate duration and dose.

The primary role of progestogens in MHT is endometrial protection. In sequential MHT regimens and following administration of estrogen, the endometrium develops progesterone receptors. Secretory differentiation occurs once these receptors are exposed to progestogens. Withdrawal of progestogens subsequently results in endometrial shedding and withdrawal bleeding. On the other hand, with continuous combined MHT intake, sustained use of progestogens results in down-regulation of the endometrial estrogen receptors, resulting in an atrophic endometrial state and a thin endometrium. This combination is often referred to as 'bleed-free' MHT.

Endometrial protection could be achieved by giving progesterone in the form of micronized progesterone or synthetic progestogens (e.g. dydrogesterone, medroxyprogesterone acetate, norethisterone or levonorgestrel).

In women who had a subtotal hysterectomy, adding progestogen to ET within MHT may be considered if there are concerns that the remnant cervical stump may contain residual endometrial tissue. In clinical practice, this could be assessed by administering sequential MHT for 3 months and if no bleeding is experienced it can be assumed that no significant endometrial tissue is present. Alternatively, if there are concerns that residual endometrial tissue is present in the remnant cervical stump, then a daily intake of progestogen by administering MHT in a continuous combined intake could be considered.

Continuous combined HRT regimens with progestogen may be considered in women following hysterectomy for severe endometriosis. This is discussed in further detail elsewhere in this book. In addition, progestogen replacement should be given as part of MHT in women who have undergone endometrial ablation.

Three classes of progestogens are utilized in MHT:

1. Progesterone derivatives (examples include medroxyprogesterone acetate, megestrol and progesterone).
2. Testosterone derivatives (norethindrone, norethindrone acetate and levonorgestrel).
3. Spironolactone-derived drospirenone.

Synthetic progestogens (also referred to as progestins) are a diverse range of molecules which have an affinity for the progesterone receptors (PR). Progestogens, however, could have an affinity towards other receptors beyond PR and this may result in agonist activity at the glucocorticoid receptors (GR), androgen receptors and mineralocorticoid receptors (MR) and may consequently result in side effects related to stimulation of these receptors.

Progestins intake could result in water retention and weight gain via its activity on the MR and GR receptors and may also affect salt and water retention. MHT containing the progestogen drospirenone as Angeliq may be considered in progestogen-intolerant women as this may be associated with less progestogenic side effects due to its anti-mineralocorticoid activity. Dydrogesterone has been noted to have a more neutral metabolic and side effect profile compared to other synthetic progestogens. These side effect profiles should be considered when counselling women to decide the optimal type of progestin to use within their MHT regimen.

Evidence from large observational studies and case control studies suggests that micronized progesterone and dydrogesterone may be associated with a lower risk of breast cancer and a lower risk of VTE and stroke compared to that noted with other progestogens.

Oral Administration

After oral administration all progestogens are rapidly metabolized in the gastrointestinal tract and liver, producing up to 30 metabolites. Low bioavailability after oral administration can be improved by micronization and then encapsulation of micronized progesterone suspended in oil in gel capsules.

The oral progestogens that are currently available to be used as adjuncts to estrogen for endometrial protection are micronized progesterone, dydrogesterone, medroxyprogesterone acetate (MPA), norethisterone or levonorgestrel.

The dose of micronized progesterone suggested in this context is 200 mg/day for 12–14 days each cycle in a sequential MHT regimen and 100 mg/day in continuous combined MHT regimens.

MPA can be given in a dose of 10 mg/day for 12–14 days in each cycle with sequential MHT or 5 mg/day in continuous combined MHT. Dydrogesterone preparations contain a dose of 10 mg/day for 12–14 days in each cycle with sequential MHT or 5 mg/day in continuous combined MHT.

Norethisterone can be given in a dose of 5 mg/day for 12–14 days in each cycle with sequential MHT or 1 mg/day in continuous combined MHT.

Alternative Methods of Administration

Transdermal progestogens are available within combined patch preparations containing norethisterone and levonorgestrel in combination with estradiol. These provide sufficient endometrial protection and are widely used in this context.

However, micronized progesterone on the other hand has variable transdermal absorption and reports on its administration in cream or gel preparations have suggested variable absorption and it may as a result not provide adequate serum concentrations for sufficient endometrial protection. It is therefore not currently recommended to administer micronized progesterone transdermally given these limitations, but to administer it orally (or vaginally) to provide sufficient endometrial protection with MHT.

The levonorgestrel-releasing intrauterine system (LNG-IUS) can be used for endometrial protection in MHT. LNG-IUS contains 52 mg of LNG, initially releasing 20 µg/day, followed by a mean release of 12 µg of LNG daily for a period of 5 years. It has a license for use within MHT for 4 years in several countries although it provides sufficient progestogen replacement for up to 5 years and can therefore be used to provide progestogen replacement for up to 5 years within MHT.

Contraindications to Estrogens and Progestogens

The following are contraindications to estrogen use:

1. Unexplained vaginal bleeding
2. Acute liver dysfunction
3. Patients with estrogen-dependent cancer as breast cancer.

Women with risk factors for stroke / VTE should be advised to take transdermal estradiol in preference to oral estradiol.

Hormonal Regimens

Cyclical Estrogen/Progestogen Regimes

Women requiring MHT who are perimenopausal would benefit from commencing a cyclical regimen of estrogen and progestogen. This would allay any concerns over unscheduled or random bleeding leading to anxiety and potentially unnecessary investigations.

Cyclical HRT generally involves taking estrogen on a continuous basis and adding 12–14 days of progestin use per calendar month. Continuous combined MHT has been reported to result in no increase in the risk of endometrial hyperplasia above background risk and to have a lower risk of hyperplasia compared to cyclical preparations. However, recent systematic reviews have shown that sequential MHT regimens taken as per recommended doses and duration of progestogen intake did not result in an increased risk of hyperplasia up to 5 years of use.

Monthly withdrawal bleeding occurs in 80–90 per cent of women after the last dose of the progestogen or during the last days of taking it.

Breakthrough bleeding is common when commencing HRT. Unscheduled bleeding beyond the first 3–6 months of starting sequential regimens should be investigated. With sequential regimens, the aim is to achieve regular withdrawal bleeding which is acceptable for the patient.

If the withdrawal bleeds are heavy, prolonged or painful, the dose of progestogen can be increased or the duration of cyclical intake increased to 21 days. Alternatively, a different progestogen preparation including the LNG-IUS may be considered.

After 1 or 2 years, women may choose to switch to a continuous combined regimen to stop as 'bleed-free' therapy, or to stay on the same regimen if they wish to have withdrawal bleeding and this is not bothersome.

Continuous Combined Regimens

Continuous daily intake of both estrogen and progestogen can be considered in women with more than 12 months of amenorrhea. The main advantage of this regimen is that it avoids withdrawal bleeding typically seen in cyclical regimens.

Studies have reported that about 40 per cent of women will notice irregular breakthrough bleeding during the first 3–6 months, however by 12 months of use, the majority will become amenorrhoeic. Some reports have shown that the duration of unscheduled bleeding with continuous combined MHT is related to the duration of amenorrhea with women who were menopausal for more than 3 years being less likely to have any bleeding during the first year of continuous combined MHT compared to women who were less than 2 years past the menopause.

Women on continuous combined MHT with unscheduled bleeding beyond the first 3–6 months of starting MHT should undergo evaluation of the endometrium to assess for and rule out endometrial pathology. If breakthrough bleeding continues, the dose of progestogen can be increased and if they have ongoing bleeding beyond that, consideration should be given to switching to a sequential regimen or having LNG-IUS as the source of progestogen within MHT.

Side Effects

Side effects with estradiol include nausea, breast discomfort and headaches. Trial data for transdermal patches delivering 75 μg/day of estradiol showed 17 per cent of women experienced headaches, 10.7 per cent noticed breast pain and nausea was reported in 5.3 per cent. Generally, the side effects with estradiol are dose dependent and so dose reduction can alleviate symptoms, but for most women symptoms did improve over time whilst remaining on the same dose.

Side effects of progestogens include alterations in mood, breast tenderness and bloating. Most of these symptoms are transient and resolve within 12 weeks. Beyond this time, if adverse symptoms persist, changing the progestogen component of MHT may be warranted.

Synthetic progestins have been shown to be more likely to cause side effects including fatigue, fluid retention, dysphoria as well as alterations in lipid levels. In the event of such symptoms, naturally derived micronized progesterone, which has a greater specificity to progesterone receptors, could be considered as this has been shown to be associated with fewer side effects.

An alternative option to reduce systemic progestogenic side effects would be to consider the LNG-IUS, especially in women experiencing ongoing unscheduled bleeding. LNG-IUS releases progestogen mainly into the endometrial cavity with little systemic absorption although some women may experience androgenic side effects with its use.

Selective estrogen receptor modulators (SERM) such as bazedoxifene can be considered as an alternative especially in women with troublesome progestogenic side effects. Alternatively, MHT containing the progestogen drospirenone as Angeliq may be considered in progestogen-intolerant women as this may be associated with less progestogenic side effects due to its anti-mineralocorticoid activity.

Compounded Bioidentical Hormones

Regulated non-compounded 'body-similar/bioidentical' estradiol , micronized progesterone and testosterone preparations are produced from plant extracts and are similar to their biological equivalents in the body. They have potential advantages over non-identical alternatives such as CEE, ethinyl estradiol or synthetic progestogens. Estradiol has been shown to have lower pro-thrombotic effect and a more neutral metabolic effect compared to CEE and ethinyl estradiol. In addition, studies have shown that estradiol administered transdermally has a neutral effect on coagulation parameters including thrombin generation and does not appear to increase the risk of stroke or VTE above baseline risk. Micronized progesterone has less side effects compared to synthetic progestogens. Furthermore, large observational studies have also suggested that micronized progesterone may be associated with a lower risk of breast cancer, VTE and stroke compared to that noted with synthetic progestogens.

A number of bioidentical hormonal products, however, are compounded by pharmacies and marketed as supplements / natural replacement and thus do not follow the same pathways applied to regulated prescribed products by Medicines and Health care products Regulatory Agency [MHRA], European Medicines Agency [EMA] and the Food and Drug Administration [FDA]. These should, therefore, be differentiated from regulated bioidentical hormones.There are concerns related to the purity, potency and safety of compounded bioidentical hormones. In addition, many such compounded products deliver progesterone transdermally in cream or gel preparations which have been shown to have variable absorption, resulting in fluctuating tissue availability and as a result may not provide sufficient endometrial protection.

Due to concerns described above, related to the use of unregulated compounded products, Advisory Bodies recommend avoiding the use of unregulated compounded bioidentical hormones and that regulated bioidentical hormones should be prescribed instead.

Counselling

Cardiovascular Risk

Coronary Artery Disease

Advice should be given to women regarding modifiable cardiovascular risk factors including achieving optimal weight and exercise as well as discussing the adverse effect of excess alcohol and smoking and other lifestyle risk factors.

The early reports from the WHI including all age groups, 50–79 years of age, suggested an increase in the risk of cardiovascular disease and possible 'early harm' in women receiving combined estrogen and progestogen. However, the long-term follow-up data, reported by the WHI study group in 2013, showed no detrimental effect with combined estrogen and progestogen replacement. This neutral cardiovascular effect was the same, regardless of the age women started combined MHT.

A number of randomised studies post-WHI have revisited the cardiovascular 'window of opportunity' concept for the primary prevention of cardiovascular disease when MHT is initiated before the age of 60.

Cochrane analysis published in 2015 showed that women who started MHT within 10 years of their menopause had lower coronary heart disease, non-fatal myocardial infarction as well as lower cardiovascular mortality compared to placebo or no treatment.

A neutral effect was noted in women who started MHT more than 10 years after the menopause, with no difference (no benefit and no harm) in mortality or coronary heart disease compared to placebo or no treatment. This is discussed in further detail elsewhere in this book.

Stroke

Modifiable lifestyle factors and risk for stroke including obesity, hypertension, elevated cholesterol levels, diabetes and smoking should be addressed in all postmenopausal women.

The risk of stroke is age related and overall the risk is low in women under the age of 60. Oral estrogen therapy may increase the risk of stroke. Transdermal estradiol is unlikely to increase the risk of stroke above the woman's own background risk and women with risk factors for stroke should therefore be advised to take transdermal estradiol in preferenceto oral estradiol.

In addition, the type of progestogen used in MHT may influence the risk of stroke with observational studies suggesting that micronized progesterone and dydrogesterone are associated with a lower risk of stroke compared to other progestogens.

Venous Thromboembolism

The risk of venous thromboembolism doubles roughly with each decade of aging. In addition to age, risk increases with obesity, immobility, presence of a thrombophilia, personal or family history of VTE.

Oral ET (with or without progestogens) results in an increased risk of VTE that is greatest in the first year after the start of therapy. In the WHI, the hazard ratio was 4.0 in year 1 and fell to 1.04 by year 6, with the risk being dose dependent.

Evidence from large observational studies and meta-analyses has shown that transdermal administration of estradiol is unlikely to increase the risk of VTE above that in non-users and is associated with a lower risk compared with oral administration of estradiol.

The risk of VTE may also be affected by the type of progestogen used within MHT with studies suggesting a greater risk with certain progestogens such as norpregnane derivatives and medroxyprogesterone acetate compared to micronized progesterone and pregnane derivatives such as dydrogesterone.

Breast Disease

Evidence from RCTs including WHI shows that estrogen-only MHT is unlikely to increase the risk of invasive breast cancer. MHT containing combined estrogen and progestogen can be associated with a small increase in the risk of invasive breast cancer but no increase in breast cancer mortality.

The type of progestogen used in MHT may also have an effect with large observational studies suggesting that micronized progesterone and dydrogesterone may be associated with a lower risk of breast cancer compared to that noted with other progestogens.

Progestogens upregulate the expression of epidermal growth factor and insulin-like growth factor receptors and as a result increase cell proliferation. The exact underlying mechanism between MHT and breast cancer risk remains unclear. MHT may act as a growth promoter as opposed to a de novo initiator of breast cancer, although further studies are needed to further assess this association and the mechanism by which MHT influences the risk of breast cancer including the type of hormones used and the effects of dose and duration of MHT use.

The WHI study reported an excess breast cancer risk of 1 per 1000 for combined HRT users each year, after 5 years of use, from the age of 50 years. This increased risk is lower than the additional risk associated with alcohol or obesity. In the absence of any breast symptoms, women do not need mammography prior to starting MHT, and MHT users do not require more frequent breast screening. Women should be informed that the risk of breast cancer with MHT is low in both medical and statistical terms and should be taken in the context of the overall benefits obtained from using MHT.

Osteoporosis

The aim of osteoporosis treatment is to reduce fracture risk and the choice of treatment should be based on safety as well as effectiveness. Randomized data from the WHI trial have shown that MHT is very effective for the prevention and treatment of osteoporosis.

At present, most advisory body statements indicate that MHT should be considered the first-line therapeutic intervention for the prevention and treatment of osteoporosis in women with premature ovarian insufficiency (POI) and menopausal women below 60 years of age, particularly those with menopausal symptoms [3]. Alternatives to MHT such as the use of bisphosphonates may be more appropriate as treatment for women over the age of 60.

Titration of Dosing

When initiating MHT, a discussion should take place to determine the therapy objectives as well as the woman's expectations from treatment. Determining the impact of the bothersome menopausal symptoms on a women's quality of life will help guide effectiveness of therapy. Women should be given advice on how they can optimize their menopausal transition and beyond, with particular reference to lifestyle and diet. Women should also be given the opportunity to discuss the advantages and disadvantages of complementary therapies as well as those of MHT.

The aim of MHT should be to establish the appropriate preparation to alleviate the symptoms of estrogen deficiency for the individual woman and no arbitrary MHT dose or duration limits should be set.

For women who do not see a response after 6–8 weeks, the dose of estrogen could be increased and if response remains suboptimal, the clinician should consider if the woman is absorbing / obtaining sufficient estrogen from her intake. If there are concerns about the latter, a serum estradiol assessment may help determine the levels obtained and assess if a different preparation / route of administration is likely to offer better control.

Assessment for other causes for vasomotor symptoms (VMS) – infection, hyperthyroidism, other endocrine causes – should take place if achieving symptom relief proves challenging with MHT. This would be particularly relevant in women who develop recent-onset symptoms a number of years after their menopause transition.

Duration of MHT

The duration of MHT usage should be based on the menopausal symptoms experienced by the woman and should not be subject to arbitrary limits and women should be informed that MHT before the age of 60 has a favourable benefit–risk profile. When prescribing MHT beyond the age of 60 consideration should be made to using the transdermal route of administration, and to using the lowest effective dose for controlling symptoms [5].

Women should be informed that the risks associated with MHT use are low overall, and these may be further lowered through appropriate selection of the appropriate regimen and route of administration. MHT should not be viewed as one intervention with set risks and side effects. The age of the woman at the time of starting treatment, the route of administration of estradiol as well as the type of progestogen used may all have a significant impact on the risk profile that women may be exposed to, and this message should be put across to women to help them make an informed choice regarding the use of MHT and the preparation that may suite them best.

Bibliography

1. National Institute for Health and Care Excellence. Menopause: diagnosis and management. NICE guideline [NG23]. November 2015.

2. International Menopause Society. IMS recommendations on women's midlife health and menopause hormone therapy. 2016.

3. Hamoda H, Panay N, Arya R, et al. British Menopause Society. The British Menopause Society and Women's Health Concern 2016 recommendations on hormone replacement therapy in menopausal women. *Post Reprod Health* 2016;22(4):165–83.

4. Hamoda H. British Menopause Society and Women's Health Concern recommendations on the management of women with premature ovarian insufficiency.

5. North American Menopause Society. The 2017 hormone therapy position statement of he North American Menopause Society.

Chapter 19

Androgen Therapy
for Postmenopausal Women

Susan R. Davis

What Is Androgen Therapy and Why Is It Sometimes Prescribed?

Traditionally, the term *androgens* refers to a group of 19 carbon steroid hormones that are associated with maleness and the induction of male secondary sexual characteristics. This is as outdated as the concept of estrogen being only a female hormone. The major androgens circulate in concentrations greater than those of the estrogens in healthy women and androgens have a critical role in female physiology.

Testosterone is the main androgen in women, with its more potent metabolite, dihydrotestosterone (DHT), being important at a cellular level. The steroids androstenedione and dehydroepiandrosterone (DHEA) are classified as preandrogens, although each exhibits very weak binding to the androgen receptor. Androstenedione and DHEA are produced by both the ovaries and the adrenals, whereas DHEA sulfate (DHEA-S) is almost exclusively a product of the adrenal glands. Dehydroepiandrosterone is a precursor for androstenedione production, which in turn can be converted to testosterone or estrone. There is increasing interest in the possible clinical importance of oxygenated C19 steroids, 11-ketestosterone (11-ketoT) and 11-ketoDHT, which are formed peripherally from the adrenal hormones 11-hydroxytestosterone and 11-androstenedione [1]. 11-ketoT and 11-ketoDHT appear to bind and activate the androgen receptor in a manner similar to that of testosterone and DHT, respectively; however, the role of these hormones in female physiology and pathophysiology is yet to be determined [1].

Androgen therapy in clinical practice refers to testosterone therapy, although DHEA is sometimes included under this heading. Androstenedione has been used as a body-building supplement, but its use as such is banned by the Food and Drug Administration of the US and international sporting bodies because of safety concerns.

There is widespread prescription of DHEA as androgen therapy for women. Clinical trials have consistently shown that systemic DHEA therapy is not effective for the treatment of female sexual dysfunction (FSD) in women with either normal or impaired adrenal function, and should not be prescribed for this purpose [2]. Dehydroepiandrosterone does not improve mood or cognitive function in healthy women. Dehydroepiandrosterone may improve the health-related quality of life and mood in women with adrenal insufficiency, although these effects have been described as trivial [3]. There are preliminary data that daily intravaginal DHEA may alleviate vulvo-vaginal atrophy, but this requires confirmation in larger studies.

Tibolone is a synthetic compound that is used as a postmenopausal hormone therapy. It is metabolized in the gut and target tissues to isomers that exhibit estrogenic, progestogenic and androgenic actions. It therefore alleviates vasomotor symptoms and urogenital atrophy but does not activate the endometrium, and so does not cause vaginal bleeding. An active metabolite of tibolone has weak androgenic action. As a result, tibolone may improve libido and arousal [4]. As tibolone is a menopausal hormone therapy, not a specific androgen therapy, it is not discussed further in this chapter. The remainder of this chapter focuses on testosterone therapy for postmenopausal women as this is the androgen therapy with a sound evidence base and the most widely used.

The primary indication for the use of testosterone therapy is for the treatment of FSD, specifically, desire-arousal disorder. Initially loss of sexual desire associated with personal distress was classified as 'hypoactive sexual desire disorder' in the *Diagnostic and Statistical Manual of Mental Disorders, Fourth Edition* (DSM–IV) [5]. Since it has been established that low sexual desire and low arousal are co-dependent, the two have been combined in DSM–5 as 'desire-arousal disorder' [6]. However, the global consensus, indicated by the International Classification of Disease 11th Revision, is that low desire and arousal dysfunction should remain as separate clinical entities [7]. Pivotal to the diagnosis of either sexual desire or arousal dysfunction is that the woman must be sufficiently bothered by the problem that it causes her some degree of distress. In clinical practice this usually translates to a woman presenting for treatment, although there is probably a large number of women troubled by low desire or low arousal who, for a range of reasons, never raise this concern with a health care provider. Treatment of a desire or arousal dysfunction may involve relationship and/or sexual counselling, or it may involve a trial of testosterone therapy. Although testosterone therapy may have other favourable effects, the evidence is not strong enough for its use for any indication other than the treatment of sexual desire dysfunction at this time.

Basic Androgen Physiology

In women, androgens exert direct actions through the androgen receptor in a range of tissues. They have anabolic actions on bone and muscle, are important for normal sexual hair growth and skin sebum production, act in the cardiovascular system with positive effects on vascular endothelial function, and influence sexual function, mood and cognitive performance.

As androgens are obligatory precursors for the production of estradiol and estrone, these steroids can be considered to exert indirect actions through the estrogen receptors. For example, an adequate intra-ovarian testosterone concentration is essential for normal cyclical follicular development.

Blood levels of testosterone and androstenedione vary across the menstrual cycle, being lowest during the early follicular phase and rising to a peak by mid-cycle. The levels then fall slightly, and remain at a plateau across the luteal phase, falling to a nadir after the onset of menstruation [8]. Testosterone may have a diurnal variation in young women in the follicular phase, with levels peaking between 0400 and midday [9]. In contrast, the levels of DHEA and DHEA-S are fairly constant across the cycle. The physiology of the ketoandrogens remains uncertain, but as adrenal products they are unlikely to change by menstrual cycle phase.

The levels of testosterone, DHT, DHEA-S, DHEA and androstenedione decline in women from the mid twenties through to the late forties, do not change across the natural menopause transition, but decline slowly with age thereafter [10]. The mechanism underpinning the decline in androgens during the reproductive years is not known, but may reflect ovarian aging.

An important aspect of testosterone physiology is that two-thirds of circulating testosterone is bound to sex hormone binding globulin (SHBG), with the remainder bound to albumin, such that only 1–2 per cent of testosterone circulates unbound to protein. As a consequence the concentration of SHBG determines how much testosterone circulates unbound. Whether this is important has been called to question in recent years. It was believed that the unbound fraction of testosterone exerts physiological effects. However, contrary to this belief the unbound fraction might be the most vulnerable to degradation and it may be SHBG-bound testosterone that is of greatest importance [11]. Women with higher SHBG levels have lower free testosterone and vice versa.

When Are Androgen Levels Low in Women?

Most women will experience a significant age-related fall in androgen levels before they reach menopause. In addition, several spontaneous and iatrogenic conditions may cause abnormally low androgen levels.

Spontaneous causes of androgen insufficiency include:

- primary ovarian insufficiency
- hypothalamic amenorrhea
- hyperprolactinaemia (which can also be iatrogenic)
- adrenal insufficiency (due to loss of DHEA, DHEA-S and androstenedione production)
- panhypopituitism.

Iatrogenic causes of androgen insufficiency include: surgical menopause at any age

- chemotherapy
- radiotherapy to the pelvis
- systemic glucocorticosteroid therapy (suppression of adrenal preandrogen production) oral estrogen, as the contraceptive pill or as menopausal hormone therapy, and exogenous thyroxine increase SHBG and lower a woman's free testosterone level.

Testosterone Therapy

How Is Testosterone Administered and Is It Effective for the Treatment of FSD?

The early studies of testosterone for the treatment of FSD used oral methyltestosterone with oral estrogen. These trials showed efficacy at the expense of lowering HDL cholesterol, apolipoprotein A1, apolipoprotein B, LDL particle size and increasing total body LDL catabolism. Other early studies involved the use of subcutaneously implanted testosterone pellets. Similarly these are highly effective, but they require a minor surgical procedure, the dissolution rate varies substantially between women, careful monitoring is required and their availability is limited.

The most extensively studied testosterone therapy for women has been a transdermal testosterone patch, which is changed twice a week, and releases approximately 300 μg of testosterone per day. The studies of this therapy have involved over 3000 women who have received active treatment for hypoactive sexual desire dysfunction (HSDD).

The transdermal testosterone patch significantly improves desire, arousal, orgasm frequency, sexual satisfaction and pleasure compared with placebo in postmenopausal women using oral or transdermal estrogen, or not on any estrogen therapy who present with HSDD. Most recently it has also been shown to increase the number of self-reported satisfactory sexual events in women with antidepressant-associated FSD. The transdermal testosterone patch was approved for use in Europe, but approval was limited to surgically menopausal women with persistently low libido despite adequate estrogen therapy. As the uptake in Europe was low, and the European regulators refused to broaden the indication for use, the patch was withdrawn from the market. Other transdermal testosterone formulations for women, including a transdermal gel and a skin spray, with demonstrated efficacy, have not progressed through the approval process. A transdermal 1 per cent testosterone cream for women is available in Australia. It has been shown to be effective and to have consistent pharmacokinetic properties in small studies.

Testosterone undecanoate, in a dose of 40 mg either daily or on alternate days, is used in many countries. Unfortunately this compound has highly variable absorption and can result in levels in the normal male range. Oral testosterone undecanoate also adversely affects lipoproteins and increases insulin resistance. Compounded testosterone implants are used by some physicians to treat women. These lack evidence of efficacy and safety and may expose women to risk of virilization.

Fundamentally, the lack of an approved testosterone formulation for women in most countries leaves many physicians with no choice but to prescribe male formulations off-label, or recommended compounded testosterone creams or lozenges. None of these approaches can be considered safe.

Is Testosterone Therapy Safe?

Approval of transdermal testosterone for use in postmenopausal women has been impeded by concerns about cardiovascular and cancer safety. No serious safety concerns were identified in studies of the transdermal testosterone patch, with use by women for up to 4 years. Transdermal testosterone therapy, in a dose appropriate for women, does not alter lipoprotein levels, haemoglobin concentration, coagulation markers, inflammatory markers, fasting insulin, glucose or insulin sensitivity.

Testosterone has favourable effects on endothelial function and is a vasodilator. In a small study of women with congestive cardiac failure, transdermal testosterone was associated with significant functional improvements in exercise capacity, muscle strength and insulin sensitivity compared with placebo [12]. This needs verification in larger studies.

Transdermal testosterone has no adverse endometrial effects and has not been associated with an increase in risk of non-gynaecologic cancer.

The main issue of contention is whether testosterone increases the risk of breast cancer. As summarized elsewhere, oral methyltestosterone has been associated with a small increase in breast cancer risk in the Nurses Health Study, but not in other studies [12]. Two Australian studies reported no increase in breast cancer risk with testosterone implants and a 1 per cent transdermal testosterone cream [12]. However, these studies

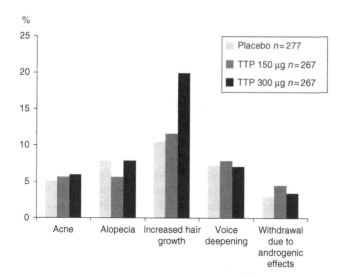

Figure 19.1 Androgenic adverse events over 52 weeks reported in a randomized controlled trial of the transdermal testosterone patch (TTP) releasing 300 µg/day or 150 µg/day. Derived from [13].

are all observational and there has been no single randomized placebo-controlled trial of sufficient size or duration to provide conclusive data. It is noteworthy that women with polycystic ovarian syndrome, who are estrogen replete and have decades of androgen excess, are not at increased risk of breast cancer.

Excessive treatment with testosterone will result in androgenic effects such as oily skin, excessive hair growth, voice change and cliteromegaly. The frequency of these effects observed with two doses of the transdermal testosterone patch, compared with placebo, in a large randomized controlled trial are shown in Figure 19.1. The use of the 300 µg/day dose patch resulted in increased hair growth, but it is of interest that withdrawals due to androgenic effects did not differ between the treatment groups [13]. These effects are not seen when a 'female-appropriate' dose is administered. The exact 'female-appropriate' dose will depend on the formulation used.

Evidence that testosterone improves mood and well-being or is a treatment for depression is lacking and it should not be prescribed for these symptoms.

The greatest risk for women with regard to testosterone therapy is the unregulated prescribing of male formulations and compounded testosterone, often described as 'bioidentical hormone therapy'. Both treatment approaches put women at serious risk of excessive exposure. The International Menopause Society and the US Endocrine Society specifically recommend against the use of male testosterone products and compounded testosterone therapy for women.

A recent large systematic review and meta-analysis has shown that androgenic side effects and risks are minimal and reversible if testosterone levels are maintained within the female physiological range[14].

The Global Consensus Position Statement on the use of testosterone therapy for women[15], formulated using much of the data from the meta analysis, concluded that

1) Testosterone therapy in doses that approximate physiological testosterone concentrations for premenopausal women, exerts a beneficial effect on sexual function above the effects of placebo/comparator therapy.

2) Testosterone therapy in doses that approximate physiological testosterone concentrations for premenopausal women, is associated with mild increases in acne and body/facial hair growth in some women, but not with alopecia, clitoromegaly or voice change and is not associated with serious adverse events.

Can I Treat My Patient with Testosterone?

Testosterone should only be prescribed if there is confidence in the formulation to be used. This leaves few options presently for clinicians. There is an urgent need for a formulation for women to be approved by the regulators.

In the interim, the only options include the 1 per cent testosterone cream available in Australia, and where available, pharmaceutically manufactured, not compounded, testosterone pellets. Before testosterone therapy is initiated, a full medical history, including sexual history, and examination should be performed. It is important to identify the duration of the problem and whether or not it is partner-specific or generalized. The patient should be asked about ability to achieve orgasm and if not, whether this has been lifelong or of new onset. If lifelong, sexual counselling is indicated.

Prior to treating a woman with HSDD with testosterone, consider and treat as indicated:

• Current circumstances.

  Relationship issues. Sexual health knowledge.

• Individual psychological factors.

  Body image and self-esteem. Experience of sexual abuse/trauma.

  Negative attitudes, inhibitions and anxieties.

• Health-related factors.

  Mental health.

  Physical health.

  Medication side effects, particularly antidepressants and antipsychotics.

Although fatigue is a common complaint amongst women, if present, this may be the cause of low desire-arousal and warrants investigation. Basic investigations should include thyroid function, iron stores and fasting blood glucose.

Absolute contraindications to testosterone therapy include evidence of androgen excess, pregnancy and lactation and a history of breast cancer.

If a woman is to be treated for desire or arousal dysfunction with testosterone, a baseline total testosterone level, as well as SHBG, should be measured. This is to avoid treating women with a normal testosterone level inappropriately and to guide therapy. Women with very high SHBG levels are unlikely to respond to treatment, and in the first instance an effort should be made to reduce their SHBG. For example, switching the woman from oral to transdermal estrogen therapy. If a woman has a very low SHBG level then the dose of testosterone should be lowered, as any exogenous testosterone is likely to be cleared rapidly from the circulation, increasing the risk of androgenic side effects.

Treated women should be monitored carefully as it is always possible for a woman to over-treat herself. Optimally, testosterone should be measured after a few weeks of initiating treatment, and if treatment is ongoing, then six monthly. When approved testosterone implants are used, a new testosterone implant should never be re-inserted without checking that the testosterone levels have fallen back into the low female range. A consistent finding in studies of transdermal testosterone has been that efficacy is not observed until after 4–6 weeks of treatment. Patients need to be made aware of this. If a woman has not experienced improvements in her sexual well-being after 6 months of therapy, then treatment should cease, as an improvement after that time is not likely. Women need to be aware that treatment is a trial, as not all women will experience a benefit.

References

1. Pretorius E, Arlt W, Storbeck KH. A new dawn for androgens: Novel lessons from 11-oxygenated C19 steroids. *Mol Cell Endocrinol* 2017;441:76–85.

2. Davis SR, Panjari M, Stanczyk FZ. DHEA replacement for postmenopausal women. *J Clin Endocrinol Metab* 2011;96:1642–53.

3. Alkatib AA, Cosma M, Elamin MB, et al. A systematic review and meta-analysis of randomized placebo-controlled trials of DHEA treatment effects on quality of life in women with adrenal insufficiency. *J Clin Endocrinol Metab* 2009;94:3676–81.

4. Nijland EA, Nathorst-Boos J, Palacios S, et al. Tibolone and transdermal E2/NETA for the treatment of female sexual dysfunction in naturally menopausal women: results of a randomized active-controlled trial. *J Sex Med* 2008;5:646–56.

5. American Psychiatric Association. *Diagnostic and Statistical Manual of Mental Disorders*, 4th ed. 1994. American Psychiatric Press.

6. American Psychiatric Association. *Diagnostic and Statistical Manual of Mental Disorders*, 5th ed. 2013. American Psychiatric Press.

7. World Health Organization. International Classification of Disease, 11th Revision. 2019. https://icd.who.int/en/

8. Sinha-Hikim I, Arver S, Beall G, et al. The use of a sensitive equilibrium dialysis method for the measurement of free testosterone levels in healthy, cycling women and in human immunodeficiency virus-infected women. *J Clin Endocrinol Metab* 1998;83:1312–18.

9. Vierhapper H, Nowotny P, Waldhausl W. Determination of testosterone production rates in men and women using stable isotope'dilution and mass spectrometry. *J Clin Endocrinol Metab* 1997;82:1492–6.

10. Davison SL, Bell R, Donath S, Montalto JG, Davis SR. Androgen levels in adult females: changes with age, menopause, and oophorectomy. *J Clin Endocrinol Metab* 2005;90:3847–53.

11. Handelsman DJ. Free testosterone: pumping up the tires or ending the free ride? *Endocr Rev* 2017;38:297–301.

12. Davis SR. Cardiovascular and cancer safety of testosterone in women. *Curr Opin Endocrinol Diabetes Obes* 2011;18:198–203.

13. Davis SR, Moreau M, Kroll R, et al. Testosterone for low libido in menopausal women not taking estrogen therapy. *N Eng J Med* 2008;359:2005–17.

14. Islam RM, Bell RJ, Green S, Page MJ, Davis SR. Safety and efficacy of testosterone for women: a systematic review and meta-analysis of randomised controlled trial data. *Lancet Diabetes Endocrinol* 2019 Oct;7(10):754–766.

15. Davis SR, Baber R, Panay N, et al Global Consensus Position Statement on the Use of Testosterone Therapy for Women. *Climacteric* 2019 Oct;22(5):429–434.

Contraception for the Perimenopausal Woman

Paula Briggs and Nicola Kersey

The World Health Organization (WHO) defines menopause as the permanent cessation of menstruation due to loss of ovarian follicular activity [1]. It is a retrospective diagnosis, which can only be made with certainty after 12 months of spontaneous amenorrhoea. The average age of menopause in UK women is 51 [2].

The perimenopause (or menopause transition) is the time leading up to the menopause and lasts until 1 year after the final menstrual period [1]. It usually begins with menstrual changes during which the menstrual cycle may shorten or lengthen and women often experience heavier bleeding. Other associated menopause-related symptoms may include vasomotor symptoms (hot flushes, night sweats), effect on mood, sleep disturbance, arthralgia, myalgia, symptoms of urogenital atrophy and loss of libido. The perimenopause typically starts in the mid forties and lasts 4–5 years [3], although this is variable.

There is a reduction in fertility with age, with a sharp decline in the late thirties. Despite this, until the postmenopause a woman is still at risk of pregnancy and requires effective contraception. Over the course of a year of unprotected sexual intercourse, the risk of pregnancy in a woman aged 40–44 years is 10–20 per cent and 12 per cent at 45–49 years, with the chance of pregnancy after the age of 50 being small [4].

There is a correlation between advancing age and an increase in peri-natal mortality and morbidity, as well as a higher incidence of miscarriage and ectopic pregnancy [5]. Women over 40 have the highest rates of spontaneous abortion compared to live births, with 28 per cent of pregnancies in this age group ending in abortion [6].

Women may not appreciate the fact that they are still at risk of pregnancy as they get older, or wrongly believe that menopausal hormone therapy (MHT) is effective as contraception, highlighting the need for appropriate counselling. It is also important to consider that some older women may still be hoping to conceive. The perimenopause is an important time to review contraceptive needs, to ensure the contraceptive method choice has the lowest risks whilst conferring the most benefit.

Contraception and MHT

MHT inhibits ovulation only in approximately 40 per cent of women, and thus cannot be relied upon for contraception [7]. Therefore, contraception is still required in woman taking MHT. Progestogen-only contraception (POC) and non-hormonal methods can be safely used alongside MHT. The Mirena intrauterine system (IUS) can be used for both contraception and endometrial protection with estrogen as MHT. However, other progestogen-only methods (including alternative intrauterine systems to the Mirena) are not licensed for endometrial protection.

Diagnosing the Menopause and Stopping Contraception

Diagnosis is usually based on a woman's symptoms and age, rather than relying on blood tests (gonadotrophin levels). However, use of hormonal contraception affects the natural menstrual cycle, and therefore symptoms including abnormal bleeding patterns cannot be used to determine the menopause. Some women experience menopause-related symptoms with progestogen-only injectable contraception, due to its hypoestrogenic effect. UK guidelines from the National Institute of Clinical Excellence (NICE) advise that women using non-hormonal methods of contraception may stop after 2 years of amenorrhoea if under 50 and 1 year if over 50 [8].

Follicle-Stimulating Hormone

The blood test follicle-stimulating hormone (FSH) is not recommended routinely for women over 45 as levels often fluctuate in the menopause transition. However, women taking hormonal contraception may wish to know when they are able to cease use [4, 8]. Women using Combined Hormonal Contraception would need to stop this 6 weeks before checking FSH. If FSH levels are to be used, two separate measurements should be taken 6 weeks apart. If both results are over 30 IU/L then contraception may be stopped after a further 2 years in women under 50 and 1 year in women over the age of 50 [4]. For women using high-dose injectable progestogens, FSH levels may be less accurate [8].

For women under the age of 50, any method of contraception can be used or continued depending upon eligibility. For women who wish to continue with contraception over the age of 50, either a non-hormonal or POC method is recommended and both can be safely continued until 55 years (Table 20.1).

Intrauterine devices are a potential source of infection and should eventually be removed.

Which Method of Contraception Is Best?

Whilst age alone does not completely contraindicate any contraceptive method, combined hormonal contraception (the pill, patch or vaginal ring) and progestogen-only injectables (Depo Provera or Sayana Press) are generally not recommended over 50 years of age [4]. It is important to consider any comorbidities when prescribing a contraceptive method, particularly as women get older. The risk of both venous thromboembolism (VTE) and arterial thromboembolism (ATE) increases with age as do common medical problems such as hypertension, diabetes, arrhythmias and hyperlipidaemia. Women should be advised of non-contraceptive benefits associated with their contraceptive method, which may help with perimenopausal symptoms, e.g. flushes, heavy menstrual bleeding.

Table 20.1 The UK Faculty of Sexual and Reproductive Health (FSRH) recommendations for women over 50

Method	Recommendation
Progestogen-only pill and implant	If amenorrhoeic for 12 months or more: – If two FSH levels taken 6 weeks apart are >30 IU/L, it is safe to stop POP after one further year. If not amenorrhoiec, continue until 55 years.
Progestogen-only intrauterine system (if fitted at the age of 45 years or older)	If amenorrhoeic for 12 months or more: – If two FSH levels taken 6 weeks apart are >30 IU/L, it is safe to remove IUS after 1 further year in women over 50 and 2 years in women under the age of 50.
DMPA[a]	Switch to a non-hormonal method and cease this after 2 years of amenorrhoea, *OR* Switch to an alternative progestogen-only method and follow the advice for the method.
CHC (COC, patch, ring)[a]	Switch to a non-hormonal method and cease this after 2 years of amenorrhoea, *OR* Switch to a progestogen-only method and follow the advice for the method.
Non-hormonal methods (copper IUD and barrier methods)	Stop after 1 year of amenorrhoea if >50.

Note. From [8].
[a] These methods are generally not recommended over the age of 50 years.

Table 20.2 Definition of UK Medical Eligibility Criteria (UKMEC) categories for contraceptive use

UK MEC 1	A condition for which there is no restriction for the use of the contraceptive method
UK MEC 2	A condition where the advantages of using the method generally outweigh the theoretical or proven risks
UK MEC 3	A condition where the theoretical or proven risks usually outweigh the advantages of using the method; the provision of the method requires expert clinical judgment and/or referral to a specialist contraceptive provider, since use of the method is not usually recommended unless other more appropriate methods are not available or not acceptable
UK MEC 4	A condition which represents an unacceptable health risk if the contraceptive method is used

Note. From [9].

The UK Medical Eligibility Criteria (UKMEC 2016) [9] is a useful method for assessing suitability of a contraceptive choice based on an individualized risk assessment (see Table 20.2).

Table 20.3 Non-contraceptive benefits of contraceptive methods

Vasomotor symptoms
Combined hormonal contraception (the pill, patch or vaginal ring).
Extended regimes are more likely to be effective.

Osteoporosis
Combined hormonal contraception may increase bone mineral density (BMD).
Depot medroxyprogesterone acetate (DMPA) may reduce BMD.

Menstrual pain, bleeding and irregularity
Combined hormonal contraception (CHC) may relieve symptoms.
Some progestogen-only methods may help or they may cause problematic bleeding.

Menstrual pain
Progestogen-only contraception may reduce symptoms.

Heavy Menstrual Bleeding
LNG-IUS is highly effective in reducing menstrual bleeding and can induce amenorrhoea.
DMPA and CHC are also recommended treatments for HMB.

Note. Adapted from NICE CKS Contraception Assessment [10].

Contraceptive Options

Combined Hormonal Contraception (CHC)

CHC acts to inhibit ovulation. It is 99 per cent effective if used as directed and is available in oral (tablet), transdermal (patch) and transvaginal (vaginal ring) delivery routes, which are all equally effective [11].

Age alone does not contraindicate CHC; however, risk of cardiovascular comorbidities increase with age, which can influence suitability. CHC is generally not recommended over the age of 50 [4, 9].

Since the early 1960s when the 'pill' first came to market, the dose of estrogen in combined oral contraception (COC) has reduced significantly, and different progestogens with unique features have improved tolerability (mostly in relation to hormonal side effects) of COC.

Benefits

There are many non-contraceptive benefits of CHC (Table 20.3). CHC can alleviate the perimenopausal symptoms of hot flushes and night sweats. CHC offers good cycle control and therefore can improve irregular and heavy menstrual bleeding (HMB) and premenstrual syndrome, more common around the menopause transition (Table 20.4). Only one COC (estradiol valerate/dienogest [Qlaira]) is currently licensed for treatment of HMB in women who require contraception, with no structural abnormality; however, NICE recommendations include use of all COC for HMB [12]. It is important to note that HMB must first be investigated based on an individualized risk assessment before initiating treatment with CHC.

Table 20.4 Non-contraceptive benefits of CHC (FSRH CHC)

Non-contraceptive benefits of CHC
Reduction in heavy menstrual bleeding
Reduction in menstrual pain
Good cycle control
Reduction in symptoms of endometriosis, PMS and PCOS
Reduced risk of endometrial and ovarian cancers
Possible positive effect on bone health, helping to maintain BMD in the perimenopause

Table 20.5 Continuous and extended regimens

Tailored Regimens
Women may prefer to use CHC with fewer, shorter or no hormone-free intervals (HFI).
Tailored regimens include

Extended regimens
– Fewer HFIs, timing can be fixed or flexible
Continuous regimens
– No HFI

Multiphasic Regimens
These COCs, e.g. Qlaira, contain varying doses of the hormones estrogen and progestogen.

Women have traditionally been advised to take CHC for 21 days with a hormone-free interval (HFI) of 7 days. Continuous and extended regimens (Table 20.5) have been shown to be more effective at conferring the non-contraceptive benefits listed in Table 20.4 and reduce hormone withdrawal symptoms during the HFI. Despite being outside of product licence, evidence has demonstrated these regimens as being safe and effective and they are recommended by the UK Faculty of Sexual and Reproductive Health (FSRH). There may, however, be associated problematic bleeding [4].

There is a reduced risk of endometrial and ovarian cancers in women using CHC. This effect lasts for decades after ceasing CHC, and longer-term use is associated with a greater reduction in risk [4]. There is some evidence that CHC has a positive effect on bone health [13].

Risks

Despite the potential benefits of CHC for perimenopausal woman, there are also serious health risks related to the use of contraceptive methods containing estrogen. CHC is associated with an increased risk of venous thromboembolism (VTE) and arterial thromboembolism (ATE) (e.g. myocardial infarction, stroke). VTE risk whilst using CHC is 5–12/10 000 women per year of use compared to non-CHC users, whose risk is 2/10 000 per year [14].

A woman over the age of 40 is more likely to have a higher baseline risk for these conditions, due to the increasing likelihood of comorbidities such as hypertension, raised BMI and diabetes that occur with advancing age [4].

Over 50, women should stop CHC and use alternative contraception if required.

UK MEC 2016 classify CHC as category 3 for women with 'multiple risk factors' and age is a relevant risk factor.

UK MEC also advises the following for women over 35 years who smoke:

- 15 or more cigarettes per day = UK MEC 4
- Less than 15 cigarettes per day = UK MEC 3

Some studies have demonstrated a slight increased risk of breast cancer in women taking COC compared to women not taking COC, with the risk decreasing after cessation [15].

Another downside of CHC is user dependency, which reduces the effectiveness of the method when 'typical user failure rates' are considered. With perfect use, the failure rate of the combined pill is less than 1 per cent. However, typical user failure rate is 9 per cent. In perimenopausal women this needs to be balanced against declining fertility [16].

When prescribing the COC, current recommendations suggest using a pill with the lowest dose of estrogen (such as 20 mcg ethinyl estradiol and levonorgestrel 100 mcg) to minimize VTE/ATE risk [17].

Recent evidence [18] has shown that Qlaira, a combined pill containing estradiol valerate and dienogest (anti-androgenic) in a quadraphasic regime, is associated with a lower risk of VTE/ATE. Studies comparing sexual function in women using Qlaira compared with women using a pill containing an androgenic progestogen show similar results. Although not considered a first-line pill, Qlaira has specific potential benefits for women in the menopause transition.

Progestogen-Only Methods

Progestogen-only methods of contraception (POC) come in different forms, and with different progestogens (Table 20.6). Most POC inhibit ovulation (with the exception of levonogestrel containing intrauterine systems (LNG-IUS)). All POC methods are a good option to use alongside HRT, with some women benefitting from non-contraceptive benefits (see Table 20.7). With the exception of injectables, POC have no age-related contraindications and have no associated increased risk of VTE or ATE.

Some women achieve amenorrhoea with POC methods, and this can be a beneficial way to manage potential problematic bleeding in the menopause transition. POC can help relieve menstrual and ovulation pain and symptoms of endometriosis [4]. Conversely, some women experience prolonged, irregular or frequent bleeding with POC. This may require investigation, particularly in women over 45 who experience a sudden change in bleeding patterns due to the increased likelihood of cervical or endometrial pathology. Mood swings, acne and breast tenderness are other reported side effects.

The most notable contraindication of POC is in patients with current breast cancer (UK MEC 4) or women with a past history of breast cancer (UK MEC 3) [9]. There is no proven association between POC and breast cancer, but a link cannot be completely excluded. Liaison with the woman's breast surgeon is important and despite the contraindication, some breast surgeons support women to use LNG-IUS. The risk associated with unplanned pregnancy is far greater and heavy menstrual bleeding can be associated with significant morbidity.

Table 20.6 Options for POC

Delivery route	Frequency	Progestogen component
Oral tablet	Once daily with no hormone-free interval	*Older ('traditional') pills*: Northisterone 350 mcg Levonogestrel 30 mcg *Newer pills*: Desogestrel 75 mcg
Implant inserted subdermally into the upper arm	Three yearly	Etonogestrel 68 mg
Injectables • Depo Provera – intramuscular injection • Sayana Press – subcutaneous	12–13 weekly	Medroxyprogesterone acetate • Depo Provera – 150 mg/1 ml • Sayana Press – 104 mg/0.6 ml
Intrauterine system	3–5 years depending on the product	Levonogestrel • Mirena 52 mg • Levosert 52 mg • Kyleena 19.5 mg • Jaydess 13.5 mg

Table 20.7 Non-contraceptive benefits of POC

May induce amenorrhoea for some women, with DMPA being the most likely (70% of women by 2 years of use)
Can help with menstrual pain
Can help with symptoms of PMS, which often worsen during the menopause transition
Can be safely used alongside MHT
A 52 mg LNG-IUS and DMPA are recommended by NICE as treatment for HMB

Progestogen-Only Pill

The progestogen-only pill (POP) is taken once daily with no hormone-free interval. The older ('traditional') pills contain northisterone or levonogestrel and have a three-hour window compared with POPs containing desogestrel, which have a 12-hour window.

For example, with an older pill, a woman who normally takes her pill at 6 pm would only have until 9 pm after missing her dose to take it to be sure that there was no reduction in efficacy. With a desogestrel POP, she would be covered until 6 am the next morning [19].

Benefits

Desogestrel-containing pills induce amenorrhoea in 50 per cent of women after 12 months of use [19]. For women taking COC who wish to remain on oral contraception over 50, the POP is a good option to continue until 55 when contraception is no longer required.

Risks

Problematic bleeding is a common reason for women ceasing this method, as it offers less cycle control than CHC and is less likely to induce amenorrhoea than DMPA and IUS [19].

The POP is user dependent and has a narrower missed pill window (three or 12 hours depending on the pill) compared to CHC, which is 24 hours.

Progestogen-Only Implant

Only one licensed product is in use in the UK at present – Nexplanon, which contains 68 mg etonogestrel and is effective for 3 years.

Benefits

This is the most effective method of contraception available [4]. Approximately 21 per cent of women experience amenorrhoea, and around one-third of women experience infrequent bleeding (the World Health Organization defines this as fewer than two episodes of bleeding over a 90 day period) [20].

Risks

Approximately 20 per cent of women experience prolonged or frequent bleeding and may discontinue use because of this [21]. There are other contraceptive methods that are more likely to induce amenorrhoea, which may be preferable for women during the perimenopause. There are some associated risks associated with insertion of the implant including infection, nerve or vascular injury, siting the implant too deep or non-insertion [20].

Progestogen-Only Injectables

Two depot medroxyprogesterone acetate (DMPA) injectables are currently available in the UK:

- Depo Provera: 150 mg/1 ml, administered intramuscularly every 12–13 weeks.
- Sayana Press: 104 mg/0.6 ml, administered subcutaneously every 13 weeks.

Benefits

Whilst women can experience problematic bleeding, most women become amenorrhoeic over time (50 per cent by 1 year of use and 70 per cent by 2 years of use [22]). NICE recommends Depo Provera as a treatment option for heavy menstrual bleeding [12] and it can therefore be particularly advantageous during the perimenopause.

DMPA is safe in women at risk of VTE and there is evidence to show that DMPA may protect against ovarian and endometrial cancer [23].

Some women prefer Sayana Press as this can be self-administered at home with only a yearly review required, reducing the reliance on health care providers.

Risks

DMPA contains high-dose progestogen, which has a hypoestrogenic effect. This can have an impact on bone health and cardiovascular risk. There is an association between DMPA and a reduction in bone mineral density, which appears to recover after discontinuation of DMPA [23]. This needs to be taken into account in women over the age of 45, with a two-yearly review of bone density, and to ensure that the benefits outweigh the risks. There is a theoretical concern about the effect of DMPA on lipid profile, and therefore DMPA is usually not advised in women with multiple risk factors for cardiovascular disease [9].

Over the age of 45 years, DMPA is a UK MEC 2, and over 50 women should consider switching method [4].

Important counselling points for the DMPA are that cessation of the method will not always resolve any potential side effects quickly, and it can delay return to fertility for up to 12 months in those women who wish to conceive in the future.

Progestogen-Only Intrauterine System

The intrauterine system (LNG-IUS) releases levonorgestrel locally within the endometrial cavity. The mode of action is to thicken cervical mucus (preventing sperm penetration) and also thin the uterine lining.

There are several devices available in the UK market (see Table 20.8). LNG-IUS confers many non-contraceptive benefits and is usually well tolerated.

Benefits

Mirena (52 mg) offers unique benefits in the menopause transition, providing contraception, management of heavy menstrual bleeding and endometrial protection in

Table 20.8 Comparing different IUS devices

Device	Levonor-gestrel dose	Licensed uses	Length of use	Non-contraceptive benefits
Mirena	52 mg	Contraception Heavy menstrual bleeding Endometrial protection	5 years (licensed for 4 years for endometrial protection but FSRH support use up to 5 years) [24] 7 years or longer in women age 45 or older at insertion (if using for contraception and amenorrhoeic)	Can be used as endometrial protection for the progestogenic arm of MHT Effective in controlling HMB and pain associated with endometriosis and adenomyosis
Levosert	52 mg	Contraception Heavy menstrual bleeding	5 years	Effective in controlling HMB and pain associated with endometriosis and adenomyosis
Kyleena	19.5 mg	Contraception	5 years	Less likely to induce amenorrhoea than higher dose IUS
Jaydess	13.5 mg	Contraception	3 years	Less likely to induce amenorrhoea than higher dose IUS

association with use of estrogen MHT delivered by any route. Levosert (52 mg) is also licensed for heavy menstrual bleeding and contraception. Kyleena (19.5 mg) and Jaydess (13.5 mg) are licensed for contraception only (see Table 20.8).

NICE recommend a 52 mg LNG-IUS as first-line treatment for HMB, although it is important to follow NICE guidelines on investigating heavy or irregular bleeding prior to insertion [12]. The IUS can reduce menstrual pain, as well as pain from endometriosis or adenomyosis.

If amenorrhoeic LNG-IUS 52 mg can be used for up to 7 years or longer if inserted at 45 years or older. The exception to this would be for women using the Mirena alongside estrogen MHT, where the device should be changed every 5 years [4] to ensure adequate endometrial protection.

Women are less likely to experience the hormonal side effects occasionally seen with other POC, such as mood swings, as only small amounts of progestogen are absorbed systemically.

There is also evidence to show that LNG-IUS 52 mg offers some protection against endometrial hyperplasia and cancer [24].

Risks

There may be some irregular or frequent bleeding for the first 3–6 months; however, this usually settles to light bleeding or amenorrhoea.

Insertion of the IUS carries some risks [24]:

- Uterine perforation (1–2/1000)
- Infection (usually during the first 3–4 weeks) (1/300)
- Expulsion (1/20)
- Risk of ectopic pregnancy compared to intrauterine pregnancy (although overall risk of pregnancy is less than the rate in women not using contraception).

It is important to undertake a risk assessment and screening for sexually transmitted infections prior to IUS insertion to reduce the risk of ascending infection [24].

Copper Intrauterine Device

The copper intrauterine device (CuIUD) is a safe and effective non-hormonal method of contraception, licensed for 5–10 years depending on the device. Copper is toxic to sperm preventing fertilization and it also causes changes in the endometrium preventing implantation should fertilization have occurred.

Benefits

This is a good option for women in whom hormonal methods are contraindicated, for example in those with current or a history of breast cancer [4].

Some women prefer using a non-hormonal method until menopause, as it easier to determine when contraception is no longer required.

The Faculty of Sexual and Reproductive Health (FSRH) recommend that a CuIUD inserted in a woman over 40 can be kept in place until menopause (2 years of amenorrhoea if under age 50 and 1 year of amenorrhoea if over age 50).

Risks

A side effect of the CuIUD is more heavy and painful periods. As menstruation around the menopause transition can be heavy, a CuIUD does nothing to improve this and actually may increase blood loss. This can impact on a woman's quality of life and even cause anaemia. CuIUD insertion carries the same risks as IUS insertion [24].

Barrier Methods

Barrier methods include male and female condoms and diaphragms. They are more effective as fertility declines with increasing age. However, regardless of age they are much less effective than other methods. Male condoms account for 10 per cent contraceptive use in perimenopausal women [25].

Benefits

Barrier methods are another good option for when hormonal contraception is contraindicated or side effects are not tolerated. In addition, women are not dependent on a health care provider for supplies and can discontinue use when menopause is reached. Male and female condoms help protect against some sexually transmitted infections (STIs), rates of which are increasing in women over the age of 40 [26].

Risks

They are a less effective method of contraception when compared to other methods. Male condoms are 98 per cent effective with perfect use, but are user dependent with 'typical use' at all ages being 82 per cent [16]. Female condoms are 95 per cent effective with perfect use. Another downside is that barrier methods can interfere with sexual intercourse, making them less acceptable for the user. Perimenopausal women may have vulvo-vaginal atrophy, making insertion of a diaphragm difficult. If using topical estrogen for vaginal dryness, condoms can weaken, increasing the risk of breakage and method failure.

Fertility Awareness Methods or Withdrawal Method

Fertility awareness methods (FAM) consist of estimating ovulation by cycle rhythm, measuring body temperature, and/or checking cervical mucus and timing intercourse with the days in the cycle where pregnancy risk is low. This method is used by 4 per cent of perimenopausal women [25]. Withdrawal is used by 5 per cent of perimenopausal women [25] and is more likely to be effective if used in conjunction with FAM.

Benefits

These methods are non-hormonal and do not require interaction with a health care professional.

Risks

Use becomes increasingly difficult for perimenopausal women due to unpredictable ovulation leading to irregular menstruation. These methods are much less effective than longer-acting methods of reversible contraception (LARCs) and require motivation. They are not recommended for women in whom pregnancy would be unacceptable. Withdrawal alone is not an effective method of contraception [4].

Male and Female Sterilization

Male sterilization (vasectomy) is a straightforward procedure, carried out under local anaesthetic, and has a failure rate of 1/2000 once azoospermia has been confirmed [26].

Female sterilization involves laparoscopic surgery under general anaesthetic. This method has a failure rate of 1/200 [27], making it less effective than LARCs.

Benefits

These options are beneficial for couples who are sure that they have completed their family. They offer choice for women who cannot use hormonal contraception.

Risks

Some couples or individuals go on to regret their decision, opting for reversal or in vitro fertilization to conceive. It is important to counsel the couple that both methods are permanent, and reversal is not always possible. If reversal is required, in the UK it is currently only available privately.

Both procedures carry risks. Fourteen per cent of men experience chronic postvasectomy pain [27].

Some women may not be fit for general anaesthetic. Women, particularly those in the menopause transition, who are unlikely to need contraception for long should be counselled regarding LARC and would benefit from the additional non-contraceptive benefits described in this chapter. Women should also be advised that menstrual periods will not change as a result of sterilization.

Summary

This chapter highlights a wealth of contraceptive choice for the older woman, with many options providing non-contraceptive benefits. The more effective LARC options in particular offer long-term additional benefits which can support the transition from reproductive to postreproductive life.

When considering contraceptive choice, it is essential to undertake an individual eligibility assessment with each woman, taking into consideration risk factors associated with advancing age. Counselling women appropriately on the risks and benefits of each method is important to ensure satisfaction with the chosen method, whilst not increasing risk of harm to the individual.

References

1. World Health Organization. *Research on the Menopause in the 1990s: Report of a WHO Scientific Group*. 1996. World Health Organization.

2. Gold EB, Crawford SL, Avis NE, et al. Factors related to age at natural menopause: longitudinal analyses from SWAN. *Am J Epidemiol* 2013 Jul;1178(1):70–83.

3. Baldwin MK, Jensen JT. Contraception during the perimenopause. *Maturitas* 2013;76:235–42.

4. Faculty of Sexual and Reproductive Healthcare. *Contraception for Women Aged over 40 Years*. 2010. Faculty of Sexual and Reproductive Healthcare. www.fsrh.org/documents/cec-ceu-gui dance-womenover40-jul-2010

5. Kenny LC, Lavender T, McNamee R, O'Neill SM, Mills T, Khashan AS. Advanced maternal age and adverse pregnancy outcome: Evidence from a large contemporary cohort. *PLoS ONE* 2013;8(2):e56583.

6. Wellings K, Jones KG, Mercer CH, Tanton C, Clifton S, Datta J, et al. The prevalence of unplanned pregnancy and associated factors in Britain: findings from the third National Survey of Sexual Attitudes and Lifestyles (Natsal-3). *Lancet* 2013;382:1807–16.

7. Gebbie AE, Glasier A, Sweeting V. Incidence of ovulation in perimenopausal women before and during hormone replacement therapy. *Contraception* 1995;52:221–2.

8. National Institute for Health and Care Excellence. Clinical knowledge summaries: menopause. 2013. http://cks .nice.org.uk/menopause

9. Faculty of Sexual and Reproductive Healthcare (FSRH). UK Medical Eligibility Criteria for Contraceptive Use (UKMEC). 2016. www.fsrh.org/standards-and-guidance/external/ukmec-2016-digital-version/

10. National Institute for Health and Care Excellence. Clinical knowledge summaries: contraception – assessment. 2016. https://cks.nice.org.uk/contracep tion-assessment

11. Lopez LM, Grimes DA, Gallo MF. Skin patch and vaginal ring versus combined oral contraceptives for contraception. *Cochrane Database Syst Rev* 2013;4: CD003552.

12. National Institute for Health and Care Excellence. *Heavy Menstrual Bleeding: Assessment and Management.* 2018. NICE. https://nice.org.uk/guidance/ng88

13. Nappi C, Bifulco G, Tommaselli GA, Gargano V, Di Carlo C. Hormonal contraception and bone metabolism: a systematic review. *Contraception* 2012;86(6):606–21.

14. European Medicines Agency. Press release: Benefits of combined hormonal contraceptives (CHCs) continue to outweigh risks. 2013. www.ema.europa.e u/en/news/benefits-combined-hormonal-contraceptives-chcs-continue-outweigh-risks-chmp-endorses- prachormonal_con traceptives/European_Commission_ nal_ decision/WC500160277.pdf

15. Beaber E, Buist DS, Barlow WE, Malone KE, Reed SD, Li CL. Recent oral contraceptive use by formulation and breast cancer risk among women 20 to 49 years of age. Cancer Res 2014;74:4078–89.

16. Trussell J. Contraceptive failure in the United States. *Contraception* 2011;83 (5):397–404.

17. Weill A, Dalichampt M, Raguideau F, et al. Low dose oestrogen combined oral contraception and risk of pulmonary embolism, stroke, and myocardial infarction in five million French women: cohort study. *BMJ Clin Res Ed* 2016;353:i2002.

18. Dinger J, Do Minh T, Heinemann K. Impact of estrogen type on cardiovascular safety of combined oral contraceptives. *Contraception* 2016;94 (4):328–39.

19. Faculty of Sexual and Reproductive Healthcare. Progestogen-only pills. 2015. www.fsrh.org/documents/ ceuguidanceprogestogenonlypills

20. Faculty of Sexual and Reproductive Healthcare (FSRH). Progestogen-only implants. 2014. www.fsrh.org/documents/ cec-ceu-guidance-implants-feb-2014/

21. Lakha F, Glasier AF. Continuation rates of implanon in the UK: data from an observational study in a clinical setting. *Contraception* 2006;74:287–9.

22. Pfizer Ltd. Depo-Provera 150 mg/ml injection. 2016. www.medicines.org.uk/e mc/medicine/11121

23. Faculty of Sexual and Reproductive Healthcare. Progestogen-only injectable contraception. 2014. www.fsrh.org/docu ments/cec-ceu-guidance-injectables-dec-2014

24. Faculty of Sexual and Reproductive Healthcare (FSRH). Intrauterine contraception. 2015. www.fsrh.org/stan dards-and-guidance/documents/ ceuguidanceintrauterinecontraception/

25. Office for National Statistics. Statistical Bulletin: conceptions in England and Wales. 2012. http://webarchive .nationalarchives.gov.uk/20160109214216

/www.ons.gov.uk/ons/rel/vsob1/concep
tion-statistics-england-and-wales/2010/20
10-conceptions-statistical-bulletin.html?
format=print

26. Public Health England. National STI
surveillance data tables 2015 – Table 20.8.
2015. www.gov.uk/government/uploads/s
ystem/uploads/attachment_data/file/5345

64/2015_Table_8_Attendances_by_gende
r__sexual_risk___age_group__2011-2015
.pdf

27. Faculty of Sexual and Reproductive
Healthcare of the Royal College of
Obstetricians and Gynaecologists. FSRH
clinical guidance: male and female
sterilisation – September 2014. 2014.

Hormone Therapy and Cancer

Anne Gompel

Aging is associated with an increase in the development of cancers. Among them some can be influenced by the gonadal hormones. Cancers which are the most hormone dependent are breast and endometrial cancer. Among breast cancer (BC) most of those occurring in postmenopausal women are estradiol (E2) receptor (ER) positive. Endometrial cancer is extremely estrogen dependent. Ovarian cancer (OC) can also mildly be influenced by hormones. Cervical adenocarcinoma (but not squamous cell carcinoma) is possibly a target of estrogen. But in addition to cancer arising from hormone-dependent organs, gonadal hormones can also impact some other cancers arising in organs which are not classically hormone dependent.

First we will address the question of the level of risk associated with MHT and cancer, and in the second part which treatment can be used in cancer survivors.

MHT and the Risk of Cancer

Breast Cancer

BC is the paradigm of hormone dependent cancer. A total 2 088 849 new cases were diagnosed in 2018 worldwide and 626 679 deaths [1]. The mortality has decreased in most of the western countries but not in eastern Europe. There are different types of BC. Most of them express ER but with different levels. They are defined by histological types, mostly ductal type (85 per cent), lobular type (15 per cent) and their content in E2, progesterone (P) receptors (PR) and HER-2 amplification. Tumours expressing high levels of ER and expressing PR correspond to Luminal A BC, have a good prognosis and are extremely hormone dependent. Luminal B contain ER but usually not PR. The prognosis of luminal B BC is less favourable. About 15 per cent of BC express also an amplification of HER-2. They are treated with antibodies against HER-2, which has significantly improved their prognosis. The last type is called triple negative (TN) BC, as they do not express ER, PR or HER-2 amplification and have the worst prognosis. The relative proportion of ER+/TN BC increases with age. After menopause, 70–80 per cent of BC contain ER and 40 per cent PR. It can thus be easily understood that MHT can feed a preexisting cancer or promote the growth of precancerous lesions or ductal carcinoma in situ (DCIS).

Evidence from most of the studies is that

- an estrogen-only treatment (ET) is associated with a lower risk than a combined (estrogen+ progestogen) therapy (CT)

- risk increases with duration and decreases after cessation of the treatment arguing for a promoter effect on preexisting lesions since the lag time to develop BC is usually 20–25 years.
- ER-positive breast cancers are associated with MHT. Luminal A type is the predominant type but luminal B is also potentially associated with MHT [2, 3]. HER-2+ and TN BC are not modified by MHT [2, 3].

Risk Associated with ET

In most observational studies, the use of ET is associated with a mild risk at long term. In the French cohort study E3 N, a small increase was observed using E2 after long-term use (>5 years) but on a small number of patients [4]. In the Nurses' Health study, a large prospective cohort study conducted in the US, the increase in the risk is observed after 10–20 years of treatment [2, 5].

The Women's Health Initiative (WHI), which has included 11 000 postmenopausal hysterectomized women randomized between conjugated estrogens (CEE) and placebo, observed no increase in the risk and even a decrease in adherent women [6]. After a mean treatment duration of 6.8 years, the relative risk (RR) of invasive breast cancer was 0.77 (0.59–1.01) in the whole population and 0.67 (0.47–0.97) in adherent women. Only women naive of treatment had a decrease in the RR [7]. Longer follow-up of the WHI population confirmed the significant decrease of BC in the whole population [8].

Difference between Observational Studies and WHI

The WHI population was different from the one included in the other studies by the fact that a majority of women were far from menopause: 45 per cent were 60–69 years old, 24 per cent were 70 or above. Observational studies include women at menopause. Clinical characteristics were different: in the WHI, mean BMI was 30.1 (6.1), and 45 per cent were obese whereas in the Nurses' and the E3 N cohort, women were much leaner and healthier. The prevalence of obesity can influence the effects of MHT on breast cancer risk. In several studies it was shown the leaner women were at higher risk than obese women using MHT. In the Nurses' the lower risk of BC was seen with 5 to 9.9 current years of ET use and to be limited to women with a BMI of 25 or higher (RR: 0.74; 0.55–1.00) [5]. Insulin resistance is decreased by estrogen. It is likely that the women in the WHI ET trial could have benefitted from the treatment by decreasing insulin resistance. Another possible explanation is that CEE which contain mixed compounds having both agonist and antagonist estrogen potencies, thereby have different impacts on the breast. The influence of type of estrogen is, however, not confirmed. In the WHI observational cohort, the dose of CEE (usual and low dose <0.625 mg) and oral and transdermal E2 were not associated with a different level of risk. In that cohort, the RR with CEE was not increased nor decreased, with an average of follow-up of 8.2 years [9]. Similarly, in a study from Finland, there was no difference in the risk of oral E2 and transdermal E2 combined with norethisterone acetate (NETA) [10].

Role of Progestogen in the Risk of Breast Cancer

There is no study which has compared head to head an ET or CT treatment, and the characteristics of women in both groups may vary. Nevertheless, in most observational studies, CT is associated with a higher risk of breast cancer than ET. The level of this risk varies with the studies and the progestogen used. The RR decreases progressively after cessation of treatment, suggesting a promoter effect on preexisting lesions. The WHI, conducted another randomized control trial (RCT) consisting of 16 000 women randomized between CEE+ medroxyprogesterone acetate (MPA) and placebo. In that trial, there was a limited increase in the RR =1.24 (1.01–1.53) of BC [8]. The characteristics of the patients were different from the observational studies: mean age at inclusion was 63.3 years, 34 per cent were obese. Observational studies in most of cases show an increase in the RR of a larger magnitude around 1.7/2 fold with CT and synthetic progestogens (SP) (Table 21.1). Different levels of risk are reported with different progestogen (for review, see [11]). Observational studies reported a lower risk of BC in women treated with progesterone/dydrogesterone compared to synthetic progestins. Micronized progesterone (P) is practically only used in France. Dydrogesterone (DYD) has some properties in common with P. There are now four studies, two from France, one from UK and one from Finland, reporting no or lower risk of BC with these two compounds, P and DYD (Table 21.1) [11].

Duration is also a factor influencing the risk, the longer the duration the more important the risk. In the French E3 N study, a small increase in the risk was observed with P/DYD after more than 6 years of use in current users (mean: 8.7 years) RR = 1.31 (1.15–1.48) compared to SP (mean use: 8.4 years) RR = 2.02 (1.81–2.26). After 3 months to 5 years of cessation, the risk disappeared in women treated by P/DYD, RR = 1.15 0.93–1.42) and for SP, the RR reached 1 after >10 years since last use [4]. In a meta-analysis the RR of BC comparing P and SP, was RR = 0.67 (0.55–0.81) [12].

The type of regimen, continuous or sequential, has also been associated with a different level of risk, the sequential treatment being at lower risk. There is no head-to-head comparison between both regimens, which precludes firm recommendations since most women prefer a continuous regimen.

Tibolone is a normethyltestosterone derivative and thus a progestogen. It is metabolized into an androgenic and two mild estrogenic metabolites. The risk associated with tibolone is likely to be in the same range as that with CT. One RCT in BC patients reported an increased risk of recurrence whereas a RCT in osteoporotic women of a mean age of 68.3 ± 5.2 years reported a decrease in the RR of BC (0.32 [0.13–0.80]), but based on six cases in the tibolone group and 19 in the placebo group and after only 3 years of use. This is a short time and those women were at lower risk of BC since osteoporotic [13, 14]. In the Million Women Study (MWS), a large observational study conducted in UK, the RR with tibolone was intermediary between ET and CT risks [15].

Levonorgestrel IUD (LnorgIUD): there are controversial data on the RR of BC with LnorgIUD. Most of the results are from its use as contraceptive. Some studies based on registers observed an increase in the risk of BC when used as contraceptive or in the menopausal transition (see [11]). At the opposite in a cohort study, in contraception use, there was no increase in the RR of BC [16]. Another observational study reported an increase in women who used LnorgIUD at the age of 40–45 years but not in women of 46–50 years old. It is thus difficult to conclude but these studies suggest that a small risk cannot be excluded.

A combination of CEE and a SERM, Bazedoxifene is available in some countries. Breast density and mastalgia are not increased by this treatment as well as the endometrial thickness, whereas breast density and mastalgia are both increased by CT. There are

Table 21.1 RR of BC with ET and CT

Study	Population	Follow-up (mean)	Risk of BC
Fournier [52]	Cohort study 80 377 Mean age: 53.1 years	8.1 years	– ET RR = 1.29 (1.02–1.65) – E2+P, RR = 1.00 (0.82–1.22) – E2 + DYD, RR = 1.16 (0.94–1.43) – E2 + SP, RR = 1.69 (1.50–1.91)
Espie [53]	Cohort study 4949 Mean age: 64.2 women with MHT 60.6 women no MHT	2.5 years	– w/o MHT = incidence of BC = 0.70% – ET = 0.28% – E2 + P = 0.40% – E2 + SP = 0.94% No increase in the risk
Cordina-Duverger [54]	– Case control study – 739 cases, 816 controls – 35–54 years (16.5%);(17.6%) – 55–64 years (47.0%); (43.6%) – >65 years – (36.5%);(38.7%)		– ET OR 1.19 (0.69–2.04) – E2 + P, OR = 0.80 (0.44–1.43) – E2 + SP, OR = 1.57 (0.99–2.49) – E2+ nortestosterone derivative, OR = 3.35 (1.07–10.4)
Schneider [55]	Case control study 1261 cases, 7566 controls Mean age 51.3 years	6.0 years	– E2 + DYD OR = 0.68 (0.38–1.20) – CEE + norgestrel, 2–4 y OR = 1.50 (1.11–2.04), ≥5 y OR = 1.34 (0.71–2.54)* – E2 + NETA, 2–4 y OR = 1.19 (0.86–1.63), ≥5 y OR = 2.85 (1.87–4.36), CEE + MPA, OR = 0.78 (0.50–1.20) Significantly less BC with DYD
Lyytinen [56]	221 551 using MHT from register 6211 cases		E2 + NET: 3–10 y RR = 1.34 (1.17–1.51) 5–10 y RR = 2.03 (1.88–2.18) >5 y RR = 3.15 (2.44–4.00) E2+MPA 3–10 y RR = 1.27 (1.09–1.48) 5–10 y RR = 1.64 (1.49–1.79) >5 y RR = 1.90 (1.07–3.07) E2 + DYD 3–5 y RR = 1.22 (0.83–1.72) 5–10 y RR = 1.13 (0.49–2.22)

Note. ET = estrogen only. CT = combined MHT. P = progesterone. DYD = dydrogesterone.

no data on breast cancer in humans and it may increase the risk of thrombosis. There may be a place for this regimen in women who develop mastalgia using standard MHT or benign breast disease but no study available.

The concept of combining an estrogen with a SERM is elegant. A randomized study (Hot study) included more than 1800 women using MHT and 5 mg of tamoxifen versus placebo demonstrated a decrease in luminal A BC [17]. The potential increase in venous thrombosis should be discussed in the risk/benefit assessment.

How to Decrease the RR of BC in Women Using MHT?

- Selecting women with a lower risk?

   Women at very high risk for BC are those belonging to a family with strong history of BC/ovarian cancer at a young age, who have an history of atypical hyperplasia at biopsies, women who have been treated by thoracic radiotherapy at a young age, and in cases of birad-d category of breast density. Those women are not the best candidates for MHT.

Other risk factors are: late first full-term pregnancy, alcohol, sedentarity, obesity, diabetes, late age at menopause, young age at menarche, biopsy with proliferative disease, mastalgia.

- Treatment with lower risk: P or DYD are associated with a lower risk. Sequential therapy seems more favourable for the breast but not for the endometrium (see below).
- Education on lifestyle.

   Physical exercise, losing weight, low breast density, low bone density are factors associated with lower risk. Several studies using models to predict the risk in their cohort showed that women who had the best score for lifestyle factors were at lower risk of BC even using MHT [18]. In the Nurses' cohort, evaluating the attributable part of BC to modifiable factors at menopause, they concluded that risk factors that are modifiable account for more than one-third of postmenopausal BC [19]. This is crucial information, and education on lifestyle may help to decrease the mild RR of BC observed with MHT.

- In practice, before prescribing a MHT, to evaluate the risk of BC is mandatory. This can be done by gathering the risk factors and, if necessary, using scores which are available online. The Gail score (https://bcrisktool.cancer.gov/) and the IBIS score (www.ems-trials.org/riskevaluator/). The last one contains more clinical items including breast density category and a detailed family history as part of the analysis to predict the probability of being a BRCA carrier. Its accuracy remains, however, about 0.70, whereas the Gail score has a lower accuracy (0.6).

Endometrial Cancer (EC)

Prevalence of EC is increased in postmenopausal women with a peak of incidence between 60 and 75 years of age. It is the sixth commonest cancer in women worldwide with 382 069 new cases and 89 929 deaths in 2018 [1]. Eighty-five per cent of endometrial cancers belong to type I: hormone dependent, well differentiated and with a good prognosis. Type II includes serous carcinoma, mixed cell and clear cell carcinoma. These are more invasive and their prognosis much less favourable. Type I is extremely sensitive to estrogen, type II can also be estrogen sensitive. The main risk factors are endogenous or exogenous estrogen, obesity, nulliparity, early menarche, late menopause, diabetes, hypertension, whereas smoking is associated with a reduced risk. It can rarely occur in the context of hereditary risk with colon cancers (Lynch syndrome). A major factor of protection is the pill with a long-term residual effect on its prevention. ET alone in women with a uterus is a high risk factor increasing with treatment duration. It progresses from hyperplasia initially, followed by hyperplasia with atypia, and then carcinoma. Sequential CT is at higher risk than continuous CT. The MWS demonstrated that obese women and overweight women were protected from EC by CT, due to the benefits of the progestogen [20]. In long-term studies, the increase in EC risk observed with ET and CT was remnant lasting up to 5–10 years after cessation of treatment [21, 22]. The duration of progestogen administration combined with estrogen is crucial [23]. In sequential administration it has to be at least 12–14 days according to the length of estrogen administration. P was suspected to be at higher risk than synthetic progestogen in the E3 N cohort but this might be due to a lack of compliance since two RCT using endometrial biopsies did not show an increase in hyperplasia in women using P nor a recent oral combination of E2+P (Lobo et al Menopause 2018) (for review, see [23]). LnorgIUD (Mirena, no data on the other IUDs) is protective of the endometrium to the same extent as an oral progestogen; they equally can reverse hyperplasia and well-differentiated adenocarcinoma [24, 25].

An uncertainty was raised about tibolone and endometrial cancer but was not confirmed in RCT [26].

Ovarian Cancer (OC)

OC occurs predominantly in postmenopausal women, with a peak in women aged 55–64 years and a median age of 63 [27]. It is the seventh most commonly diagnosed cancer among women in the world with 295 414 new cases in 2018 and 184 799 deaths [1]. The percentage surviving at 5 years is 30–40 per cent [28]. The most frequent belong to the epithelial group and among them high-grade and low-grade serous tumours represent 70 per cent. Clear cell carcinoma, endometrioid and mucinous types are the other differentiations. Other types are germ cell, stroma cell and small cell carcinomas. Borderline tumours can be of the same type, but with a lower potential of evolution.

Risk factors are a family history of OC (and BC) or colon cancer (CC) (Lynch syndrome), infertility, endometriosis (for the clear cell and endometrioid carcinoma), obesity. A major factor for protection is the pill (with a long-term remnant effect on prevention) and tubal ligation. There are only data from observational studies. No data were obtained in the WHI on OC, due to its relative low frequency. In the MWS, an increased risk was reported as well as in a meta-analysis which included 52 studies but with a high weight for the MWS itself [29]. There was a RR = 1·43 (1·31–1·56). Not all the risk or protective factors were available in part of the population, in particular hormonal contraception, which is a strong factor suggesting that bias could be present in that study. In most observational studies, ET appeared to be associated with a mildly higher risk than CT. In this meta-analysis ET and CT were equivalent. The mucinous type is not influenced either by MHT or by hormonal contraception.

Cervical Cancer

Cervical cancers belong to squamous small cell carcinoma (SSCC) (over 90 per cent) and adenocarcinoma. Worldwide, 569 847 new cases were diagnosed in 2018 and 311 365 deaths occurred. It is the fourth commonest cancer in women, predominant in countries with low income (no screening). The main risk factor is HPV infection. The SSCC is not dependent on hormones and thus not influenced by MHT. Adenocarcinoma is considered as estrogen dependent. However, there are few data on adenocarcinoma and its risk factors. A publication suggested that the pill could increase the risk of adenocarcinoma in a larger instance than for SSCC [30] but not MPA when used as a contraceptive [31]. In postmenopausal women, ET was associated with an increase of adenocarcinoma but based on a very small number of cases (14).

Colon Cancer (CC)

CC represents 520 812 new cases in women worldwide and 260 760 deaths [1]. Colon is not considered a hormone-dependent organ but the normal epithelium contains ERβ. The main risk factors are genetic, obesity, processed meat, sedentary and alcohol. Exercise and healthy diet help to decrease the risk. Both the oral contraceptive pill (OCP) and MHT are reported to be associated with a decrease in CC in most but not all of the studies. In the WHI, a significant decrease in CC was observed in the CT trial, but not in the ET trial (more obesity?, role of MPA?) [8]. Several case control and observational studies also reported less CC in women using MHT [32, 33]. One possible bias is the prevalence of screening and colonoscopy in different populations, which may vary and is an effective means of CC prevention. In the E3 N cohort ET use was associated with a decrease risk of CC but an increase in adenomas, which could indicate colonoscopy and thus prevention of cancer [34].

Lung Cancer

Lung cancer has an increasing incidence in women and will be in most countries the first cause of death by cancer in women [1]. New cases in women represent 725 352 and 576 060 deaths, just after BC [1]. The main risk factor is smoking: 80 per cent of lung cancers occur in smokers. Lung cancer may contain ERα, ERβ and PR and their contents have been associated with prognosis [35, 36]. The prognosis in women is more favourable than in men. In the WHI CT trial, there were less lung cancers but a higher mortality [8], whereas there was no effect in the ET trial. The effect in the CT trial decreased after stopping CT [37]. The results from other studies are contradictory. Smoking is a confounding factor since it may modulate ER and PR status in lung cancer [36]. There are different kinds of lung cancer and the effect of hormones may vary according to their biology. A recent meta-analysis did not observe increase in mortality in women using MHT [38].

Melanoma

It represents 137 025 new cases and 25 881 deaths [1]. Melanomas are more prevalent in women before menopause than in men of same age. The main factor is sun exposure. The effect of MHT is controversial showing no effect in a meta-analysis nor increase by ET and decrease by CT in a more recent cohort study performed in Norway [39].

Non-Hodgkin Lymphoma (NHL)

A total of 224 877 new cases of NHL are diagnosed in women worldwide and 102 755 deaths occur. A recent pooled analysis showed that NHL (diffuse large B-cell [DLBCL] and follicular lymphoma [FL]) were less frequent in women using MHT. The HR was 0.79 (0.69–0.90) [40]. Only current users were at lower risk. Five years after stopping the benefit disappeared [40]. The rest of the literature reviewed in that publication has provided mixed results but this pooled analysis has gathered the higher number of cases. There were no data on ET or CT, only on hysterectomy or not. DLBCL were decreased in both groups, FL only in non-hysterectomized women.

Hormone Therapy in Cancer Survivals

Breast Cancer

As stated previously, BC is predominantly hormone dependent and thus all MHT are contraindicated. There are two randomized trials on the use of MHT in BC survivors. The first one, HABITS trial, included 442 women randomized between ET or CT and no hormone. The mean duration of MHT was 2 years with a median of 4 years of follow-up. The study was terminated early because of a recurrence rate higher in the MHT group. Thirty-nine of the 221 women in the MHT arm and 17 of the 221 women in the control arm experienced a new breast cancer event HR = 2.4 (1.3–4.2) [41]. The Stockholm study randomized 378 women for a mean duration of 2.1 years with the aim to use less progestogen. There were no more recurrences after 10 years of follow-up. The treatment was E2+MPA when one was used [42]. The main difference is that in the Stockholm trial there were more women on tamoxifen, which can help to prevent BC.

Recommendations for BC Survivors

Non-hormonal therapy is recommended to alleviate climacteric symptoms in these patients [43].

Can vaginal estrogens be used in patients on aromatase inhibitors (AI)? There are no RCTs on vaginal estrogens in BC patients. A recent review reported on all the trials ongoing with different vaginal estrogens in women with BC but only one addresses the question of recurrence [44]. The usual recommendations are to use non-hormonal vaginal products for vaginal dryness in patients using AI [43]. In patients using tamoxifen in case of failure of non-hormonal treatments, an occasional administration of vaginal estrogens can be discussed [43].

Endometrial Cancer

Estrogens are drivers for EC. Retrospective studies, two prospective studies and a RCT did not find more recurrences among treated women (Table 21.2). A meta-analysis looked differentially at the risk according to ET or CT. There was no increase with ET and a significant decrease with CT [45].

It is likely that in low grades of EC, MHT will not worsen the course of endometrial cancer, but the data are too limited to recommend MHT as first line in these women. As progestogen

Table 21.2 Risk of recurrence of endometrial cancer using MHT

Authors	Studies	TRT/no TRT	Stage	Follow-up (months)	Recurrence TRT/no TRT
Creasman [57]	Case control retrospective	47/174 ET	I	25–150	1/26
Bryant [58]	Cohort retrospective	20	I–II	42–168	0
Lee [59]	Case control retrospective	44/99 ET	I	24–84	0/8
Chapman [60]	Case control retrospective	62/61 ET	I–II	57 (median)	2/8
Suriano [61]	Cohort retrospective	75/75 51% ET, 49%CT	I–III	83 (median)	2/11
Ayhan [62]	Case control prospective	50/52 CT	I–II	49 (median)	0/1
Barakat [63]	RCT	618/618 ET	I–II	57 months (median)	12/14
Felix [64]	Cohort prospective	392/498	I–IV	8.8 years (median)	EPT (deaths) 11/169 0.51 (0.26, 0.98) ET(deaths) 11/72 1.34 (0.66, 2.71)
Cho [65]	Cohort	847/4820 ET 22%, CT16% Tibolone 32% Progestogen 30%		48 months	HR = 0.62 (0.46–0.83) Multivariate HR = 0.81 (0.31–2.10)

can alleviate vasomotor symptoms and help sleep disorders (P) we would recommend checking their efficacy as first line. In case of failure in grade Ia, a CT could be discussed.

There is also some concern about using vaginal estrogens in those women. The localization of recurrence is frequently the vaginal section. There are no data to evaluate their use in women after an endometrial cancer.

Ovarian Cancer

Epithelial Tumour

Several retrospective and prospective studies reported no increase in the risk of recurrence after an invasive epithelial OC.

Three randomized trials are available and all reassuringly show no increase or even a decrease in recurrence and deaths (Table 21.3). They are based on a relatively small

Table 21.3 Risk of ovarian cancer and MHT, RT

Study	TRT/no TRT	Follow-up	Type of ovarian cancer	Recurrence
Guidozzi [66]	75/75 <59 years	>48 months		32 on ET vs 41 RR: 1.13 (055–2.31)
Li [67]	31/45 CT	Duration TT 6–43 months	47 serous 28 mucinous	RR: 0.88 (0.35–2.32)
Eeles [68]	75/75 38 CEE, 19 CEE+norgestrel 14 E2 patch 1 E2 implant	19.1 years (if alive) Mean duration of TRT: 1.4 years	39.3% serous 14.7% mucinous 10% endometroid 10% clear cell	0.67 (0.47–0.97) recurrence 0.63 (0.44–0.90) survival

number of cases. A meta-analysis published before the last RT has pooled the prospective observational studies and the first two RTs. For overall survival, RR : 0.83 (0.64–1.07); for grades 1, 2, 3 and grades 2–3, RR: 0.74 (0.57–0.96). Stages I–II and stages III–IV, RR: 0.65 (0.33–1.25) and RR: 0.94(0.73–1.20) [38].

Endometrioid cancer represented a minority of cases in these studies. It is considered to be hormone dependent and caution may be indicated in women with this type of cancer. In high-grade serous and mucinous, the data strongly suggest that MHT can be used. It is not clear so far if ET or CT are recommended. In low-grade serous cancer, there are insufficient data to recommend any attitude, but the high content in hormone receptors suggest avoiding MHT in those patients [46].

Concerning germ cell tumours, most of them can be treated by MHT except granulosa cell tumours. High doses of SP have been reported to improve the prognosis and thus can be used in symptomatic patients. The attitudes were recently reviewed and recommendations made by a group of ovarian cancer experts [46].

Cervical Cancer

Only adenocarcinoma is considered as estrogen dependent. The same rules that were stated for an endometrial cancer should be applied.

Colon Cancer

Four prospective cohorts reported lower risk of recurrence and deaths in women treated for colon cancer and who use MHT for within the 5 years of diagnosis [47–50]. No data are available on the kind of MHT to choose.

Lymphoma

There are no specific studies on using MHT after lymphoma. However, there is no evidence for an increase in recurrence in particular in young women treated after a bone marrow transplantation and experiencing a premature ovarian failure (see below).

Melanoma

There is one study which looked at recurrence after surgical treatment of melanoma and treated with MHT. The treated patients showed improved survival with MHT. MHT is considered as acceptable in women with low-grade melanoma but caution is recommended for invasive cases [51].

Premature Ovarian Failure (POF) and MHT in Cancer Survivors

Because of the evidence for an increase in cardiovascular diseases, cognitive disorders, osteoporosis and mortality in women experiencing POF below the age of 45 years, MHT should be recommended as frequently as possible. In addition, the quality of life will clearly improve. This is especially the case after treatment for hematologic disorders with or without bone marrow transplantation.

Specific Conditions

- In women with BC carriers of BRCA mutation, prophylactic oophorectomy is usually performed at the age of 35, if the woman is parous, or 40. Most of the recommendations concerning those women are to prescribe a MHT up to the age of natural menopause.
- In case of hormone-dependent cancer and POF, MHT is contraindicated. If quality of life being is extremely disabled, a discussion with the oncologist can be taken in order to better evaluate the balance of benefit/risk.
- Lynch Syndrome: EC and OC are increased and prophylactic hysterectomy and oophorectomy are usually proposed at the age of 40–45. There is no contraindication for these patients to use MHT, since there is no clear increase in BC.

Conclusions

Women at high risk of BC should not be prescribed MHT. Obese women could benefit from progestogen treatment as a preventive strategy for the EC. Management of climacteric symptoms is especially important in cancer survivors where ovarian failure may occur. Hormone therapy or non-hormonal therapy have to be chosen acknowledging the influence of estrogen and progestogen on each cancer.

References

1. Bray F, et al. Global cancer statistics 2018: GLOBOCAN estimates of incidence and mortality worldwide for 36 cancers in 185 countries. *CA Cancer J Clin* 2018;68:394–424.

2. Sisti JS, et al. Reproductive risk factors in relation to molecular subtypes of breast cancer: Results from the nurses' health studies. *Int J Cancer* 2016;138:2346–56.

3. Ellingjord-Dale M, et al. Parity, hormones and breast cancer subtypes – results from a large nested case-control study in a national screening program. *Breast Cancer Res BCR* 2017;19:10.

4. Fournier A, et al. Risk of breast cancer after stopping menopausal hormone therapy in the E3 N cohort. *Breast Cancer Res Treat* 2014;145:535–43.

5. Chen WY, et al. Unopposed estrogen therapy and the risk of invasive breast cancer. *Arch Intern Med* 2006;166:1027–32.

6. Anderson GL, et al. Effects of conjugated equine estrogen in postmenopausal women with hysterectomy: the Women's Health

Initiative randomized controlled trial. *JAMA* 2004;291:1701–12.

7. Stefanick ML, et al. Effects of conjugated equine estrogens on breast cancer and mammography screening in postmenopausal women with hysterectomy. *JAMA* 2006;295:1647–57.

8. Manson JE, et al. Menopausal hormone therapy and health outcomes during the intervention and extended poststopping phases of the Women's Health Initiative randomized trials. *JAMA* 2013;310:1353–68.

9. Shufelt C, et al. Estrogen-alone therapy and invasive breast cancer incidence by dose, formulation, and route of delivery: findings from the WHI observational study. *Menopause NY* 2018;25:985–91.

10. Lyytinen H, Pukkala E, Ylikorkala O. Breast cancer risk in postmenopausal women using estradiol-progestogen therapy. *Obstet Gynecol* 2009;113:65–73.

11. Gompel A, Plu-Bureau G. Progesterone, progestins and the breast in menopause treatment. *Climacteric J Int Menopause Soc* 2018;21:326–32.

12. Asi N, et al. Progesterone vs. synthetic progestins and the risk of breast cancer: a systematic review and meta-analysis. *Syst Rev* 2016;5:121.

13. Kenemans P, et al. Safety and efficacy of tibolone in breast-cancer patients with vasomotor symptoms: a double-blind, randomised, non-inferiority trial. *Lancet Oncol* 2009;10:135–46.

14. Cummings SR, et al. The effects of tibolone in older postmenopausal women. *N Engl J Med* 2008;359:697–708.

15. Beral V, Million Women Study Collaborators. Breast cancer and hormone-replacement therapy in the Million Women Study. *Lancet* 2003;362:419–27.

16. Jareid M, et al. Levonorgestrel-releasing intrauterine system use is associated with a decreased risk of ovarian and endometrial cancer, without increased risk of breast cancer: results from the NOWAC Study. *Gynecol Oncol* 2018;149:127–32.

17. DeCensi A, et al. A phase-III prevention trial of low-dose tamoxifen in postmenopausal hormone replacement therapy users: the HOT study. *An Oncol* 2013;24:2753–60.

18. Maas P, et al. Breast cancer risk from modifiable and nonmodifiable risk factors among white women in the United States. *JAMA Oncol* 2016;2:1295–302.

19. Tamimi RM, et al. Population attributable risk of modifiable and nonmodifiable breast cancer risk factors in postmenopausal breast cancer. *Am J Epidemiol* 2016;184:884–93.

20. Beral V, Bull D, Reeves G, Million Women Study Collaborators. Endometrial cancer and hormone-replacement therapy in the Million Women Study. *Lancet* 2005;365:1543–51.

21. Shapiro S, et al. Risk of localized and widespread endometrial cancer in relation to recent and discontinued use of conjugated estrogens. *N Engl J Med* 1985;313:969–72.

22. Weiderpass E, et al. Risk of endometrial cancer following estrogen replacement with and without progestins. *J Natl Cancer Inst* 1999;91:1131–7.

23. Gompel A. Progesterone, progestins and the endometrium in perimenopause and in menopausal hormone therapy. *Climacteric J Int Menopause Soc* 2018;21:321–5.

24. Roberti L, Maggiore U, et al. Efficacy and fertility outcomes of levonorgestrel-releasing intra-uterine system treatment for patients with atypical complex hyperplasia or endometrial cancer: a retrospective study. *J Gynecol Oncol* 2019;30:e57.

25. Gallos ID, Krishan P, Shehmar M, Ganesan R, Gupta JK. LNG-IUS versus oral progestogen treatment for endometrial hyperplasia: a long-term comparative cohort study. *Hum Reprod* 2013;28:2966–71.

26. Formoso G, et al. Short-term and long-term effects of tibolone in postmenopausal women. *Cochrane Database Syst Rev* 2016;10:CD008536.

27. Bray F, et al. Global cancer statistics 2018: GLOBOCAN estimates of incidence and mortality worldwide for 36 cancers in 185 countries. *CA Cancer J Clin* 2018;68:394–424.

28. Reid BM, Permuth JB, Sellers TA. Epidemiology of ovarian cancer: a review. *Cancer Biol Med* 2017;14:9–32.

29. Collaborative Group on Epidemiological Studies of Ovarian Cancer, et al. Menopausal hormone use and ovarian cancer risk: individual participant meta-analysis of 52 epidemiological studies. *Lancet* 2015;385:1835–42.

30. Lacey JV, et al. Oral contraceptives as risk factors for cervical adenocarcinomas and squamous cell carcinomas. *Cancer Epidemiol Biomark Prev* 1999;8:1079–85.

31. Thomas DB, Ray RM. Depot-medroxyprogesterone acetate (DMPA) and risk of invasive adenocárcinomas and adenosquamous carcinomas of the uterine cervix. WHO Collaborative Study of Neoplasia and Steroid Contraceptives. *Contraception* 1995;52:307–12.

32. Mørch LS, Lidegaard Ø, Keiding N, Løkkegaard E, Kjær SK. The influence of hormone therapies on colon and rectal cancer. *Eur J Epidemiol* 2016;31:481–9.

33. Symer MM, Wong NZ, Abelson JS, Milsom JW, Yeo HL. Hormone replacement therapy and colorectal cancer incidence and mortality in the Prostate, Lung, Colorectal, and Ovarian Cancer Screening Trial. *Clin Colorectal Cancer* 2018;17:e281–8.

34. Morois S, Fournier A, Clavel-Chapelon F, Mesrine S, Boutron-Ruault M-C. Menopausal hormone therapy and risks of colorectal adenomas and cancers in the French E3 N prospective cohort: true associations or bias? *Eur J Epidemiol* 2012;27:439–452.

35. Hsu L-H, Chu N-M, Kao S-H. Estrogen receptor and lung cancer. *Int J Mol Sci* 2017;18.

36. Ishibashi H, et al. Progesterone receptor in non–small cell lung cancer–a potent prognostic factor and possible target for

37. Chlebowski RT, et al. Estrogen plus progestin and lung cancer: follow-up of the Women's Health Initiative Randomized Trial. *Clin Lung Cancer* 2016;17:10–17.

38. Li W, et al. Hormone therapy and lung cancer mortality in women: systematic review and meta-analysis. *Steroids* 2017;118:47–54.

39. Botteri E, et al. Menopausal hormone therapy and risk of melanoma: do estrogens and progestins have a different role? *Int J Cancer* 2017;141:1763–70.

40. Kane EV, et al. Postmenopausal hormone therapy and non-Hodgkin lymphoma: a pooled analysis of InterLymph case-control studies. *Ann Oncol Off J Eur Soc Med Oncol* 2013;24:433–41.

41. Holmberg L, et al. Increased risk of recurrence after hormone replacement therapy in breast cancer survivors. *J Natl Cancer Inst* 2008;100:475–82.

42. Fahlén M, et al. Hormone replacement therapy after breast cancer: 10 year follow up of the Stockholm randomised trial. *Eur J Cancer* 1990;49:52–9.

43. Santen RJ, et al. Managing menopausal symptoms and associated clinical issues in breast cancer survivors. *J Clin Endocrinol Metab* 2017;102:3647–61.

44. Sulaica E, et al. Vaginal estrogen products in hormone receptor-positive breast cancer patients on aromatase inhibitor therapy. *Breast Cancer Res Treat* 2016;157:203–10.

45. Shim S-H, Lee SJ, Kim S-N. Effects of hormone replacement therapy on the rate of recurrence in endometrial cancer survivors: a meta-analysis. *Eur J Cancer* 2014;50:1628–37.

46. Rousset-Jablonski C, et al. Fertility preservation, contraception and menopause hormone therapy in women treated for rare ovarian tumours: guidelines from the French national network dedicated to rare gynaecological cancers. *Eur J Cancer* 2019;116:35–44.

47. Slattery ML, et al. Hormone replacement therapy and improved survival among postmenopausal women diagnosed with colon cancer (USA). *Cancer Causes Control CCC* 1999;10:467–73.

48. Mandelson MT, Miglioretti D, Newcomb PA, Harrison R, Potter JD. Hormone replacement therapy in relation to survival in women diagnosed with colon cancer. *Cancer Causes Control CCC* 2003;14:979–84.

49. Calle EE, Miracle-McMahill HL, Thun MJ, Heath CW. Estrogen replacement therapy and risk of fatal colon cancer in a prospective cohort of postmenopausal women. *J Natl Cancer Inst* 1995;87:517–23.

50. Chan JA, et al. Hormone replacement therapy and survival after colorectal cancer diagnosis. *J Clin Oncol Off J Am Soc Clin Oncol* 2006;24:5680–6.

51. Kuhle CL, et al. Menopausal hormone therapy in cancer survivors: a narrative review of the literature. *Maturitas* 2016;92:86–96.

52. Fournier A, Berrino F, Clavel-Chapelon F. Unequal risks for breast cancer associated with different hormone replacement therapies: results from the E3 N cohort study. *Breast Cancer Res Treat* 2008;107:103–11.

53. Espie M, Daures JP, Chevallier T, Mares P, Micheletti MC, De Reilhac P. Breast cancer incidence and hormone replacement therapy: Results from the MISSION study, prospective phase. *Gynecol Endocrinol* 2007;23:391–397.

54. Cordina-Duverger E, et al. Risk of breast cancer by type of menopausal hormone therapy: a case-control study among post-menopausal women in France. *PloS ONE* 2013;8:e78016.

55. Schneider C, Jick SS, Meier CR. Risk of gynecological cancers in users of estradiol/dydrogesterone or other HRT preparations. *Climacteric* 2009;12:514–24.

56. Lyytinen H, Pukkala E, Ylikorkala O. Breast cancer risk in postmenopausal women using estradiol-progestogen therapy. *Obstet Gynecol* 2009;113:65–73.

57. Creasman WT, Henderson D, Hinshaw W, Clarke-Pearson DL. Estrogen replacement therapy in the patient treated for endometrial cancer. *Obstet Gynecol* 1986;67:326–30.

58. Bryant GW. Administration of estrogens to patients with a previous diagnosis of endometrial adenocarcinoma. *South Med J* 1990;83:725–6.

59. Lee RB, Burke TW, Park RC. Estrogen replacement therapy following treatment for stage I endometrial carcinoma. *Gynecol Oncol* 1990;36:189–91.

60. Chapman JA, et al. Estrogen replacement in surgical stage I and II endometrial cancer survivors. *Am J Obstet Gynecol* 1996;175:1195–200.

61. Suriano KA, et al. Estrogen replacement therapy in endometrial cancer patients: a matched control study. *Obstet Gynecol* 2001;97:555–60.

62. Ayhan A, Taskiran C, Simsek S, Sever A. Does immediate hormone replacement therapy affect the oncologic outcome in endometrial cancer survivors? *Int J Gynecol Cancer Off J Int Gynecol Cancer Soc* 2006;16:805–8.

63. Barakat RR, et al. Randomized double-blind trial of estrogen replacement therapy versus placebo in stage I or II endometrial cancer: a Gynecologic Oncology Group Study. *J Clin Oncol Off J Am Soc Clin Oncol* 2006;24:587–92.

64. Felix AS, et al. Menopausal hormone therapy and mortality among endometrial cancer patients in the NIH-AARP Diet and Health Study. *Cancer Causes Control CCC* 2015;26:1055–63.

65. Cho HW, Ouh YT, Lee JK, Hong JH. Effects of hormone therapy on recurrence in endometrial cancer survivors: a nationwide study using the Korean Health Insurance Review and Assessment Service database. *J Gynecol Oncol* 2019;30:e51.

66. Guidozzi F, Daponte A. Estrogen replacement therapy for ovarian carcinoma survivors: A randomized controlled trial. *Cancer* 1999;86:1013–18.

67. Li L, et al. Impact of post-operative hormone replacement therapy on life quality and prognosis in patients with ovarian malignancy. *Oncol Lett* 2012;3:244–9.

68. Eeles RA, et al. Adjuvant hormone therapy may improve survival in epithelial ovarian cancer: results of the AHT Randomized Trial. *J Clin Oncol Off J Am Soc Clin Oncol* 2015;33:4138–44.

Chapter 22

Menopausal Hormone Therapy (MHT) and Venous Thrombosis

Sven O. Skouby and Johannes J. Sidelmann

Venous thromboembolism (VTE) is a specific reproductive health risk for women. In pregnancy, the relative risk of VTE is increased approximately 5-fold and in the puerperium it is increased by as much as 60-fold. Additionally, large numbers of women worldwide are exposed to an increased relative risk of VTE as a result of using combined hormonal contraception (CHC), in particular combined oral contraceptives (COCs). Even women undergoing infertility treatment may be exposed to situations of significantly increased risk of VTE [1]. Users of menopausal hormone therapy (MHT) have a two- to four-fold increased risk of VTE compared with non-users [2], comparable to the attributable risk of CHC. The risk for VTE induced by MHT is, however, higher in absolute figures because of the age factor per se, but is also dependent on the composition of the MHT used, since users of estrogen-only preparations have lower risk of VTE than women receiving combined estrogen-progestin preparations [3]. Also the dose and route of administration seems of importance, as women treated with transdermal MHT have lower risk of VTE than women receiving orally administered MHT, as consistently demonstrated in clinical studies [2]. Moreover, epidemiological and pharmacological factors may contribute to the precipitation of VTE among MHT users. The pharmacodynamics of MHT on the haemostatic system may be of particular interest [4], because MHT changes the inhibitory potential of coagulation significantly. Consequently, the choice of MHT may translate into clinical manifestations in thrombosis-prone individuals. Venous thrombosis mostly manifests in the deep veins of the leg, but may occur in other sites, such as the upper extremities, cerebral sinus, liver and portal veins or retinal veins. Major complications of VTE are a disabling post-thrombotic syndrome or acute death from a pulmonary embolus (PE) occurring in 1–2 per cent of patients [5].

Risk Factors

The risk factors for VTE fit into a contemporary and extended version of Virchow's triad (stasis, hypercoagulability, endothelial damage) changing the haemostatic balance towards clot formation (thrombophilia). The change can be achieved by decreasing blood flow and lowering oxygen tension, activation of the endothelium, inborn or acquired immune responses and blood platelets, increasing the number of platelets and red blood cells, or modifying the concentrations of pro- and anticoagulant proteins in the blood. Numerous genetic and acquired risk factors are known (Table 22.1). For details, see [6]. An extended multiple-hit hypothesis implies that more than one risk factor is present at any one time. Superficial vein thrombosis combined with an acquired thrombotic risk factor increases the

223

Table 22.1 Prevalance of congenital thrombophilias

Genetic			Acquired		
Risk factor	Prevalence	Relative risk	Risk factor	Prevalence	Relative risk
Factor V Leiden heterocygote	6%	5	Age > 30 years	50%	2.5
Factor V Leiden homocygote	0.2%	50	Adiposity (BMI > 25 g/m²)	30%	2
Protein C deficiency[a]	0.2%	>10	COC and HRT	30%	2–6
Protein S deficiency[a]	<0.1%	>10	Varicose veins	8%	2
Antithrombin deficiency[a]	0.02%	>10	Pregnancy	4%	8
Prothrombin G20210A mutation	2%	2–3	Medical diseases	5%?	2–5
Hyperhomocysteinemea	3%	3	Immobilization/trauma	?	2–10

[a] Heterozygous.

risk of venous thrombosis 10–100-fold [7], but one of the most well-known acquired risk factors is the use of exogenous sex steroids such as COCs and MHT.

Gender Differences and Age

Younger women during the child-bearing years have higher incidence of VTE than men at similar age. With advancing age, however, risk is higher in men than women. A relative risk (RR) of 1.3 in men with an age between 60 and 69 years versus women in the same age group is reported. Also the risk of recurrent venous thrombosis is two-fold higher in men than in women [8]. Venous thromboembolism has an annual incidence of 1–3 per 10 000 individuals per year (global background rate). It is uncommon in young individuals, but becomes more frequent with advancing age. The risk is doubled between the ages of 20 and 40. The incidence is estimated to be approximately 5 per 10 000 per year in women in their forties, 6–12 per 10 000 per year in women in their fifties, 30–40 per 10 000 per year in women aged 70–80 years, and approximately 70 per 10 000 in women above 80 [9, 10]. Similarly, in the Women's Health Initiative Study (WHI), users of combined MHT in the sixth, seventh and eighth decades of life had a two-, four- and seven-fold VTE risk, respectively [11]. An analogous though less pronounced effect of age was seen in the estrogen-only arm of the WHI [12].

Obesity

Obesity has been suggested to be a risk factor for fatal pulmonary embolism for a long time, but whether obesity is an independent risk factor for pulmonary embolism or VTE has not been fully determined until recently [13]. Investigations on increased risk because of obesity have been criticized because they failed to control for hospital confinement or other risk factors. Although high proportions of patients with venous VTE have been found to be obese, the importance of the association is diminished because of the high proportion of obesity in the general population. To date, however, there is notable and consistent evidence of an association of obesity with VTE, more so in women compared with men. The risk appears to be at least double that for normal weight subjects (BMI 20–24.9) [14]. In the WHI, VTE risk increased in both over-weight and obese (BMI > 30) MHT users when compared with normal weight placebo users. The risk of venous thromboembolism may be additive when using MHT, and with the continuous and global rise in obesity, this interaction will become a more prevalent risk issue.

Specific Risk of MHT

A number of different estrogen and progestin preparations in both sequential and continuous combined products are available. They differ according to the chemical structure of the estrogen as well as the progestin component, daily dose and route of administration. The estrogen compound of combined MHT consists of either natural 17β-estradiol (E2), including estradiol valerate (E2V), or the conjugated equine estrogens (CEE). E2 can be administered orally or transdermally. CEE is always orally adminis-tered. CEE and E2, administered alone, are associated with different risks of major thrombotic events. Compared with current use of oral E2, current use of oral CEE is associated with a doubling of the risk of deep vein thrombosis (DVT) [15]. The associa-tion of VTE risk with the different pharmacological classes of progestins has not been elucidated in detail, despite many clinical and epidemiologic investigations. Progestins include progesterone, the physiologic molecule synthesized and secreted by the ovary, as well as synthetic compounds named progestins, derived from either progesterone or testosterone. To date, the only desired effect in relation to MHT is endometrial protec-tion [16]. An indirect comparison within the WHI clinical trials showed that the combination of estrogens plus progestins was more thrombogenic than unopposed estrogens. Indeed, compared with placebo, the VTE risk was doubled in the opposed clinical trial and not significantly elevated among MHT users in the estrogen-alone clinical trial. Similarly, the WISDOM trial provided a direct comparison of the effect of CEE alone and CEE plus medroxyprogesterone (MPA) on VTE risk among postmeno-pausal hysterectomized women [3]. Users of CEE plus MPA had a doubling in throm-botic risk compared with women treated with CEE alone [17]. While MPA may have a thrombogenic effect among postmenopausal women using estrogens, micronized progesterone could be safe with respect to thrombotic risk [3]. The effects of the different types of progestins on VTE risk have to be further investigated.

Tibolone, a testosterone-derived progestin, has estrogenic, progestogenic and andro-genic properties and can be used alone for treatment of climacteric symptoms. The available studies, although limited in types and number, show that tibolone is not associated with an increased risk of VTE [3, 18].

Route of Administration

In general, investigations of the relationship of venous thromboembolism and MHT have focused on oral administration. Orally administered estrogen may exert a pro-thrombotic effect through the hepatic induction of haemostatic imbalance, as observed with COCs. The pro-thrombotic effect is possibly related to high concentrations of estrogen in the liver due to the 'first-pass' effect. Studies comparing oral and transdermal estrogen administration have demonstrated that transdermally administered estrogen has little or no pro-thrombotic effect and may have beneficial effects on pro-inflammatory markers, including C-reactive protein. The EStrogen and THromboEmbolism Risk (ESTHER) Study Group demonstrated that oral but not transdermal estrogen is associated with a four-fold increased VTE risk. They also noted that norpregnane progestins may be thrombogenic, whereas micronized progesterone and pregnane derivatives appear safe with respect to thrombotic risk [19].

Smoking and Length of Use

No interaction between smoking and MHT was found in the WHI clinical trial [11], although smoking is a weak risk factor for incident VTE. Smoking further increases the risk of VTE in women using CHC [20].

The risk of VTE in users of MHT decreases with length of use. There is a marked increased risk of VTE during the first year of use with the odds ratio as high as 8 ('the timing effect') [21]. This is likely to be caused by the presence of pro-thrombotic/thrombophilic abnormalities in these women, as has been shown for COCs. Besides the type and route of administration, comparisons of the thrombosis risks between MHT regimens must therefore also account for length of use. With time, the risk of thrombosis decreases, but the risk remains always higher than in non-users. This VTE risk disappears during the first months after stopping treatment.

Thrombophilia

Thrombophilia describes conditions with increased tendency for excessive clotting, including inherited conditions, based on genetic mutation such as Factor V Leiden, antithrombin, protein C and S deficiencies and the prothrombin G20210A mutation; or an acquired condition, such as lupus anticoagulant or antiphospholipid syndrome. The presence of an inherited thrombophilia is a major modifier of thrombosis risk in users of both CHC and MHT. The absolute risk of venous thrombosis in factor V Leiden heterozygous carriers is estimated as being 0.15 per 100 person-years, whereas in antithrombin-, protein C- or protein S-deficient persons, these estimates range from 0.7 to 1.7 per 100 person-years, indicating a considerably higher degree of risk. Risk estimates for thrombophilic women using MHT are less precise compared with estimates performed in CHC users, because fewer women on MHT have been included in retrospective studies informative for this situation. In principle, the known relative risks for the various thrombophilias should be multiplied by the MHT baseline risk in the relevant age category. The route of administration as well as the progestin component has been clearly shown to modulate/decrease the risk. In general, thrombophilic women or women with a positive first-degree family history of VTE should refrain from oral MHT. However, as part of the shared decision-making process, the gynecologist should weigh the risks against the benefits when prescribing MHT and counsel the patient accordingly, taking into consideration the possible thrombosis-sparing properties of transdermal administration and tibolone.

The Pharmacodynamics of MHT on the Haemostatic System

The pharmacodynamics of MHT on haemostatic proteins has been addressed in intervention studies performed two or three decades ago and include a variety of MHT-formulations, concentrations, applications, duration of treatment and study designs. Thus, the results of the studies should be interpreted with care, also because the effect of MHT on many of the haemostatic factors has been investigated in few studies only. The paragraph focuses on the effect of oral MHT on the plasma concentration of coagulation factors and inhibitors, measures of fibrinogen-fibrin turnover and fibrinolytic factors and inhibitors with particular attention to the formulation, i.e. unopposed estrogen and opposed formulations. The effects of ultra-low-dose MHT preparations, transdermal MHT and tibolone, are not addressed because these treatment modalities are apparently without increased risk of VTE, and only few studies have addressed their effect on haemostasis. A detailed description of the biochemistry of the haemostatic system is beyond the scope of this paragraph with the reader referred to a previous review [22] and Figure 22.1.

The Surface-Induced Pathway of Coagulation

Very few studies have investigated the effect of MHT on the proteins involved in the surface-induced pathway of the coagulation system, i.e. coagulation factor XII, prekallikrein, high molecular weight kininogen, coagulation factor FXI and IX (Figure 22.2). Consistent results are not obtained and firm conclusions regarding the pharmacodynamics of MHT on these factors cannot be drawn. The effect on coagulation factor VIII (FVIII), which is a cofactor of FIX in the activation of coagulation factor X (FX), however,

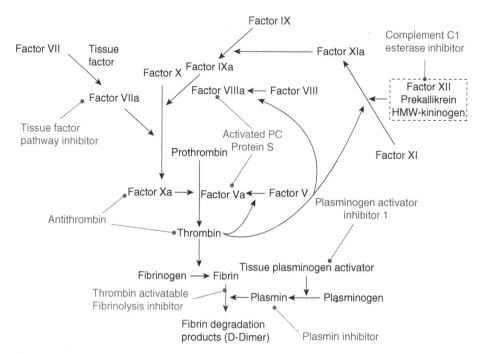

Figure 22.1 The haemostatic system.

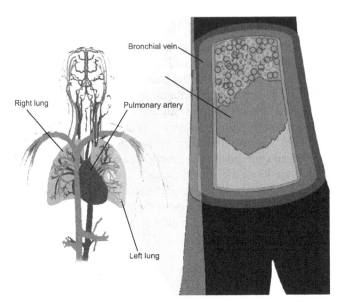

Figure 22.2 Pulmonary embolus.

Bronchial vein

Right lung

Pulmonary artery

Left lung

has been addressed in some studies (Figure 22.1), but the impact of MHT on FVIII is uncertain. While oral unopposed estrogen does not change FVIII levels significantly, inconsistent results are obtained regarding the effect of opposed estrogen where increased, decreased or no effects are reported. Studies performed in human endometrial endothelial cells challenge these findings demonstrating increased synthesis of FVIII in cells exposed to estrogen but no effect of progestin. Moreover, genetic studies using erythroleukaemic human cell lines suggest that also the levels of FIX are estrogen related. In line with these observations, animal studies have failed to demonstrate a significant effect of progestin on the plasma levels of FIX and FVIII. Thus, the lacking effect of oral unopposed estrogen on plasma levels of FVIII is surprising. However, the dosage and metabolism of the hormones may play specific roles with respect to the pharmaco-dynamics of MHT in relation to FIX and FVIII.

The Tissue Factor–Induced Pathway of Coagulation

The tissue factor (TF) driven pathway of coagulation is initiated upon vascular injury releasing TF from the damaged tissue. TF subsequently binds and activates coagulation factor VII (FVII) into FVIIa (Table 22.1). FVII is one of the most studied coagulation factors with respect to the pharmacodynamics of MHT. Most studies on unopposed estrogen demonstrate a significant increase in FVII. This finding is in line with gene expression studies in human hepatocytes demonstrating that estrogen upregulates VII mRNA expression 2–4 fold. Progestin increases TF mRNA expression and protein concentration, suggesting a pro-coagulant role of progestin. These findings suggest that opposed estrogen may increase the protein concentration and induce activation of FVII. Clinical studies, however, demonstrate decreased concentrations of FVII in women treated with opposed estrogen or no effect on the plasma levels of FVII. Moreover, the plasma levels of FVIIa are not affected by oral treatment with opposed estrogen. Thus, extrapolation of the results on TF and FVII obtained from in vitro studies to the in vivo situation is challenging. The role of regulatory proteins, i.e. tissue factor pathway inhibitor (TFPI), may have substantial influence on the effect of MHT on the TF-driven coagulation pathway. This issue will be discussed later in this paragraph.

The contact-induced pathway and the TF-driven pathway of coagulation merge into the common coagulation pathway by the activation of FX. The activation can be induced by FIXa as well as FVIIa (Table 22.1). The pharmacodynamics of FX induced by MHT is, however, only sparsely studied, and conclusive results are not obtained. Studies employing hepatoma HepG2 cells demonstrate, however, no significant estrogen-induced effect on the expression of FX suggesting that the estrogen component of HMT is without effect on the plasma measures of FX. Coagulation factor V (FV) is a cofactor for the FXa-induced activation of prothrombin into thrombin (Figure 22.1). The effect of MHT on the plasma levels of FV and prothrombin has been addressed in few inconclusive studies. Notably, however, human cell culture studies demonstrate no effect of estrogen on prothrombin, whereas progestin down-regulates prothrombin expression, underscoring the discrepancies between the protein expression in in vitro studies and the plasma measures observed in clinical studies.

Cell culture studies indicate that fibrinogen is upregulated by estrogen and down-regulated by progestin. Surprisingly, however, unopposed estrogen reduces in some studies the plasma levels of fibrinogen, while other studies report no significant effect of unopposed estrogen. Also the effect of opposed estrogen on plasma fibrinogen is controversial. Thus, the pharmacodynamics of MHT in relation to plasma fibrinogen is inconclusive.

Inhibition of Coagulation

In contrast to the pharmacodynamics of MHT on the coagulation factors, the effect of MHT on the inhibitory proteins of coagulation is more consistent and straightforward. No studies, however, have addressed the effect of MHT on complement C1-esterase inhibitor, which is the most important regulator of the surface-induced pathway of coagulation.

Antithrombin is a major regulator of coagulation with particular inhibitory effect on FXa and thrombin (Figure 22.1). Most studies on antithrombin demonstrate a significant reduction in the plasma levels of antithrombin irrespective of the MHT formulation used. Hence, unopposed oral estrogen and opposed oral estrogens impair the plasma measures of antithrombin.

Protein C regulates the velocity of the coagulation process by degradation of the cofactors FVIIIa and FVa (Figure 22.1). Protein S is an important cofactor for the protein C-induced cleavage of FVIIIa and FVa. The effect of MHT on the plasma concentration of protein C is more unclear than the effect on antithrombin. Unopposed oral estrogen is reported to increase, to reduce, or to be without effect on protein C levels. Opposed oral estrogen either decreases protein C or is without significant effect and studies indicate that the effect of opposed estrogen on plasma protein C depends on the progestin formulation.

MHT-induced reduction in plasma protein S is consistently reported in studies with unopposed and opposed oral estrogen, while only few studies demonstrate no effect on protein S levels. Protein S does not only contribute to the efficacy of activated protein C, but is also a cofactor for tissue factor pathway inhibitor (TFPI). TFPI is mainly produced in the vascular endothelium, and can be released from endothelial cells upon stimulation [23]. Estrogen inhibits TFPI production in endothelial cells, and in line with this observation, both unopposed and opposed oral estrogens decrease the plasma concentration of TFPI. Long-cycle treatment with opposed estrogen is apparently without effect on plasma TFPI.

Measures of Coagulation Activation

The previous paragraphs have focused on the effect of MHT on specific coagulation factors and anticoagulant proteins. A more general measure of the influence of MHT on coagulation can be achieved by determination of prothrombin fragment 1+2 (F1+2) and thrombin-antithrombin complex (TAT).

FXa-induced activation of prothrombin leads to release of F1+2 from the prothrombin molecule and augmentation of the plasma concentration of F1+2 indicates activation of the coagulation system in general. Intervention studies have demonstrated that unopposed oral estrogen increases the plasma levels of F1+2. Opposed oral estrogen is also reported to increase F1+2 in most studies, while unaffected levels of F1+2 are observed in other trials.

Coagulation activation induces formation of complexes between thrombin and its major inhibitor antithrombin. The plasma level of TAT, however, is essentially unaffected by MHT, irrespective of the formulation and application of the hormones.

The Fibrinolytic System and Fibrin Turnover

Fibrinolysis is initiated by activation of plasminogen induced primarily by tissue plasminogen activator (tPA) (Figure 22.1). The activation results in formation of plasmin, which degrades fibrin into fibrin degradation products, e.g. D-dimer. The activity of tPA is regulated by plasminogen activator inhibitor 1 (PAI-1), while plasmin inhibitor is an efficient inhibitor of plasmin. Thrombin activatable fibrinolysis inhibitor (TAFI) regulates fibrinolysis by removing lysine residues from the fibrin surface. The residues are prerequisite for the binding of plasminogen to fibrin and consequently the action of TAFI reduces the efficacy of the fibrinolytic system (Figure 22.1) [24].

Genetic in vitro experiments have revealed a promoting effect of estrogen on the expression of plasminogen. In line with this finding, orally administered MHT is reported to increase plasma plasminogen. Many studies have addressed the effect of both opposed and unopposed oral MHT on the plasma levels of PAI-1, reporting either reduced concentrations or no effect of MHT.

Here it should be noticed that the majority of PAI-1 circulates in blood in complex with tPA, while the amount of free and active PAI-1 is low. The studies reporting a decreasing effect of MHT on plasma levels of PAI-1 employ assays determining the antigen levels of PAI-1, which predominantly represent the PAI-1-tPA complexes. Other studies have focused on the effect of MHT on plasma measures of active PAI-1, demonstrating no significant changes in PAI-1 levels.

In parallel, studies addressing the effect of oral MHT on tPA measures report decreased or unchanged levels of tPA. Again, the antigen methods used for determination of tPA in most studies determine the concentration of tPA-PAI-1 complexes and report decreased concentrations of tPA, whereas the very few studies determining free and active tPA report no significant changes.

Thus, treatment with oral MHT decreases the plasma levels of tPA-PAI-1 complexes, while the active forms of tPA and PAI-1 are unaffected by the treatment, suggesting that oral MHT is without significant effect on the plasma fibrinolytic capacity.

Studies on the plasma levels of plasmin-plasmin inhibitor complexes support this notion. Activation of the fibrinolytic system, i.e. the conversion of plasminogen into plasmin, will in turn lead to inhibition of plasmin by plasmin inhibitor (Figure 22.1). Hence, elevated plasma levels of plasmin-plasmin inhibitor complexes indicate increased fibrinolytic activity. Oral MHT, however, has no significant effect on plasma measures of plasmin inhibitor or plasmin-antiplasmin complexes indicating that MHT is without significant effect on the fibrinolytic capacity in women treated with MHT. An elevated concentration of TAFI is a risk factor for VTE, but oral unopposed estrogen induces no significant changes in the plasma levels of TAFI, whereas opposed oral estrogen decreases TAFI concentrations in plasma.

Conclusion

MHT is known to increase the risk of DVT and pulmonary embolism, though the absolute risk for a given patient is very small. The risk of DVT appears to be greatest soon after the initiation of MHT and returns to the baseline level after discontinuation. There are inconsistent data about whether estrogen-only or combined estrogen-progestin MHT products are associated with similar VTE risk. There is compelling evidence for a differential effect of estrogens according to route of administration, with impaired inhibition of coagulation among oral estrogen users and definite haemostatic balance among transdermal estrogen users. This difference depends on neither the estrogen compound nor the daily dose. Retrospective analyses suggest that transdermal MHT is not as pro-thrombotic as oral MHT, though this has not been evaluated in randomized clinical trials. Some, but not all, clinical studies have suggested that progestins could be an important determinant of thrombotic risk, but no clear effect of the different progestins on haemostasis has been highlighted. Increasing age and weight further promote MHT's VTE risk. Some studies have investigated whether pro-thrombotic combinations may increase MHT's DVT risk. However, no benefit to screening prospective MHT users has been described, yet.

The current literature provides no clear picture of the pharmacodynamics of oral MHT on coagulation factors. Many of the intervention studies addressing this issue include only few individuals, questioning the power of the results obtained. Statistical type II errors, i.e. failing to observe a difference when in truth there is one, cannot be excluded. More significant and consistent results demonstrate that oral MHT reduces the plasma measures of antithrombin, protein S and TFPI. This reduction may potentially contribute to the increased risk of venous thromboembolism (VTE) observed in women treated with MHT. Studies have shown that even a modest reduction of the plasma levels of these anticoagulant proteins may increase the risk of VTE significantly [25]. Notably, lowering of the plasma concentration of antithrombin to levels below the mean reference range increases the risk of VTE approximately 1.5 times. A reduction of the plasma levels of protein S is also thrombogenic and the lowering effect of MHT on protein S may be of particular importance. Besides being an essential cofactor for protein C in the degradation of FVa and FVIIIa [22], protein S is an important cofactor for TFPI, and contributes by this action to TFPI-induced down-regulation of the tissue factor–driven pathway of coagulation [23]. The MHT-induced decrease in protein S combined with the very substantial decrease in TFPI may therefore contribute significantly to the increased risk of VTE induced by MHT, in particular in patients with thrombophilia.

The reduced coagulation inhibitory capacity may explain the MHT-induced elevated concentration of F1+2 persistently reported for both unopposed and opposed estrogen when administered orally. The concentration of TAT, another marker of coagulation activation, however, is unaffected questioning the coagulation activating features of MHT. The values of F1+2 and TAT as risk markers for VTE are, however, debatable. More dynamic tests, such as the thrombin generation test, may be considered to elucidate the pharmacodynamics of MHT on the coagulation system. Only one intervention study has demonstrated increased thrombin generation capacity after opposed oral estrogen so far.

The plasma concentration of the fibrinolytic proteins plasminogen, tPA, PAI and TAFI is not significantly affected by MHT. It should be noted that only few studies have employed assays capable of measuring the active forms of t-PA and PAI-1. The studies on plasmin-plasmin inhibitor complexes, demonstrating no significant activation of the fibrinolytic system though, discourage further studies on MHT and fibrinolysis.

Advanced proteomic and genomic studies may hold promise in the future for better elucidating which MHT users are at highest risk for VTE. Presently, physicians and prospective MHT users should discuss the potential risks and benefits for the individual patient, acknowledging there is no way to fully mitigate the risk of VTE. Shared decision-making is mandatory and the clinician should weigh the risks against the benefits when prescribing MHT and counsel the patient accordingly, taking into consideration the possible thrombosis-sparing properties associated with the route of administration and the preparation used.

References

1. Chan WS, Dixon ME. The 'ART' of thromboembolism: a review of assisted reproductive technology and thromboembolic complications. *Thromb Res* 2008;121:713–26.

2. 556 Acon. Postmenopausal estrogen therapy: route of administration and risk of venous thromboembolism. *Obstet Gynecol* 2013;121:887–90.

3. Canonico M, Plu-Bureau G, Scarabin PY. Progestogens and venous thromboembolism among postmenopausal women using hormone therapy. *Maturitas* 2011;70:354–60.

4. Canonico M. Hormone therapy and hemostasis among postmenopausal women: a review. *Menopause* 2014;21:753–62.

5. Rosendaal FR. Venous thrombosis: a multicausal disease. *Lancet* 1999;353:1167–73.

6. Rosendaal FR, Reitsma PH. Genetics of venous thrombosis. *J Thromb Haemost* 2009;7 Suppl 1:301–4.

7. Roach RE, Lijfering WM, Helmerhorst FM, et al. The risk of venous thrombosis in women over 50 years old using oral contraception or postmenopausal hormone therapy. *J Thromb Haemost* 2013;11:124–31.

8. Anderson FA, Jr., Wheeler HB, Goldberg RJ, et al. A population-based perspective of the hospital incidence and case-fatality rates of deep vein thrombosis and pulmonary embolism. The Worcester DVT Study. *Arch Intern Med* 1991;151:933–8.

9. Tsai AW, Cushman M, Rosamond WD, et al. Cardiovascular risk factors and venous thromboembolism incidence: the longitudinal investigation of thromboembolism etiology. *Arch Intern Med* 2002;162:1182–9.

10. White RH. The epidemiology of venous thromboembolism. *Circulation* 2003;107 Suppl 1:14–8.

11. Cushman M, Kuller LH, Prentice R, et al. Estrogen plus progestin and risk of venous thrombosis. *JAMA* 2004;292:1573–80.

12. Curb JD, Prentice RL, Bray PF, et al. Venous thrombosis and conjugated equine estrogen in women without a uterus. *Arch Intern Med* 2006;166:772–80.

13. Ageno W, Becattini C, Brighton T, et al. Cardiovascular risk factors and venous thromboembolism: a meta-analysis. *Circulation* 2008;117:93–102.

14. Allman-Farinelli MA. Obesity and venous thrombosis: a review. *Semin Thromb Hemost* 2011;37:903–7.

15. Smith NL, Blondon M, Wiggins KL, et al. Lower risk of cardiovascular events in postmenopausal women taking oral estradiol compared with oral conjugated equine estrogens. *JAMA* 2014;174:25–31.

16. Skouby SO, Jespersen J. Progestins in HRT: sufferance or desire? *Maturitas* 2009;62:371–5.

17. Smith NL, Heckbert SR, Lemaitre RN, et al. Esterified estrogens and conjugated equine estrogens and the risk of venous thrombosis. *JAMA* 2004;292:1581–7.

18. Skouby SO, Sidelmann JJ, Nilas L, et al. The effect of continuous combined conjugated equine estrogen plus medroxyprogesterone acetate and tibolone on cardiovascular metabolic risk factors. *Climacteric* 2008;11:489–97.

19. Canonico M, Oger E, Plu-Bureau G, et al. Hormone therapy and venous thromboembolism among postmenopausal women: impact of the route of estrogen administration and progestogens: the ESTHER study. *Circulation* 2007;115:840–5.

20. Blondon M, Wiggins KL, Van Hylckama Vlieg A, et al. Smoking, postmenopausal hormone therapy and the risk of venous thrombosis: a population-based, case-control study. *Br J Haematol* 2013;163:418–20.

21. Eisenberger A, Westhoff C. Hormone replacement therapy and venous thromboembolism. *J Steroid Biochem Mol Biol* 2014;142:76–82.

22. Sidelmann JJ, Gram J, Jespersen J, et al. Fibrin clot formation and lysis: basic mechanisms. *Semin Thromb Hemost* 2000;26:605–18.

23. Hackeng TM, Sere KM, Tans G, et al. Protein S stimulates inhibition of the tissue factor pathway by tissue factor pathway inhibitor. *Proc Natl Acad Sci U S A.* 2006;103:3106–11.

24. Urano T, Castellino FJ, Suzuki Y. Regulation of plasminogen activation on cell surfaces and fibrin. *J Thromb Haemost* 2018. doi 10.1111/jth.14157

25. Bucciarelli P, Passamonti SM, Biguzzi E, et al. Low borderline plasma levels of antithrombin, protein C and protein S are risk factors for venous thromboembolism. *J Thromb Haemost* 2012;10:1783–91.

The Risk–Benefit Analysis of Menopausal Hormone Therapy in the Menopause

Elizabeth Stephenson and Tim Hillard

The menopausal hormone therapy (MHT) risk–benefit profile has been at the centre of the debate that polarizes opinion between those who advocate the use of MHT and those who oppose it even before the publication of the original Women's Health Initiative (WHI) study in 2001. Whilst there is broad agreement around some of the key benefits of MHT there remains considerable difference about the interpretation of the risks in taking it. Revised data from the WHI and other randomized clinical trials since the publication of WHI together with various recent authoritative international position statements and recommendations since the last edition have helped to clarify some of the uncertainties and provide more robust evidence for clinical decision-making.

The available evidence suggests that MHT should be offered to well-informed peri- or early postmenopausal women to control moderate to severe menopausal symptoms, as the benefits outweigh the risks in otherwise healthy women in this age group [1, 2]. Whilst many women remain fearful of the risks of MHT, the revised findings of the WHI trial analyses and subsequent analyses such as the NICE (National Institute for Health and Care Excellence) guidelines should reassure healthy women who require symptom control [3]. Whilst there is currently less evidence for the widespread use of MHT for long-term chronic disease prevention, MHT is a proven effective treatment for the prevention of osteoporosis and appears to also reduce cardiovascular disease risk if started in the early postmenopause. An individualized and rational approach to commencing and continuing MHT is recommended, as the risk–benefit balance will differ for each woman and for any individual woman over time. A variety of factors can influence an individual's risk–benefit ratio (Table 23.1). This chapter aims to review the current evidence for the benefits and risks of MHT as a guide to clinical decision-making.

Benefits of MHT

For young, healthy menopausal women (below the age of 60) with bothersome symptoms the benefits of MHT generally outweigh the risks. However the risk–benefit profile for a particular woman is not static, therefore regular clinical reviews are necessary. In their comprehensive review of menopause management NICE recommends that review should take place after commencing treatment for short-term menopausal symptoms at 3 months to assess efficacy and tolerability, and annual review thereafter unless there are clinical indications for earlier review. We will briefly

Table 23.1 Factors influencing an individual's risk–benefit ratio for hormone replacement therapy

- Relevant personal or family history
- Lifestyle (weight, diet, exercise, smoking and alcohol use)
- Severity of menopausal symptoms
- Age and time of HRT initiation in relation to onset of menopause ('critical therapeutic window')
- Type of MHT (combined or estrogen only)
- Dose of MHT preparation
- Route of MHT administration and length of MHT use

discuss the main known benefits of MHT; many of these are discussed in more detail elsewhere in the book.

Vasomotor Symptoms

Vasomotor symptoms – often described as hot flushes or flashes and night sweats – affect 60–80 per cent of menopausal women to some extent. The severity of these symptoms peaks in the late perimenopause and early postmenopause, but there is a large individual and ethnic variation in their prevalence, severity, frequency and duration (mean of 7–10 years) and some women continue to experience them well into their sixties and beyond [4].

MHT remains the most effective treatment for vasomotor symptoms. A Cochrane review reported a 75 per cent reduction in the frequency and an 87 per cent reduction in severity of hot flushes in MHT users [5]. As these symptoms can be debilitating in a significant proportion of women, managing them effectively should have an important positive impact on their quality of life. Although this seems obvious, clear data on the benefits of MHT on quality of life are lacking, primarily because randomized placebo-controlled trials of symptomatic women are not considered ethical in many countries. The addition of progestogen to estrogen as part of MHT did not show any change in results. The lowest effective estrogen dose should be used and increasingly lower and lower doses have proven to be effective.

Whilst there is little doubt that MHT is the most effective treatment for vasomotor symptoms many clinicians have been wary of prescribing it and have instead been offering women alternatives such as anti-depressants and clonidine. Following their comprehensive review of the data NICE recommended that selective serotonin reuptake inhibitors (SSRIs), serotonin and norepinephrine reuptake inhibitors (SNRIs) or clonidine should not be offered as first-line treatment for vasomotor symptoms alone [3].

Urogenital Symptoms

The symptoms of vulvo-vaginal atrophy (VVA) such as vaginal dryness, soreness, dyspaerunia, urinary frequency, urgency and nocturia are extremely common amongst postmenopausal women. Topical vaginal estrogen therapy provides effective symptom relief and improvement in the cytological composition and physiology of the vaginal epithelium. Vaginal estrogens are also effective in reducing the number of episodes of recurrent urinary tract infections in postmenopausal women [6].

As topical vaginal estrogens have minimal systemic absorption, they are considered safe and are not associated with the risks associated with MHT discussed later. Systemic MHT preparations offer no therapeutic advantages over low-dose local estrogens in the management of VVA, indeed meta-analyses suggest that bladder symptoms such as sensory urgency respond better to topical rather than systemic preparations. Women taking topical vaginal estrogen preparations should be reassured of their safety and that there is no requirement to take additional progestogens. Topical estrogens can be continued safely long term to maintain healthy vaginal function and to prevent symptom relapse, which frequently occurs if they are stopped. Because they have no significant systemic absorption they can also be considered in women where systemic MHT is contraindicated, e.g. breast cancer patients, although this is off-label and requires careful consideration.

Whilst women taking systemic MHT for other indications are likely to gain beneficial effects on VVA, for women with just symptoms of VVA and no other symptoms, there is no advantage in taking systemic MHT. Approximately 15–20 per cent of women taking systemic MHT may not get complete relief of their VVA symptoms and in these women topical estrogens can be used in addition to systemic MHT.

Female Sexual Function

Sexual dysfunction is common amongst postmenopausal women and its correction can lead to improved quality of life for women and their partners.

Systemic and topical MHT improves the superficial and sometimes deep dyspaerunia associated with VVA in postmenopausal women, which is often the first step to improve sexual function [6]. Vaginal lubricants and moisturizers can be added to topical estrogen or used alone to improve symptoms further. Restoring libido is altogether a more complex challenge. For some women correction of underlying menopausal symptoms and improvements in sleep and mood can all have a positive impact. The addition of testosterone therapy has been shown to improve sexual desire and satisfaction in surgically and naturally menopausal women, provided appropriate doses are used so androgenic and virilizing side effects do not occur. The use of transdermal testosterone for women both on and not on estrogen/progestin therapy in the short term is thought to be effective and not associated with serious complications when treating hypoactive sexual desire disorder [7].

Mood, Depression and Anxiety

Peri- and postmenopause are associated with an increase in mood and depressive disorders. Estrogen interacts with mood-regulating brain mechanisms through a number of neurotransmitters and the serotonin system. Randomized trials have shown significant beneficial associations between MHT and mood; 68–80 per cent of women using estrogen-only MHT reported decreased mood symptoms, compared with only 20–22 per cent of women using placebo [2]. In a double-blinded randomised controlled trial women taking placebo were 2.5 times more likely to have high depression scores than those on MHT. MHT and CBT (cognitive behavioural therapy) improve low mood for some women and MHT can and should be considered in women experiencing these symptoms [3]. For some women the additional progestogen can have a negative impact on these symptoms. This may vary with the type, dose and route of progestogen so careful selection of combination therapy is required. SSRIs do not appear to improve low mood in women who are not clinically depressed. MHT use is also associated with a significant improvement in sleep quality.

Osteoporosis and Fractures

The relationship between menopause, the decline in bone density and an increased risk of osteoporotic fractures is well established [2, 8]. Equally numerous studies, including the WHI, have shown that MHT is effective in preventing bone loss and reducing the incidence of all osteoporotic fractures even in low-risk women. A Cochrane review demonstrated a 30 per cent reduction in osteoporotic fractures (hip, vertebrae and overall) among women taking estrogen-only or combined MHT compared with placebo.

Thus hormone replacement therapy should be considered one of the first-line choices of therapy in postmenopausal women below the age of 60 with a significant fracture risk and for those women with premature ovarian insufficiency. Women taking MHT primarily for menopausal symptoms will also derive benefit. The protective effect of MHT on bone mineral density may remain for a variable length of time after cessation of therapy before an inevitable gradual decline in bone density occurs, emphasizing the importance of ongoing bone conservation strategies. Initiating MHT after the age of 60 for the sole purpose of osteoporosis prevention is not recommended as a first-line therapy although it may still be effective.

Degenerative Arthritis

Estrogen has a regulatory role in the metabolism of cartilage. Declining estrogen levels after menopause is associated with thinning of intervertebral discs and osteoarthritic joint changes. Most of these changes occur in the first 5 years after the menopause. Timely hormone replacement initiation can have a protective effect on intervertebral discs and articulated joint cartilage. In the WHI Study, women treated with estrogen alone had significantly lower rates (RR 0.84, 95 per cent CI 0.70–1.00) of arthroplasty than those in the placebo group. These benefits, however, were not evident in the WHI continuous combined MHT arm. It thus seems possible that progestogens may neutralize the chondro-protective actions of estrogen, although whether this varies with type of progestogen is not known [2].

Skin and Muscle Mass

Estrogens play an important role in skin physiology. The hypo-estrogenic state of the menopause accelerates age-related skin changes (thinning and dryness of the skin, increase in the number and depth of wrinkles, decrease in skin elasticity). Several randomized, double-blind, placebo-controlled trials have shown a 30 per cent increase in dermal thickness in postmenopausal women after 12 months of estrogen therapy, as well as an overall increase in collagen content and a decrease in facial wrinkling.

Sarcopenia, which is associated with declining estrogen levels after the menopause, is one of the major factors responsible for declining motor function and increased propensity to falls in the elderly. Whilst MHT may help improve muscle mass and strength, women should be encouraged to adopt an active lifestyle with regular weight-bearing exercise to help maintain a healthy musculoskeletal system.

Cognition

Estrogen receptors are widespread throughout the central and peripheral nervous systems and estrogens facilitate autonomic regulation and cognitive functions. Early untreated surgical menopause is associated with an increased incidence of dementia and other neurologic conditions.

The impact of MHT on cognitive function depends on the woman's age and timing of MHT initiation [2]. Several studies have revealed cognitive benefits of MHT if commenced around the time of menopause, i.e. during a 'critical therapeutic window' period. Early MHT initiators have demonstrated improved memory, stronger global cognition and executive function. In an observational study there was a 30 per cent reduction of Alzheimer's disease risk in women who initiated MHT within 5 years of menopause and used it for 10 years, but later MHT initiation, as in the WHI Study, does not appear to have the same positive effect, indeed may even have a negative effect. This view is also supported by a case control study in Finland, which found Alzheimer's sufferers were slightly more likely to have used MHT.

Further well-designed trials are necessary to explore the neuro-protective effects of various MHT preparations and their potential use in prevention of neurodegenerative conditions but at this stage the impact of MHT on the risk of dementia is unclear [3].

Cardiovascular Disease

Cardiovascular disease is the leading cause of death in women over 50 years of age worldwide. Considerable evidence suggests that atherosclerotic changes are delayed by estrogen – whether endogenous in the premenopause, or exogenous in the form of MHT after the onset of menopause. Estrogens are associated with reduction in endothelial injury, as well as plaque formation through lowering total and LDL cholesterol and raising HDL cholesterol levels.

There is strong and consistent evidence that Estrogen therapy started around the time of menopause may be cardioprotective but may be harmful if started more than 10 years after menopause (the 'critical therapeutic window' theory) [2]. Observational studies have shown a 40 per cent decrease in cardiovascular disease rates, as well as cardiovascular disease-related and all-cause mortality rates, in women who commenced MHT in early menopause vs non-users. This cardioprotective effect was not observed in women starting MHT after the age of 60 (Table 23.2). A Cochrane review of 19 RCTs concluded that whilst MHT has little or no benefit in the prevention of cardiovascular events overall, for those within 10 years of menopause at the time of initiation there was a significant reduction in all-cause mortality and cardiovascular disease [9]. A 10-year randomized trial of women receiving MHT started early after menopause showed that the MHT group had a significantly reduced risk of mortality, heart failure and stroke compared with the untreated group [2]. Data from the Finnish database have also demonstrated a reduction in cardiovascular disease and all-cause mortality in both long-term estrogen and combined estrogen/progestogen users.

A double-blind RCT of 643 healthy postmenopausal women showed timing of commencing MHT may affect the development of atherosclerosis but whether this correlates with clinically relevant endpoints has yet to be demonstrated. Current evidence suggests that estrogen-only regimens may offer greater cardioprotection than combined regimens, and a transdermal route of administration may provide further additional benefits of lowering the blood pressure and preventing athero-sclerotic plaque rupture and thrombosis as compared with oral estrogen preparations [2]. Treatment seems to be duration dependent and becomes effective after at least 6 years of use. More research is needed on the role of cardiovascular effects of progestogens in combined MHT preparations.

Table 23.2 Relative risk (RR) for cardiovascular events by age and time since onset of menopause in the WHI study

	CEE	CEE + MPA
Age (years)		
50–59	0.63	1.29
60–69	0.94	1.03
70–79	1.13	1.48
Time since menopause (years)		
<10	0.48	0.88
10–19	0.96	1.23
20	1.12	1.66

Note. CEE = conjugated equine estrogens. MPA = medroxyprogesterone acetate.

Type II Diabetes

Type II diabetes is a multifactorial condition with an increased incidence in the mid-life. Decline in estrogen levels during menopause transition and MHT may play a role in insulin sensitivity; however, insufficient evidence is currently available [2, 8]. A large RCT indicated a lower incidence (by 7.5 cases per 1000 women per 5 years of use) of type II diabetes among women using combined MHT in comparison with the placebo group. Taking MHT does not appear to increase the risk of developing type II diabetes nor does it affect blood glucose control (NICE). The effects of MHT may depend on baseline metabolic status and abdominal obesity, and women with larger waist circumferences are more likely to benefit from MHT use [8]. Women with type 2 diabetes are more likely to have other comorbidities which may influence the type and dose of MHT used.

Colorectal Cancer

Epidemiologic studies have consistently shown up to a 20 per cent reduction in colon cancer incidence in ever-users of MHT compared with never-users [2, 8]. The WHI randomized trial reported a smaller decrease in risk in women taking combined MHT; the absolute risk decreased from 9 per 1000 in the control group to 6 per 1000 in the MHT group. However estrogen-only therapy did not have any effect on the risk of colorectal cancer. There are no current data on the effects on colorectal cancer of non-oral preparations. Despite these consistent observations there is no clear explanation as to why MHT should lower colon cancer risk, and MHT should not be used solely for the prevention of colon cancer.

Other Benefits

Long-term estrogen therapy appears to reduce the risk of nuclear lens opacities that form the cataract by 60–80 per cent. A small absolute reduction in the risk of developing glaucoma has also been reported in some studies.

Estrogen seems to protect the teeth and reduce edentia (RR 0.6), possibly through preserving jaw bone density. Menopausal hormone therapy users may also have a reduced incidence of stomach cancer (RR 0.48, 95 per cent CI 0.29–0.79) [2].

Risks of MHT

Breast Cancer

The potential risk of breast cancer associated with MHT remains one of the principal reasons for anxiety among patients and health care professionals about prescribing MHT. The baseline risk of developing breast cancer is individual and varies according to underlying risk factors [1–3]. Women should be reassured that the absolute increase in breast cancer risk associated with MHT use is small, and is overall less than the increase in risk associated with obesity, nulliparity or consumption of three alcoholic drinks per day (Table 23.3).

The WHI reported a RR of 1.26 (95 per cent CI 1.02–1.56) after a mean of 5.6 years of continuous combined MHT use, which is less than a 0.1 per cent increase in risk per year. This equates to 4–5 extra breast cancers/1000 women over 5 years' usage. In a more recent but smaller Danish study there was no significant increase in breast cancer with 10 years of MHT usage. NICE guidelines add that any additional risk reduces after stopping combined MHT [3] although a recent meta-analysis suggests the risk may continue for up to 10 years [10].

Among women taking estrogen alone there was a non-statistically significant decrease in the risk of breast cancer at 10.7 years follow-up in the WHI Study (RR 0.78, 95 per cent CI 0.63–0.96) [2, 8]. The NICE guidelines conclude that there is little or no change in the risk of breast cancer in women on unopposed estrogen [3]. It has been hypothesized that estrogen causes apoptosis of breast cancer cells and the available data now point to the progestogen component being responsible for the small increase in breast cancer risk seen with combined MHT. Not all progestogens have the same effect;

Table 23.3 Comparison of relative risk (RR) for different breast cancer risk factors

Breast cancer risk factors	RR of breast cancer
No MHT	1.0
Combined MRT (E + P)	1.26
More than 5 years of MHT use	1.35
Unopposed estrogen (E-only)	07.78
Aged > 50 with a BMI > 35	2.0
Alcohol, two units per week	1.5–2.0
Early menarche (<12 years)	1.3
Late menopause (>55 years)	1.2–1.5
First pregnancy after the age of 30	1.9
Combined oral contraceptive pill use in the past 10 years	1.07–1.24

data such as those from the French EPIC Cohort suggest that whilst the nortestosterone derivatives are associated with a small increase in breast cancer risk, the natural progesterone-based preparations are not [8].

Breast cancer is relatively common in the menopausal age group. At the time of initiation of MHT, it is likely that a proportion of women harbour a 'reservoir' of occult undiagnosed breast tumours. Combined results from studies in women of all ages indicate that this could be the case in 0–14.7 per cent of women. It is likely that MHT promotes the growth of these preexisting lesions to a level at which they are detected and therefore diagnosed earlier in MHT users than in non-users. Thus newly detected breast cancers in the RCTs could be either *de novo* tumours, or preexisting tumours promoted by MHT use, which can affect the outcome data. This may also explain why women diagnosed with breast cancer on MHT seem to have a better outcome than those not [8]. Breast cancer risk with MHT has recently been evaluated in a meta analysis published in the Lancet (10). The overall finding are felt to be in keeping with the current NICE guidance. The findings did indicate a higher incidence of breast cancer in both combined and to a lesser extent oestrogen only preparations although no information was collected on breast cancer mortality. The risk was found to be greatest with combined continuous preparations and with the type of progesterone used although it is important to point out that continuous combined preparations do reduce the risk of endometrial cancer. The meta analysis did also show that the risk of breast cancer diagnosis remains elevated for 10 years after discontinuing MHT which is longer than previously thought. The limitations of the study and individual risk should be taken into account when counseling women about MHT.

Cardiovascular Disease

The beneficial cardioprotective effects of MHT in women under the age of 60 are discussed above. There seems to be little or no increase in cardiovascular disease risk with either unopposed estrogen or combined MHT if commenced in women under the age of 60. For women starting MHT after the age of 60 there appears to be an increased risk of cardiac events during the first few years of use (HR 1.47, 95 per cent CI 1.12–1.92) [2]. However, other data suggest that cardiac morbidity declines in a population of older healthy women after taking MHT for 2 years (HR 0.79, 95 per cent CI 0.67–0.93). Estrogen is a potent vasodilator and it is hypothesized that when MHT is initiated in women with established coronary disease, estrogen may promote atherosclerotic plaque rupture and thrombosis. This effect seems to be dose dependent and may not be seen with lower doses.

These potential risks should be borne in mind when weighing up the risks and benefits in women wishing to start MHT over the age of 60, and low or ultra-low doses should be used where possible, at least initially.

Stroke

Stroke is the second leading cause of mortality among females worldwide. It is a rare event in women under 60 but its incidence increases with age and is associated with hypertension, obesity and other risk factors. In the WHI trial, estrogen use, with or without progesterone, increased the risk of ischaemic stroke by about one-third (RR 1.31, 95 per cent CI 1.02–1.68 and RR 1.37, 95 per cent CI 1.09–1.73, respectively) across all the age groups [2]. However, 13-year follow-up demonstrated no increased incidence in those who started MHT within 10 years of menopause. There does appear to be an increased risk in those initiating HRT > 60 years which increases with age. Any increased risk is likely to be dose and route dependent with lower or no additional risk seen with low-dose transdermal preparations [2, 3, 8]. Overall the risk of stroke is very small in the population most likely to be taking MHT. The most likely mechanism is thrombotic so as with VTE (below) low-dose transdermal therapy is preferred for those with risk factors.

Venous Thromboembolism

Because of its background prevalence and potentially serious consequences, the risk of venous thromboembolism (VTE) is one of the most important factors in the risk–benefit equation of MHT decision-making. The absolute risk of thromboembolism for any individual will depend on co-existent risk factors, such as age, obesity, immobility, previous history and presence of hereditary thrombophilias.

It is estimated that in women aged 50–59 years there are an additional two thromboembolic events per 1000 women with 5 years of unopposed estrogen, and 5 additional events per 1000 over 5 years with combined MHT [8]. The risk of thromboembolism in women taking oral HRT seems to be higher in the first years of use and disappears once MHT is stopped. These risks may be magnified in women with co-existent risk factors and thrombophilias. However, the route of estrogen administration as transdermal therapy avoids the first-pass effect on coagulation factors. Transdermal estrogen appears to convey no additional VTE risk and is recommended in those with risk factors [2, 3]. Conversely oral estrogens should be avoided in those with a high risk, particularly personal history of VTE.

The type and dose of progestogen too is important in combined regimens. Micronized progesterone or pregnane derivatives have a lower thromboembolic risk than the other progestogens used in MHT and should be preferred for those with co-existent risk factor. For those with a very high risk, e.g. factor V Leiden, even transdermal estrogens maybe associated with a significantly increased risk. In such women with very severe symptoms, MHT may be prescribed in conjunction with thromboprophylaxis.

Ovarian Cancer

Eighty per cent of ovarian cancers occur in women after the age of 50. Some observational studies reported a RR of 1.6 (95 per cent CI 1.2–2.0) with estrogen-only MHT with a 7 per cent increase in risk per year of use, with the risk declining to average population risk 2–4 years after cessation of therapy [2]. However, these results have not been consistently reproduced and the WHI trial observed a non-significant RR of 1.58 (95 per cent CI 0.77–3.24) for continuous combined MHT vs placebo [2, 8]. In women with epithelial ovarian cancer, studies have either shown no difference or an improvement in survival rate with the use of MHT. A more recent meta-analysis involving principally prospective follow-up studies of over 12 000 women reported a small increase risk of one extra ovarian cancer per 1000 users in women over 5 years' MHT use. This analysis has been robustly challenged but even at face value this is a very small absolute risk. At present the association between ovarian cancer risk and MHT is unclear [2].

Endometrial Cancer

Ninety per cent of endometrial cancers develop after the age of 50. Unopposed estrogen therapy has long been associated with a dose- and duration-dependent increase in risk of premalignant and malignant endometrial conditions. Estrogen-only MHT used for 10 years increases the risk of endometrial cancer by 9.5 times. The risk tends to persist for many years after cessation of therapy, with an RR of 1.9 12 years after stopping estrogen compared with non-users [8]. The addition of cyclical or continuous progestogen eliminates the increased risk. Combined MHT regimes do not increase endometrial cancer risk in RCTs and observational studies. The WHI, for example, quote an RR of 0.81 (95 per cent CI 0.48–1.06) in the continuous combined HMT arm versus placebo. Continuous progestogen regimens are associated with a lower risk than sequential ones and it is recommended that women change to a no-bleed preparation once they are clearly postmenopausal. A recent Cochrane review concludes that there is no significant harm in women taking MHT even after surgical treatment for early endometrial cancer. However, there is no evidence available to inform women with higher-stage endometrial cancer.

Other Gynaecologic Cancers

There is no evidence that MHT increases the risk of other gynecologic cancers such as cervix or vulva [2]. Equally a history of such a cancer does not preclude the use of subsequent MHT if appropriate.

Lung Cancer

The WHI reported a small overall increase in death from non–small cell lung cancer with MHT use compared with placebo (RR = 1.87, 95 per cent CI 1.22–1.88) [8]. This was not seen in women in the 50–59 age group, was more pronounced in smokers and was not seen in the estrogen-alone arm. Epidemiologic studies have not identified any association between MHT and lung cancer.

Gallbladder Disease

Both estrogen-only and combined MHT increase the risk of gallbladder disease (cholecystitis and cholelithiasis) and cholecystectomy. The WHI showed a gallbladder disease or surgery hazard ratio (HR) of 1.67 in the estrogen-alone arm and an HR of 1.59 in the combined MHT arm when compared with the non-users [2]. The risk tends to persist for many years after MHT cessation and may be altered with the type and dose of estrogen as well as the route of administration. Transdermal estrogen preparations are associated with a significantly lower gallbladder disease risk. Shorter duration of MHT use also minimizes this risk.

Conclusion

Careful counselling about the risks and benefits of MHT is essential prior to commencing treatment, and an annual reappraisal of the individual risk–benefit profile thereafter should be conducted to ensure the safest effective management of symptoms. Most women seeking hormone therapy are in their late forties or early fifties and are likely to use MHT for a few years only, so it is important that the relevant figures for the risks and benefits pertinent to that age group are used to aid the consultation (Table 23.4).

Table 23.4. Number of excess benefit or risk cases per 1000 women for 5 years of combined estrogen and progesterone (E + P) or unopposed estrogen (E-only) use in women starting hormone replacement therapy between the ages of 50 and 59 years

Benefits and risks (±cases per 1000 women per 5 years)	50–59 years old E + P	50–59 years old E-only
Coronary heart disease	−0.9	−3.8
Fractures	−4.9	−5.9
Breast cancer	+6.8	−1.5
Type II diabetes	−11	−11
Colorectal cancer	−1.2	N/A
Stroke	+1.0	+1.2
Thromboembolism	+5	+2
Cholecystitis	+9.6	+14.

For the majority of healthy postmenopausal women below the age of 60 with moderate to severe menopausal symptoms, the benefits of MHT will outweigh the risks (NICE). Appropriate hormone replacement therapy commenced in the 'critical therapeutic window' period may also provide additional protective cardiovascular and cognitive benefits, as well as osteoporosis prevention. For women who have premature ovarian insufficiency (POI) the potential benefits are such that the risk–benefit balance is likely to be heavily in favour of taking MHT [1–3, 8]. Women who have been hysterectomized and only require estrogen therapy are likely to have a more beneficial risk analysis at all ages than those who require combined therapy.

Women over the age of 60 or those who wish to continue to use MHT longer term should not be denied treatment provided there is careful consideration and discussion about the potential risks. The absolute risks of many relevant conditions such as breast cancer, cardiovascular disease, stroke and thromboembolism increase with age. However, provided women make a well-informed choice, MHT can still be initiated or continued. It is important to distinguish between the risks of starting MHT over 60 (as reported in the WHI) and continuing MHT into the sixties, which would appear to have fewer risks, particularly with regard to cardiovascular disease. For this group of patients, using lower or ultra-low doses, using the transdermal route, and minimizing or eliminating the progesterone component may all help reduce the potential risk. Careful documentation of the discussion should be made and regular reappraisal of benefits vs risks is advised at least once a year.

Over the last few years many of the high-profile concerns about the safety of MHT raised by the WHI and other studies around that time have been addressed and put into context. Women deserve an honest evaluation of the risks and benefits associated with any treatment to help them maintain their quality of life through the menopause and to prevent the potentially devastating long-term consequences of the menopause. Further research is needed to develop an individual evidence-based calculator model for the risk–benefit equation taking into account all the relevant variables which would help guide both women and their health care professionals.

References

1. Shufelt C, Bairey Merz CN. Reassurance for many Healthy Women Considering HRT. *BMJ* 2017;359:4652.

2. Baber RJ, Panay N, Fenton A. IMS recommendations on women's midlife health and menopause hormone therapy. *Climacteric* 2016;19(2):109–50.

3. Menopause: diagnosis and management NICE guideline [NG23]. November 2015. www.nice.org.uk/guidance/ng23

4. Avis NE, et al. Duration of menopausal vasomotor symptoms over the menopause transition study of Women's Health. *JAMA Intern Med* 2015;175(4):531–9.

5. Maclennan AH, Broadbent JL, Lester S, Moore V. Oral oestrogen and combined oestrogen/progestogen therapy versus placebo for hot flushes. *Cochrane Database Syst Rev* 2004;4.

6. Pitkin J. Urogenital atrophy. British Menopause Society consensus statement. *Post Reprod Health* 2018;24(3):133–8.

7. Davis S, Baber R, Panya N, et al. Global Position Statement on the use of testosterone therapy for women. *Climacteric* 2019;104:4660–6.

8. Santen RJ, Allred DC, Ardoin SP, et al. Postmenopausal hormone therapy: an Endocrine Society Scientific statement. *J Clin Endocrinol Metab* 2010;95:S7–66.

9. Boardman HMP, Hartley L, Eisinga A, Main C, Roquéi, Figuls M, Bonfill Cosp X, Gabriel Sanchez R, Knight B. Hormone therapy for preventing cardiovascular disease in post-menopausal women. *Cochrane Database Syst Rev* 2015;3.

10. Collaborative Group on Hormonal Factors in Breast Cancer. Type and timing of menopausal hormone therapy and breast cancer risk: individual participant meta-analysis of the worldwide epidemiological evidence. *Lancet* 2019. doi 10.1016/S0140-6736(19)31709-X

Selective Estrogen Receptor Modulators (SERMs) and Menopausal Hormone Therapy (MHT)

Steven R. Goldstein

SERMs (selective estrogen receptor modulators) are unique synthetic compounds that bind to the estrogen receptor and, depending on their unique conformational change, will either initiate estrogen agonistic activity or antagonistic activity. There are many that have come to market and others that have not. The first, for all practical purposes, was **tamoxifen** (although, clomiphene citrate is often considered a SERM). Approved in the US for treatment of breast cancer in 1978, tamoxifen became the most widely prescribed anti-cancer drug worldwide. When news of its ability to cause a small number of endometrial carcinomas surfaced, there was renewed interest in the SERM **raloxifene**, whose preclinical work suggested that, in experimental animals, it behaved differently in the uterus. In the US, raloxifene was approved for prevention of osteoporosis in 1997, treatment of osteoporosis in 1999, and breast cancer risk reduction in 2009. Tamoxifen is also currently approved for breast cancer risk reduction.

Any more in-depth analysis of these and other SERMs is beyond the scope of this chapter. Specifically, this chapter seeks to address the use of SERMs in menopausal hormone therapy (MHT). Currently, there are two such SERMs: **ospemifene**, approved as an oral agent to treat moderate to severe dyspareunia as well as vaginal dryness due to vulvo-vaginal atrophy of menopause, and **bazedoxifene**, used as a stand-alone drug for osteoporosis as well as in combination with conjugated estrogen for prevention of osteoporosis and treatment of moderate to severe vasomotor symptoms.

Ospemifene and Urogenital Atrophy

Estrogen and androgen deficiency from menopause causes vulvo-vaginal and urogenital changes and a plethora of symptoms, most prominently dyspareunia. The nomenclature recently has been expanded to genitourinary syndrome of menopause (GSM).

Reproductive hormone deficiency leads to vulvar and vaginal thinning, loss of rugal folds, diminished elasticity, diminished vaginal glycogen, and decreased acidity (increased pH) of the vaginal secretions, thereby reducing the vagina's natural defences [1].

Few women with GSM report their symptoms to their health care professionals [2], and conversely most health care professionals do not sufficiently query patients or inform them of their therapeutic options. Furthermore, class labelling of most available treatments has emphasized unsubstantiated risks [3] (i.e. increased endometrial cancer, stroke, myocardial infarction [MI], deep vein thrombosis [DVT], pulmonary embolism [PE], probable dementia, and invasive breast cancer), thus resulting in only 7 per cent of symptomatic women using any pharmacologic agent [4].

Clinical Development of Ospemifene

Until recently, all available vulvo-vaginal atrophy (VVA)/GSM treatments were systemic or local steroid hormones (estradiol, conjugated estrogens, dehydroepiandrosterone [DHEA]). Fear of estrogens from the 'class labelling' and the nuisance of vaginal administration undermines utilization for some women.

Ospemifene, a third-generation SERM originally developed for osteoporosis, has estrogenic effects on bone, lipids and vaginal tissue while remaining antiestrogenic or neutral in the breast and endometrium, respectively [5]. Multiple phase 3, placebo-controlled, clinical trials were conducted [6, 7]. Compared to placebo, ospemifene improved superficial cells and reduced parabasal cells as seen on a maturation index; lowered vaginal pH, and improved most bothersome symptoms (original studies for dyspareunia). This resulted in US Food and Drug Administration (FDA) approval for moderate to severe dyspareunia from vulvo-vaginal atrophy of menopause. Subsequent studies allowed for the indication to be broadened to include moderate to severe dryness due to menopause [8]. The American College of Obstetricians and Gynecologists (ACOG) endorsed ospemifene (Level A evidence) as first-line therapy for dyspareunia noting absent endometrial stimulation [9]. The most common adverse reactions in these ospemifene trials versus placebo were hot flashes and sweating (9.1 per cent vs 3.2 per cent), and muscle spasms (3.2 per cent vs 0.9 per cent), mostly leg cramps [6, 7]. Only 1 per cent of participants discontinued due to hot flashes, and there were no differences in rates of bleeding or breast tenderness.

Endometrial Safety

There is a boxed warning in the ospemifene label that says, 'in the uterus, ospemifene has estrogenic agonist effects' [10]. Despite the fact that ospemifene is not an estrogen (it's a SERM), it goes on to state, 'there is an increased risk of endometrial cancer in a woman with a uterus who uses unopposed estrogen'. This statement actually caused *The Medical Letter* to initially suggest that patients receiving ospemifene also should receive a progestational agent (something they later retracted) [11, 12]. In trying to understand why the labelling might possibly be worded in such a way, one has to review the actual data and understand the error the FDA made in response to the poorly named entity, 'weakly proliferative endometrium'. If one combines any proliferative endometrium (weakly + actively + disordered) in the clinical trial, 86.1 per 1000 in the ospemifene-treated patients (versus 13.3 per 1000 for those taking placebo) had any one of the proliferative types. The problem is that actively proliferating endometrial glands will have mitotic activity in virtually every nucleus of the gland as well as abundant glandular progression, whereas 'weakly proliferative' is actually closer to inactive or atrophic endometrium with just an occasional mitotic figure in just a few of the nuclei of each gland.

Furthermore, at 1 year, the incidence of active proliferation with ospemifene was 1 per cent [13]. Compare this finding with the Uterine Safety Study for raloxifene – both doses of that agent had an incidence of active proliferation at 1 year of 3 per cent [11]. Furthermore, that study had an estrogen-only arm in which, at endpoint, the incidence of proliferative endometrium was 39 per cent and hyperplasia, 23 per cent [14]! Thus, it is evident that, in the endometrium, ospemifene is much more like the SERM raloxifene than it is like estrogen.

Other Effects of Ospemifene

Ospemifene was originally approved for use in the US in 2013. Since that time a great deal of clinical and preclinical work has been brought to the attention of clinicians. As a SERM, based on class effects, one would expect it to be an estrogen antagonist in breast and estrogenic in bone. Additionally, improvement in overactive bladder (OAB) symptoms as well as prevention of recurrent lower urinary tract infections have been reported.

Previous data have demonstrated that ospemifene inhibits breast cancer cell growth in in vitro cultures as well as experimental animals [15] and inhibits proliferation of human breast tissue epithelial cells [16], with such breast effects similar to tamoxifen and raloxifene. Thus, although one would not choose ospemifene as a primary treatment, or risk-reducing agent, for breast cancer, the *direction* of its activity in breast tissue is indisputable and is likely the reason that in the European Union, unlike in the US, it is approved to treat dyspareunia from VVA of menopause in women *with* a prior history of breast cancer.

Furthermore, with increased aging, the morbidity and mortality associated with osteoporotic fractures becomes increasingly important. Ospemifene effectively reduced bone loss in ovariectomized rats, with activity comparable to estradiol and raloxifene [17]. Clinical data from three phase 1 or 2 clinical trials found ospemifene 60 mg/day to have a positive effect on biochemical markers for bone turnover in healthy postmenopausal women with significant improvements relative to placebo and effects comparable to raloxifene [18]. Actual fracture or bone mineral density (BMD) data in postmenopausal women are lacking but it is known that there is a good correlation between biochemical markers for bone turnover and occurrence of fracture [19]. Once again, women needing treatment for osteoporosis should not be treated with ospemifene but women using ospemifene for dyspareunia can expect positive activity on bone metabolism.

Shiavi and colleagues [20] reported on 46 postmenopausal women with VVA and OAB syndrome who were evaluated at baseline and after 12 weeks of treatment with 60 mg/day of ospemifene. There was a statistically significant decrease in detrusor overactivity, mean number of voids, nocturia and urinary incontinence episodes.

That same research group [21] studied 39 women (mean age, 59) with a history of recurrent urinary tract infections (UTIs). Twenty-one of the 39 reported being sexually active. After treatment for 6 months with ospemifene 60 mg/day, only two of these women had a UTI confirmed by culture. Thus, the ospemifene behaved like estrogen, which has been shown to reduce recurrent UTIs [22].

Summary

Ospemifene is an oral SERM approved for treatment of moderate to severe dyspareunia as well as dryness from VVA due to menopause. The label currently states that, 'because ospemifene has not been tested in women with breast cancer, it should not be used in women with a history of breast cancer', although preclinical in vitro, experimental animal in vivo and human in vitro testing all point to antagonistic activity in the breast, similar to other SERMs. The preclinical animal data and human markers of bone turnover all support the antiresorptive action of ospemifene on bones. Thus, it appears, one can safely surmise that the *direction* of activity of ospemifene in bone and breast is virtually indisputable. The *magnitude* of that activity is, however, unstudied. Therefore, in trying to choose an agent to treat women with dyspareunia or vaginal dryness from VVA of menopause, determination of any potential add-on benefit for that particular patient in either bone and/or breast is appropriate. There is also promising preliminary data that suggest a positive effect of ospemifene in patients with OAB or recurrent UTIs. Clearly, further study for both of these is necessary.

Bazedoxifene and Combined Bazedoxifene/Conjugated Estrogen

Osteoporosis is widespread in postmenopausal women because the decrease in estrogen production can accelerate bone loss [23]. High morbidity and mortality of osteoporosis-related fractures impose a heavy economic burden for patients and society [24]. Bazedoxifene is a SERM that has been shown to prevent bone loss and reduce the risk of new vertebral fractures in postmenopausal women with an increased risk of fracture and has a favourable safety/tolerability profile with no adverse effects on the reproductive system [25–27]. A meta-analysis of four randomized, placebo-controlled trials [28] showed that bazedoxifene can significantly decrease the incidence of vertebral fracture at follow-up of 5–7 years as well as confirming the long-term favourable safety/tolerability of bazedoxifene with no increase in adverse events, serious adverse events, myocardial infarction, stroke, venous thromboembolic event and breast carcinoma using bazedoxifene. However, bazedoxifene may result in an increased incidence of hot flushes and leg cramps across 7 years.

In summary, bazedoxifene shows an important ability to reduce the risk of vertebral fracture, and increase spine BMD at 3 and 7 years in postmenopausal women as well as showing long-term favourable safety/tolerability.

TSEC (Tissue-Specific Estrogen Complex)

The rationale for developing a tissue-specific estrogen complex is the partnering of a SERM with one or more estrogens to achieve pharmacologic results based on their blended tissue-selective activity profile [29]. The desire to pursue this grows mainly out of data derived from the two arms of the Women's Health Initiative. In the arm that combined conjugated estrogen with medroxyprogesterone acetate through 11.3 years, there was a 25 per cent increase in the incidence of invasive breast cancer, which was statistically significant [30]. Contrast that with the arm in hysterectomized women who received only *conjugated* estrogen (often inaccurately referred to as the 'estrogen-only' arm of the WHI). In that study, the relative risk of invasive breast cancer was reduced 23 per cent and was also statistically significant. Thus, it appears that the culprit in the breast cancer incidence difference in these two arms was the addition of the progestogen medroxyprogesterone acetate. It is well known that a progestogen is only added to confer endometrial protection to those patients with a uterus who are receiving any estrogenic therapy. Thus, the question arises, can one protect the endometrium with a non-progestogen substance (i.e. a SERM) and, thus, avoid the negative consequences especially in the breast (as well as bleeding) seen with the combination of estrogen plus a progestogen in the WHI? As further evidence of the above, Manson and colleagues [31] looked at mortality outcomes in the Women's Health Initiative trials with 18-year cumulative follow-up. Although, all-cause mortality, cancer mortality, cardiovascular mortality were not significantly different in either arm, when one drills down on breast cancer mortality alone, there is a difference between conjugated estrogen plus medroxy-progesterone versus placebo in conjugated estrogen alone versus placebo. In the CEE plus MPA arm, there was a 44 per cent increase, which, although trending towards statistical significance ($p = 0.07$), was not quite statistically significant. On the other hand, the CE-only arm had a 45 per cent reduction in breast cancer mortality, with $p = 0.02$ and was thus statistically significant. Various SERMs were looked at in preclinical trials and bazedoxifene was chosen because of its potent uterine protective qualities. In fact, bazedoxifene is the only SERM that has actually been shown to decrease endometrial thickness compared to placebo in a clinical trial [32]. Preclinical trials showed that a combination of BZA/CE in various doses of estrogen resulted in uterine wet weight in an ovariectomized rat model that was no different than placebo [33]. In terms of effects on breast, preclinical models showed that conjugated estrogen resulted in less mammary duct elongation and end bud proliferation than estradiol by itself [34] and that the combination of CE/BZA resulted in mammary duct elongation and end bud prolifera-tion that was similar to the ovariectomized animal and considerably less than a combination of estradiol with bazedoxifene [34].

Five phase 3 studies known as the SMART (Selective estrogens, Menopause, And Response Therapy) trials were then conducted. Collectively they looked at frequency and severity of vasomotor symptoms, bone mineral density, bone turnover markers, lipid profiles, sleep, quality of life, breast density and endometrial safety [35]. On the basis of these trials in over 7500 women, the US Food and Drug Administration approved this conjugated estrogen 0.45 mg/bazedoxifene 20 mg compound in 2013 and it was branded as Duavee in the US and Duavive outside the US.

In terms of frequency of vasomotor symptoms (VMS) there was a 74 per cent reduc-tion from baseline at 12 weeks, which, compared to placebo, had a p-value of < 0.001 as well as a 37 per cent reduction in VMS severity score ($p < 0.001$) [36]. There were statistically significant improvements in lumbar spine and hip BMD ($p < 0.01$) for women 1–5 years since menopause as well as those greater than 5 years since menopause [37].

The incidence of endometrial hyperplasia at 12 months was consistently less than 1 per cent, which is the FDA guidance for approval of hormone therapies. The incidence of bleeding or spotting in each 4-week interval over 12 months mirror-imaged placebo and ranged from 3.9 per cent in the first 4-week interval to 1.7 per cent in the last 4 weeks, compared to CE 0.45 mg/MPA 1.5 mg, which had a 20.8 per cent incidence of bleed or spotting in the first 4-week interval and was still 8.8 per cent in the last 4 weeks [38]. This is extremely relevant in clinical practice. There was no difference from placebo in breast cancer incidence, breast pain or tenderness, abnormal mammograms, or breast density at month 12 [39–41].

Realize that all of these data were for this particular estrogen (conjugated estrogen) with this particular SERM (bazedoxifene). Others have tried to combine raloxifene and 17 beta-estradiol to obtain similar results [42]. That study was meant to be a 52-week treatment study with either raloxifene 60 mg alone or in combination with 17 beta-estradiol 1 mg/day on vasomotor symptoms and endometrial safety. The study was stopped early because signs of endometrial stimulation were observed in the raloxifene plus estradiol group. Thus, one cannot combine *any* estrogen with *any* SERM and expect similar results.

In summary, this particular combination of conjugated estrogen/bazedoxifene is approved for treatment of vasomotor symptoms of menopause as well as prevention of osteoporosis. Although not approved for treatment of moderate to severe vulvo-vaginal atrophy, it should allow the prevention of younger women who initiate treatment from developing moderate to severe symptoms of VVA. Finally, this drug should be protective of breast. As discussed above conjugated estrogen has clearly shown a reduction in breast cancer incidence and mortality and bazedoxifene is a SERM. All SERMs have been shown, as a class effect, to be antiestrogens in breast tissue as well as abundant preclinical data that point in that direction. Thus, this combination of conjugated estrogen/bazedoxifene may well provide a new paradigm of hormone therapy that is progestogen free, in whom the benefit/risk ratio is severely tilted towards its benefits.

References

1. Wilson JD, Lee RA, Balen AH, Rutherford AJ. Bacterial vaginal flora in relation to changing oestrogen levels. *Int J STD AIDS* 2007;18(5):308–11.

2. Parish SJ, Nappi RE, Krychman ML, et al. Impact of vulvovaginal health on postmenopausal women: a review of surveys on symptoms of vulvo-vaginal atrophy. *Int J Womens Health* 2013;5:437–47.

3. Crandall CJ, Hovey KM, Andrews CA, et al. Breast cancer, endometrial cancer, and cardiovascular events in participants who used vaginal estrogen in the Women's Health Initiative Observational Study. *Menopause* 2018;25(1):11–20.

4. Kingsberg SA, Krychman M, Graham S, et al. The Women's EMPOWER Survey: identifying women's perceptions on vulvar and vaginal atrophy and its treatment. *J Sex Med* 2017;14(3):413–24.

5. Berga SL. Profile of ospemifene in the breast. *Reprod Sci* 2013;20(10):1130–6.

6. Bachmann GA, Komi JO, Ospemifene Study Group. Ospemifene effectively treats vulvovaginal atrophy in postmenopausal women: results from a pivotal phase 3 study. *Menopause* 2010;17(3):480–6.

7. Portman DJ, Bachmann GA, Simon JA, Ospemifene Study Group. Ospemifene, a novel selective estrogen receptor modulator for treating dyspareunia associated with postmenopausal vulvar and vaginal atrophy. *Menopause* 2013;20 (6):623–30.

8. Archer DF, Goldstein SR, Simon JA, Waldbaum AS, Sussman SA, Altomare C, Zhu J, Yoshida Y, Schaffer S, Soulban G. Efficacy and safety of ospemifene in postmenopausal women with moderate-to-severe vaginal dryness: a phase 3, randomized, double-blind, placebo-controlled, multicenter trial. *Menopause* 2019;26(6):611–21.

9. ACOG Practice Bulletin No. 141: management of menopausal symptoms. *Obstet Gynecol* 2014;123(1):202–16.

10. Osphena [package insert]. 2018. Shionogi Inc.

11. Ospemifene (Osphena) for dyspareunia. *Med Lett Drugs Ther* 2013;55(1420):55–6.

12. Addendum: Ospemifene (Osphena) for dyspareunia (*Med Lett Drugs Ther* 2013;55:55). *Med Lett Drugs Ther* 2013;55 (1427):84.

13. Goldstein SR, Bachmann G, Lin V, et al. Endometrial safety profile of ospemifene 60 mg when used for long-term treatment of vulvar and vaginal atrophy for up to 1 year [abstract]. *Climacteric* 2011;14 Suppl 1:S57.

14. Goldstein SR, Scheele WH, Rajagopalan SK, et al. A 12-month comparative study of raloxifene, estrogen, and placebo on the postmenopausal endometrium. *Obstet Gynecol* 2000;95 (1):95–103.

15. Qu Q, Zheng H, Dahllund J, et al. Selective estrogenic effects of a novel triphenylethylene compound, FC1271a, on bone, cholesterol level, and reproductive tissues in intact and

ovariectomized rats. *Endocrinology* 2000;141(2):809–20.

16. Eigeliene N, Kangas L, Hellmer C, et al. Effects of ospemifene, a novel selective estrogen-receptor modulator, on human breast tissue ex vivo. *Menopause* 2016;23 (7):719–30.

17. Kangas L, Unkila M. Tissue selectivity of ospemifene: pharmacologic profile and clinical implications. *Steroids* 2013;78 (12–13):1273–80.

18. Constantine GD, Kagan R, Miller PD. Effects of ospemifene on bone parameters including clinical biomarkers in postmenopausal women. *Menopause* 2016;23(6):638–44.

19. Gerdhem P, Ivaska KK, Alatalo SL, et al. Biochemical markers of bone metabolism and prediction of fracture in elderly women. *J Bone Miner Res* 2004;19 (3):386–93.

20. Schiavi MC, Zullo MA, Faiano P, et al. Retrospective analysis in 46 women with vulvovaginal treated with ospemifene for 12 weeks: improvement in overactive bladder symptoms. *Gynecol Endocrinol* 2017;33(12):942–5.

21. Schiavi MC, Di Pinto A, Sciuga V, et al. Prevention of recurrent lower urinary tract infections in postmenopausal women with genitourinary syndrome: outcome after 6 months of treatment with ospemifene. *Gynecol Endocrinol* 2018;34 (2):140–3.

22. Brostrøm S, Lose G. Oestrogen for prevention of recurrent urinary tract infections in postmenopausal women – a survey of a Cochrane review [in Danish]. *Ugeskr Laeger* 2009;171(36):2568–71.

23. Unni S, Yao Y, Milne N, et al. An evaluation of clinical risk factors for estimating fracture risk in postmenopausal osteoporosis using an electronic medical record database. *Osteoporos Int* 2015;26:581–7.

24. Silverman SL, Kupperman ES, Bukata SV, Members of IOFFWG. Fracture healing: a consensus report from the International Osteoporosis Foundation Fracture

Working Group. *Osteoporos Int* 2016;27:2197–206.

25. Silverman SL, Chines AA, Kendler DL, et al. Sustained efficacy and safety of bazedoxifene in preventing fractures in postmenopausal women with osteoporosis: results of a 5-year, randomized, placebo-controlled study. *Osteoporos Int* 2012;23:351–63.

26. de Villiers TJ, Chines AA, Palacios S, et al. Safety and tolerability of bazedoxifene in postmenopausal women with osteoporosis: results of a 5-year, randomized, placebo-controlled phase 3 trial. *Osteoporos Int* 2011;22:567–76.

27. Silverman SL, Christiansen C, Genant HK, et al. Efficacy of bazedoxifene in reducing new vertebral fracture risk in postmenopausal women with osteoporosis: results from a 3-year, randomized, placebo-, and active-controlled clinical trial. *J Bone Miner Res* 2008;23:1923–34.

28. Peng L, Luo Q, Lu H. Efficacy and safety of bazedoxifene in postmenopausal women with osteoporosis: a systematic review and meta-analysis. *Medicine* 2017;96(49): e8659.

29. Komm BS, Mirkin S. Incorporating bazedoxifene/conjugated estrogens into the current paradigm of menopausal therapy. *Int J Womens Health* 2012;4:129–40.

30. Anderson GL, Chlebowski RT, Aragaki AK, et al. Conjugated equine oestrogen and breast cancer incidence and mortality in postmenopausal women with hysterectomy: extended follow-up of the Women's Health Initiative Randomized Trial. *Lancet Oncol* 2012;13:476–86.

31. Manson JE, Aragaki AK, Rossouw JE, et al. Menopausal hormone therapy and long-term all-cause and cause-specific mortality: The Women's Health Initiative Randomized Trials. *JAMA* 2017;318:927–38.

32. Ronkin S, Notthington R, Baracat E, et al. Endometrial effects of bazedoxifene acetate, a novel selective estrogen receptor

modulator, in postmenopausal women. *Obstet Gynecol* 2005;105:1397–404.

33. Kharode Y, Bodine PV, Miller CP, Lyttle CR, Komm BS. The pairing of a selective estrogen receptor modulator, bazedoxifene, with conjugated estrogens as a new paradigm for the treatment of menopausal symptoms and osteoporosis prevention. *Endocrinology* 2008;149:6084–91.

34. Song Y, Santen RJ, Wang JP, Yue W. Effects of the conjugated equine estrogen/bazedoxifene tissue-selective estrogen complex (TSEC) on mammary gland and breast cancer in mice. *Endocrinology* 2012;153:5706–15.

35. Umland EM, Karel L, Santoro N, et al. Bazedoxifene and conjugated equine estrogen: a combination product for the management of vasomotor symptoms and osteoporosis prevention associated with menopause. *Pharmacotherapy* 2016;36:548–61.

36. Pinkerton JV, Utian WH, Constantine G, Oliver S, Pickar JH. Relief of vasomotor symptoms with the tissue-selective estrogen complex containing bazedoxifene/conjugated estrogens: a randomized, controlled trial. *Menopause* 2009;16:1116–24.

37. Lindsay R, Gallagher JC, Kagan R, Pickar JH, Constaine G. Efficacy of tissue-selective estrogen complex of bazedoxifene/conjugated estrogens for osteoporosis prevention in at-risk postmenopausal women. *Fertil Steril* 2009;92:1045–52.

38. Kagan R, Goldstein SR, Pickar JH, Komm BS. Patient considerations in the management of menopausal symptoms: role of conjugated estrogens with bazedoxifene. *Ther Clin Risk Manag* 2016;12:549–62.

39. Komm BS, Mirkin S, Jenkins SN. Development of conjugated estrogens/bazedoxifene, the first tissue selective estrogen complex (TSEC) for management of menopausal hot flashes and postmenopausal bone loss. *Steroids* 2014;90:71–81.

40. Mirkin S, Pinkerton JV, Kagan R, et al. Gynecologic safety of conjugated estrogens plus bazedoxifene: pooled analysis of five Phase 3 trials. *J Women's Health* 2016;25:431–42.

41. Pinkerton JV, Harvey JA, Pan K, et al. Breast effects of bazedoxifene-conjugated estrogens: a randomized controlled trial. *Obstet Gynecol* 2013;121:959–68.

42. Stovall DW, Utian WH, Gass MLS, et al. The effects of combined raloxifene and oral estrogen on vasomotor symptoms and endometrial safety. *Menopause* 2007;14:510–17.

Chapter 25

Non-hormonal Treatments for Menopausal Symptoms

Jenifer Sassarini

There are a number of symptoms associated with perimenopause and decreasing estrogen levels, although some women will experience none of these. They include hot flashes and night sweats (vasomotor symptoms), vaginal symptoms, depression, anxiety, irritability and mood swings (psychological effects), joint pains, migraines or headaches, sleeping problems and urinary incontinence.

With improved health care and increased life expectancy, women spend a considerable proportion of their lives (30 years on average) after the menopause. At present 36 per cent of women in the UK are over 50 years of age, and it is estimated that approximately 75 per cent of women will experience some symptoms related to estrogen deficiency during the menopausal transition. The most commonly reported symptoms are vasomotor symptoms, and recent evidence suggests that these may last on average 7.4 years [1]. The British Menopause Society has long held the belief that HRT is safe and effective, and has published the affirmation of this in the light of data from the Danish and KEEPS trials; however, there is still concern amongst general practitioners and women that the risks of HRT far outweigh the benefits and for this reason there is an interest in non-hormonal alternatives.

Care must be taken though when recommending non-hormonal alternatives as first-line therapy with the belief that they are more effective than HRT, as selective interpretation of data and personal sentiments can cloud objective evaluation of the literature. There are of course a group of women for whom hormonal therapy is not suitable and, for this reason, increasing our understanding of alternative treatments is vital.

Pathophysiology of a Hot Flash

The exact pathophysiology of flashing is not known, although it is generally accepted that falling estrogens play a main role; flashes generally occur at times of relative estrogen withdrawal and replacing it will result in improvement in most women. However, whilst estrogen concentrations remain low after the menopause, most vasomotor symptoms will diminish with time, and therefore a fall in estrogen concentration does not seem to provide the complete answer. It has also been found that circulating levels of estrogen do not differ significantly between symptomatic and asymptomatic postmenopausal women.

Furthermore, it is thought that withdrawal of estrogen, rather than low circulating estrogen levels, is the central change that leads to hot flashes and there are several observations to support this theory. The abrupt estrogen withdrawal due to bilateral oophorectomy in premenopausal women is associated with a higher prevalence of flashes than in those women who experience a gradual physiological menopause, and young

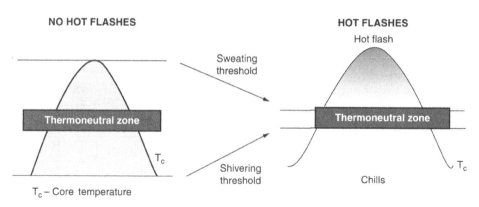

Figure 25.1 Thermoregulatory zone in women with flashes compared with postmenopausal women who do not have flashes.

women with gonadal dysgenesis, who have low levels of endogenous estrogen, do not experience hot flashes unless they receive several months of estrogen therapy and then abruptly discontinue its use.

Hot flashes are characterized by a feeling of intense warmth, often accompanied by profuse sweating, anxiety, skin reddening and palpitations, and sometimes followed by chills. In this respect, flashes resemble a systemic heat dissipation response, which is controlled, in humans, by the medial preoptic area of the hypothalamus.

Studies using an ultrasensitive temperature probe suggest that hot flashes are triggered by small elevations in core body temperature acting within a narrowed thermoneutral zone in symptomatic postmenopausal women [2, 3]. Those studies found that small but significant elevations in T_c precede most hot flash episodes and that postmenopausal women with hot flashes had a narrower thermoregulatory zone compared with postmenopausal women who do not flash (see Figure 25.1). This narrowing was mainly due to a lowering of the sweating threshold in symptomatic women, and estrogen replacement has been shown to elevate this threshold, with reduced hot flash occurrence.

Changes in core temperature may also be associated with alterations in neuroendocrine pathways involving steroid hormones, noradrenaline (NA), the endorphins and serotonin (Figure 25.2). Noradrenaline and serotonin, particularly, are thought to play a key role.

Over recent years, our understanding of the kisspeptin-neurokinin B (NKB)- dynorphin (KNDy) signalling system in the hypothalamus has increased. It has become clear that these KNDy neurons act as the proximate stimulus of GnRH secretion, and as such are responsible for the control of the reproductive axis, via GnRH. NKB neurons also project into the medial preoptic area, the hypothalamic site of thermoregulation, and there is evidence that these neurons may play a key role in vasomotor symptoms seen at the time of menopause.

Non-hormonal Pharmacological Preparations

Clonidine

Clonidine is an α2-adrenergic agonist licensed for the treatment of hypertension, migraines and postmenopausal vasomotor symptoms.

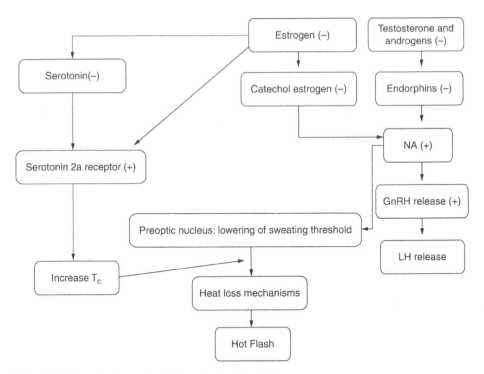

Figure 25.2 Postulated neurochemical mechanism of hot flashes.

Monoamines have been shown to play an important role in the control of thermo-regulation, and animal studies have shown that noradrenaline (NA) acts to narrow the thermoregulatory zone. Noradrenergic stimulation of the medial preoptic area of the hypothalamus in monkeys and baboons causes peripheral vasodilatation, heat loss and a drop in core temperature, similar to changes which occur in women during hot flashes.

It has also been shown that plasma levels of a noradrenaline metabolite are significantly increased both before and during hot flash episodes in postmenopausal women.

The hypotensive effect of clonidine is thought to be mediated mainly through selective stimulation of presynaptic α-adrenergic receptors in the region of the vasomotor centre in the medulla; however, it has a dual action. When first administered, clonidine stimulates peripheral α1-adrenoceptors (ARs) resulting in vasoconstriction, but subsequently acts on the central ARs to inhibit sympathetic drive resulting in vasodilatation.

It has also been shown to widen the thermoregulatory zone in humans. Clonidine is used for postoperative shivering because it is thought that, like general anesthetic agents and sedatives, it decreases shivering thresholds by a generalized impairment of central thermoregulatory control. It has also been demonstrated to increase the sweating threshold.

A meta-analysis [4] has examined 10, poor-to-fair-quality, trials in which clonidine (0.1 mg/day) demonstrated a moderate, but statistically significant, reduction in hot flash frequency and severity at 4 and 8 weeks. This suggests that clonidine is an effective alternative to hormonal therapy; however, adverse effects, including dry mouth, insomnia and drowsiness, were noted in 8 out of 10 trials.

Selective Serotonin (and Noradrenaline) Reuptake Inhibitors

Serotonin is involved in many bodily functions including mood, anxiety, sleep, sexual behaviour and thermoregulation. Estrogen withdrawal is associated with decreased blood serotonin levels, and short-term estrogen therapy has been shown to increase these levels. Selective serotonin reuptake inhibitors (SSRIs) are a group of drugs typically used as antidepressants, which are thought to function by blocking the reuptake of serotonin to the presynaptic cell. This increases the amount of serotonin in the synaptic cleft available to bind to the postsynaptic cell. Selective serotonin reuptake inhibitors were commonly prescribed for the treatment of depression in women undergoing treatment for breast cancer. Anecdotally, these same women were noted to have an improvement in their vasomotor symptoms, which occurred as a side effect of treatment. Studies were then carried out to determine the efficacy of these as an effective treatment for flashing.

A meta-analysis [4] assessed two double-blind randomized placebo-controlled trials (fair and good quality) comparing paroxetine to placebo and concluded that paroxetine was more effective than placebo in reducing the frequency and severity of hot flashes. One study included predominantly women with breast cancer using tamoxifen. Doses used varied from 10 mg/day to 25 mg/day, and although efficacy did not vary with dose, those on higher doses experienced more side effects, including nausea, headaches, drowsiness or insomnia.

This same meta-analysis assessed a further two randomized controlled trials comparing venlafaxine and placebo. In one fair-quality trial, an improvement in quality of life (51 per cent with venlafaxine compared with 15 per cent placebo users) was demonstrated despite no reduction in frequency of flashes. In the second, a good-quality trial, venlafaxine at doses of 37.5, 75, 150 mg/day decreased hot flash frequency compared with placebo. Improvement appeared to be greater with the two higher doses, although adverse effects included dry mouth, constipation, decreased appetite, nausea and sleeplessness. Nausea typically improves in 2–3 days, and can be improved by titrating the dose slowly. Venlafaxine was also found to be superior to clonidine, decreasing flashes by 57 per cent compared with 37 per cent in clonidine users.

Fluoxetine (20–30 mg/day) and citalopram (30 mg/day) were no better than placebo for flash frequency or score improvement.

Two further studies, published following the meta-analysis by Nelson, and included in a Cochrane systematic review examining non-hormonal treatments in women with breast cancer [5], demonstrated a reduction in the number and severity of flashes with venlafaxine at low dose and at 75 mg/day when compared with placebo.

Desvenlafaxine is a novel serotonin-norepinephrine reuptake inhibitor, highly selective for serotonin and norepinephrine transporters, with weak or no affinity for dopamine receptors and transporters. Desvenlafaxine restored thermoregulatory function more rapidly than estrogen replacement in two rodent models of vasomotor symptoms and in two double-blind randomized placebo-controlled trials [6, 7]; 100 and 150 mg were found to decrease number of hot flashes after 12 weeks compared with placebo.

Use of these drugs in women with breast cancer using tamoxifen is common; therefore consideration must be given to potential interactions. Tamoxifen must be metabolized by the cytochrome P450 enzyme system, predominantly cytochrome P450 isoenzyme 2D6 (CYP2D6), to become active, and CYP2D6 is inhibited to varying degrees by SSRIs. Paroxetine is an exceptionally potent inhibitor, whereas sertraline inhibits to a lesser degree and citalopram and escitalopram are only weak inhibitors. Evidence is conflicting on the success rates of tamoxifen in preventing recurrence of breast cancer when using a concurrent SSRI. For those women who need to begin treatment with an SSRI for depression, citalopram or escitalopram may be the safest choice, however improvements in flashing are better with venlafaxine and desvenlafaxine, and these appear to be safe choices.

Gabapentin

The mechanism of action of gabapentin in the amelioration of vasomotor symptoms is unknown, but it is thought to involve a direct effect on the hypothalamic thermoregulatory centre.

Two double-blind randomized placebo-controlled trials, examined in a meta-analysis [4], both conducted in women with breast cancer, showed a significant reduction in frequency and severity of hot flashes when taking gabapentin 900 mg/day, but not when taking 300 mg/day. Titrated to 2400 mg/day continued to be superior to placebo but was not significantly different to estrogen 0.625 mg/day. However, dizziness, unsteadiness and fatigue were reported in the gabapentin-treated group and resulted in a higher dropout rate than in the control group.

Non-pharmacological Therapies

Phytoestrogens

Phytoestrogens are chemicals that resemble estrogen and are present in most plants, vegetables and fruits. There are three main types of phytoestrogens; soy isoflavones (the most potent), coumestans and lignans. Soyabean and red clover are also rich in phytoestrogens. These compounds are converted into weak estrogenic substances in the gastrointestinal tract.

Isoflavones are the most researched, and Nelson's meta-analysis included 17 RCTs. From six trials comparing Promensil (red clover isoflavone) with placebo, only one fair-quality trial found a reduction in flash frequency with Promensil, although there was no overall reduction in the meta-analysis, and no improvement in flash severity was demonstrated in any of the included trials.

Soy isoflavones were compared with placebo in the remaining 11 trials. The meta-analysis revealed an improvement in hot flashes after 12–16 weeks (four trials) and after 6 months (two trials), but were not significantly decreased in studies examining 4–6 weeks' use.

A systematic review [8] was also carried out by the Cochrane Collaboration. They included five trials in a meta-analysis, which demonstrated no significant decrease in the frequency of hot flashes with phytoestrogens.

Thirty trials were also studied comparing phytoestrogens with control. Some of the trials found that phytoestrogens alleviated the frequency and severity of hot flashes and night sweats when compared with placebo but many of the trials were of low quality or were underpowered. The great variability in the results of these trials may result in part from the difference in efficacy of the various types of phytoestrogens used, the exact treatment protocol and the fraction of equol producers in the cohort. It is claimed that only 30–40 per cent of the US population possess the gut microflora responsible for converting isoflavones to the active estrogenic equol. It should be noted that there was also a strong placebo response in most trials, ranging from 1 per cent to 59 per cent.

Black Cohosh

Black cohosh is a native American herb that is thought to behave as a selective estrogen receptor modulator (SERM) with mild central estrogenic effects.

A meta-analysis of several short-term and relatively small RCTs comparing black cohosh use with placebo 'revealed a trend towards reducing vasomotor symptoms', but only in cases of mild to moderate symptoms [9]. This was particularly notable when hot flashes were associated with sleep and mood disturbances. This was confirmed in another 12-week study of 304 women in addition to improvements in mood, sleep disorders, sexual disorders and sweating. In contrast, however, the recent Herbal Alternatives for Menopause Trial (HALT) [10], which compared black cohosh to both placebo and estrogen replacement over 12 months, suggested that black cohosh was ineffective in relieving vasomotor symptoms.

Whilst there has been no confirmation of its efficacy, many women, both cancer-free as well as breast cancer patients and survivors, will use black cohosh to relieve vasomotor symptoms. Nevertheless, it is important to exercise caution as there is limited information on its potential to influence breast cancer development or progression. No effect has been seen on mammary tumour development, which would suggest that black cohosh would not influence breast cancer risk if given to women before tumour formation, but there has been an increase in the incidence of lung metastases in tumour-bearing animals when compared with mice fed with an isoflavone-free control diet. Additional studies will be needed to correlate these findings to women taking different black cohosh products at various times during breast cancer development; however, these results suggest caution for women using black cohosh, especially for extended periods of time.

Hepatotoxicity has also been associated with black cohosh; however, a recent critical analysis and structured causality assessment has shown no causal relationship between treatment by black cohosh and liver disease.

Vitamin E

Only one randomized placebo-controlled trial involving vitamin E is available, in which 105 women with a history of breast cancer received placebo and vitamin E 800 IU daily for 4 weeks in a crossover design [11]. There was no improvement in frequency or severity of hot flashes with vitamin E when compared with placebo, and care must be taken when a toxic vitamin is ingested in excessive amounts.

Evening Primrose Oil

This is a widely used product for the treatment of menopausal symptoms, although the exact mechanism of action is not fully understood. Its effectiveness has been analysed in a double-blind randomized placebo-controlled trial. This trial used a combination of evening primrose oil (2000 mg/day) with vitamin E (10 mg/day) versus placebo and showed a significantly greater reduction in daytime flashes in the placebo group than in the treatment group. Unsurprisingly, there was a high dropout rate due to unrelieved symptoms, and this precluded reliable conclusions.

Lifestyle Modifications

There is evidence that body mass index (BMI), smoking, alcohol consumption and sedentary lifestyle are associated with reports of vasomotor symptoms; however, there are few papers reporting the direct effect that modifications have on flashes.

Data from the WHI trial in healthy women, however, demonstrate a reduction in hot flashes as a result of weight loss [12]. This is supported by a pilot study, suggesting that weight loss in overweight or obese healthy women is associated with a reduction in HFs [13, 14], although this study was designed to examine weight loss in women with urinary incontinence.

Smoking cessation has numerous health benefits, not exclusively alterations of endothelial function, which may be involved in the hot flash mechanism [15].

Exercise

As well as having significant physiologic benefits (for example cardiovascular and bone health), exercise may be one of the promising alternatives to HRT and if demonstrated to be effective in the treatment of vasomotor symptoms, is an inexpensive intervention that typically has few known side effects.

The Cochrane Collaboration carried out a systematic review [16] to examine the effectiveness of any type of exercise intervention in the management of vasomotor symptoms in symptomatic perimenopausal and postmenopausal women. Only one very small trial was considered suitable for inclusion, which found, not unexpectedly, that HRT was more effective than exercise.

However, a recent study reported that improvements in fitness mediated by exercise training may reduce the severity of physiological symptoms that occur during a post-menopausal hot flash [17].

An RCT by Cramer et al. [18], suggested that yoga was effective in reducing meno-pausal symptoms in breast cancer survivors. In a systematic review and meta-analysis of 13 RCTs on 1306 women, yoga compared with no treatment reduced total menopausal symptoms, HFs, psychological and urogenital symptoms without serious adverse events, and reduced hot flashes when compared to exercise controls [19].

CBT

Cognitive behavioural therapy (CBT) focuses on the links between physical symp-toms, thoughts, feelings and behaviour, and has been shown to reduce the problem rating score associated with hot flashes in healthy women and women with breast cancer [20].

The MENOS 1 RCT demonstrated improvements with CBT after 9 weeks compared with usual care. The improvement was maintained at 26 weeks from randomization and additional benefits to mood, sleep and quality of life were observed [21].

Improvements have been noted with both group and self-help CBT.

An Alternative Treatment: Stellate Ganglion Blockade

Stellate ganglion blocks have been carried out safely for more than 60 years, for pain syndromes and vascular insufficiency; 0.5 per cent bupivicaine is injected on the right side of the anterolateral aspect of the C6 vertebra under fluoroscopy and an effective block confirmed by the presence of Horner's syndrome.

A case report was published in 1985 of a 77-year-old man with flashing after orchiectomy. He was treated with a stellate ganglion blockade, based on the belief that the flashing centre has a sympathetic outflow to the stellate ganglion, and his attacks of flashing ceased. A pilot study of 13 women (age range 38–71 years), with a history of breast cancer, who suffered with severe hot flashes, demonstrated reductions in flash episodes and an improvement in sleep quality following stellate ganglion blockade. A more recent study revealed a benefit in only half of the 20 women in the study [22].

The first randomized, sham-controlled trial of SGB demonstrated improvements in moderate to severe HF, as well as objectively measured HF, but no overall reduction in frequency of vasomotor symptoms [23]. Whilst studies are limited and small, there were no adverse events reported in this trial, and it is thought that SGB may be considered to be safe when performed by experienced practitioners.

On the Horizon: NKB Antagonists

Two randomized placebo-controlled trials have evaluated the effects of oral neurokinin B receptor antagonists on hot flashes [24]. Both agents (MLE 4901 and fezolinetant) reduced hot flash frequency and severity by 40–50 per cent over placebo in postmenopausal women, with negligible side effects. As these inhibitors act on specific hot flash mediating pathways, they show promise as effective, non-hormonal agents to treat hot flashes, particularly useful in survivors of hormone-dependent gynaecological cancers. Long-term safety data for these drugs are still awaited.

Conclusion

Clonidine, SSRIs and gabapentin have all shown a significant improvement in flashing, whilst vitamin E and evening primrose oil have been shown to be of no benefit. Adverse effects may limit the use of clonidine and gabapentin, but SSRIs and SNRIs have a well-established safety profile and appear to have only minor adverse effects.

The evidence surrounding the efficacy of phytoestrogens and black cohosh is contradictory. Soy isoflavones may be more effective with longer-term use than other phytoestrogens, but black cohosh, or any compound with estrogenic properties, should be used with extreme caution in women with a history of breast cancer or any other estrogen-dependent disease.

Lifestyle modifications, exercise and CBT may be effective alternatives to prescribed and over-the-counter therapies, and should be discussed with women.

The effectiveness of stellate ganglion blockade for vasomotor symptoms is unconfirmed, therefore further studies are required. It is also worth considering that the uptake of this treatment may be limited as it is costly, invasive and the short-term side effects of Horner's syndrome may be unacceptable to some.

Long-term safety data are awaited for novel non-hormonal therapies, but are a potentially exciting prospect.

References

1. Avis NE, Crawford SL, Greendale G, Bromberger JT, Everson-Rose SA, Gold EB, Hess R, Joffe H, Kravitz HM, Tepper PG, Thurston RC1, Study of Women's Health Across the Nation. Duration of menopausal vasomotor symptoms over the menopause transition. *JAMA Intern Med* 2015 Apr;175(4):531–9.

2. Freedman RR. Biochemical: metabolic, and vascular mechanisms in menopausal hot flashes. *Fertil Steril* 1998;70:332–7.

3. Freedman RR, Krell W. Reduced thermoregulatory null zone in postmenopausal women with hot flashes. *Am J Obstet Gynecol* 1999;181:66–70.

4. Nelson HD, Vesco KK, Haney E, et al. Nonhormonal therapies for menopausal hot flashes: systematic review and meta-analysis. *JAMA* 2006;295:2057–71.

5. Rada G, Capurro D, Pantoja T, et al. Non-hormonal interventions for hot flushes in women with a history of breast cancer. *Cochrane Database Syst Rev* 2010;9: CD004923.

6. Speroff L, Gass M, Constantine GD, Olivier S, Study 315 Investigators. Efficacy and tolerability of desvenlafaxine succinate treatment for menopausal vasomotor symptoms: a randomized controlled trial. *Obstet Gynecol* 2008;111:77–87.

7. Archer DF, Dupont CM, Constantine GD, Pickar JH, Olivier S, Study 319 Investigators. Desvenlafaxine for the treatment of vasomotor symptoms associated with menopause: a double-blind, randomized, placebo-controlled trial of efficacy and safety. *Am J Obstet Gynecol* 2009;200:238e1–e10.

8. Lethaby A, Marjoribanks J, Kronenberg F, et al. Phytoestrogens for vasomotor menopausal symptoms. *Cochrane Database Syst Rev* 2007;4:CD001395.

9. Wong VC, Lim CE, Luo X, Wong WS. Current alternative and complementary therapies used in menopause. *Gynecol Endocrinol* 2009;25:166–74.

10. Newton KM, Reed SD, LaCroix AZ, et al. Treatment of vasomotor symptoms of menopause with black cohosh, multibotanicals, soy, hormone therapy, or placebo: a randomized trial. *Ann Intern Med* 2005;145:869–79.

11. Barton DL, Loprinzi CL, Quella SK, et al. Prospective evaluation of vitamin E for hot flashes in breast cancer survivors. *J Clin Oncol* 1998;16:495–500.

12. Kroenke CH, Caan BJ, Stefanick ML, Anderson G, Brzyski R, Johnson KC, LeBlanc E, Lee C, La Croix AZ, Park HL, Sims ST, Vitolins M, Wallace R. Effects of a dietary intervention and weight change on vasomotor symptoms in the Women's Health Initiative. *Menopause* 2012 Sep;19 (9):980–8.

13. Thurston RC, Ewing LJ, Low CA, et al. Behavioral weight loss for the management of menopausal hot flashes: a pilot study. *Menopause* 2015;22:59–65.

14. Huang AJ, Subak LL, Wing R, et al. An intensive behavioral weight loss intervention and hot flushes in women. *Arch Intern Med* 2010;170:1161–7.

15. Sassarini J, Fox H, Ferrell W, Sattar N, Lumsden MA. Vascular function and cardiovascular risk factors in women with severe flushing. *Clin Endocrinol* 2011 Jan;74(1):97–103.

16. Daley A, Stokes-Lampard H, Mutrie N, MacArthur C. Exercise for vasomotor menopausal symptoms. *Cochrane Database Syst Rev* 2007;4:CD006108.

17. Bailey TG, Cable NT, Aziz N, et al. Exercise training reduces the acute physiological severity of post-menopausal hot flushes. *J Physiol* 2016;594:657–67.

18. Cramer H, Rabsilber S, Lauche R, Kümmel S, Dobos G. Yoga and meditation for menopausal symptoms in breast cancer survivors – a randomized controlled trial. *Cancer* 2015 Jul 1;121 (13):2175–84.

19. Cramer H, Peng W, Lauche R. Yoga for menopausal symptoms—a systematic review and meta-analysis. *Maturitas* 2018;109:13–25.

20. Ayers B, Smith M, Hellier J, et al. Effectiveness of group and self-help

cognitive behavior therapy in reducing problematic menopausal hot flushes and night sweats (MENOS 2): a randomized controlled trial. *Menopause* 2012;19:749–59.

21. Mann E, Smith MJ, Hellier J, et al. Cognitive behavioural treatment for women who have menopausal symptoms after breast cancer treatment (MENOS 1): a randomised controlled trial. *Lancet Oncol* 2012;13:309–18.

22. van Gastel P, Kallewaard J-W, van der Zanden M, de Boer H. Stellate-ganglion block as a treatment for severe postmenopausal flushing. *Climacteric* 2013;16:41–7.

23. Walega DR, Rubvvbounoussin LH, Banuvar S, et al. Effects of stellate ganglion block on vasomotor symptoms: findings from a randomized controlled clinical trial in postmenopausal women. *Menopause* 2014;21(8):807–14.

24. Prague JK, Roberts RE, Comninos AN, Clarke S, Jayasena CN, Nash Z, Doyle C, Papadopoulou DA, Bloom SR, Mohideen P, Panay N, Hunter MS, Veldhuis JD, Webber LC, Huson L, Dhillo WS. Neurokinin 3 receptor antagonism as a novel treatment for menopausal hot flushes: a phase 2, randomised, double-blind, placebo-controlled trial. *Lancet* 2017;389 (10081):1809–20.

Chapter

26

Alternative Therapies for the Management of Menopausal Symptoms

Edzard Ernst and Paul Posadzki

Prevalence of Alternative Therapies: Use by Menopausal Women

For the purpose of this chapter, we operationally define alternative therapies (ATs) as medical interventions which are not usually used in conventional medicine. Other terms frequently employed to describe this sector include complementary, holistic, folk, traditional, natural or integrative (integrated) therapies/ medicine.

Our systematic review (SR) of 26 surveys including 32 465 menopausal women found that on average 50.5 per cent of them reported using ATs specifically for their menopausal symptoms [1]. The 12-month prevalence of use was on average 47.7 per cent (range: 33.1–56.2). Nearly one-third of the surveyed women declared themselves to be current/regular AT users. Fifty-five per cent did not disclose their use of ATs to their conventional health care team. The majority of women sought information about ATs from the Internet, i.e. doctors or other health care professionals were often not considered as a source of information about ATs. The most popular AT was herbal medicine, followed by relaxation therapies and yoga. Alternative therapies were perceived as effective by 60.5 per cent of all women using them (range: 42–98.8).

Expectations of Patients Using Alternative Therapies

For many health care professionals, this popularity of ATs is somewhat puzzling. They point out that conventional medicine is today more effective than it ever has been, and that turning to uncertain alternatives is therefore less than rational. The reasons for the present boom in ATs are certainly not easy to define, and numerous factors are likely to play a role:

- Incessant media hype
- Disappointment with conventional medicine
- Fear of side effects / hope for a cure without risk
- Affluence

In this context, it is relevant to ask what patients expect from ATs. We have attempted to answer this question by conducting a systematic review of all 73 surveys that addressed this issue [2]. A wide range of expectations emerged. In order of prevalence, they included:

- Hope to influence the natural history of the disease
- Disease prevention and health/general well-being promotion
- Being in control over one's health
- Symptom relief; boosting the immune system
- Emotional support
- Holistic care
- Improving quality of life
- Relief of side effects of conventional medicine
- Good therapeutic relationship
- Obtaining information
- Supporting the natural healing process
- Availability of treatment

Claims Made by Proponents of Alternative Therapies

Many patients with menopausal symptoms search the Internet in the hope of finding a safe and effective treatment for their condition. A woman using the Google search engine for 'alternative treatments for menopause' would currently be inundated by more than 5 million websites. Disappointingly, very few of these sources offer reliable information. Many seem to promote unproven or disproven treatments and some even discourage the use of proven conventional therapies.

Further evidence seems to confirm the assumption that women are frequently misled: after identifying the seven best-selling lay books on ATs, we assessed which treatments their authors recommended for a range of specific conditions. For menopausal symptoms, they advised 68 different ATs. There was very little consensus amongst the seven authors as to which treatments were recommendable, and the vast majority of the recommended therapies were not supported by sound evidence [3].

The Evidence for Alternative Therapies

Effectiveness

In an overview of the evidence from Systematic Reviews, randomized controlled trials (RCTs) and epidemiologic studies of ATs for the management of menopausal symptoms, we attempted to assess the existing data critically [4]. We found that some promising evidence was available for phytosterols and phytostanols for reducing increased low-density lipoprotein (LDL) and total cholesterol levels in postmenopausal women. Similarly, regular fibre intake seemed to be effective in reducing serum total cholesterol in hypercholesterolemic postmenopausal women. Black cohosh seemed to be effective therapy for relieving menopausal symptoms, primarily hot flashes, in early menopause. Phytoestrogens, including isoflavones and lignans, appeared to have only minimal effect on hot flashes but may have other positive health effects, e.g. on plasma lipid levels and bone loss [5]. Promising evidence also existed for the effectiveness of vitamin K, a combination of calcium and vitamin D as well as for a combination of walking combined with other weight-bearing exercise in reducing bone mineral density loss and the incidence of osteoporosis/fractures in postmenopausal women [6, 7]. In premenopausal women, encouraging evidence for the effectiveness of vitamin B6 supplementation has been found [8].

Relaxation therapies seem to have positive effects on menopausal symptoms [3]. For other commonly used ATs including probiotics, prebiotics, acupuncture, homeopathy and dehydroepiandrosterone sulfate (DHEA-S), placebo-controlled RCTs are scarce and the evidence was thus unconvincing [3]. Similarly, there is insufficient evidence for the effectiveness of other popular modalities such as yoga [4] or ginseng [9]. Our findings were confirmed in more recent reviews.[1]

Safety

Direct Risks

Consumers often assume that ATs are inherently safe, not least because the media incessantly promote this notion. However, the assumption is clearly not correct. As there are no (or very few) systems to monitor adverse effects of ATs, it is plausible that the documented risks merely represent the tip of a much bigger iceberg. In particular, oral supplements can cause adverse effects through

- The toxicity of an ingredient
- Interactions with prescribed medications
- Contamination
- Adulteration

Alternative therapies and therapists are usually not tightly regulated, which can increase their risks considerably. Table 26.1 summarizes the known risks of the types of ATs mentioned above.

Indirect Risks

Even if an AT is entirely safe, such as a highly diluted homeopathic remedy, there are indirect risks to consider [10]. The most obvious of those is that a curable condition might get treated for prolonged periods of time with a therapy that is ineffective. In fact, even the most harmless but ineffective AT can become life-threatening, if it is used as an alternative for treating a serious condition.

The Risk–Benefit Balance

It is often argued by proponents of ATs that the risks of their treatments are far less than those of conventional therapies. This may well be true, but it is fairly irrelevant for judging the value of any given intervention. Therapeutic decisions should never be guided by their effectiveness or their safety in isolation but by balancing the two factors. If a treatment has no or little demonstrable benefit, as seems to be the case for many ATs, then even relatively small risks would tilt this balance into the negative, and the treatment in question cannot be recommended

---

[1] www.ncbi.nlm.nih.gov/pubmed/28561959

Table 26.1 Risks of particular alternative treatments for menopause

Type of alternative treatment	Examples of adverse effects reported in medical literature
Acupuncture	Bleeding, infections, pneumothorax, nerve injury and death
Black cohosh	Gastrointestinal upset, rash, acute hepatitis, multiorgan failure
Dietary supplements (general)	Overdosing, toxicity, interactions with prescribed drugs
Ginseng	Anxiety, burning sensation, flu, headache, insomnia, pain, skin problem, gastrointestinal upset
Herbal remedies (general)	Adulteration, contamination, toxicity, herb/drug interactions
Homeopathy	Delay of effective therapy
Prebiotics	Bloating, abdominal pain, diarrhea, increase in gastroesophageal reflux
Probiotics	Sepsis, altered metabolism, or immune system functioning, increased sensitivity to allergens
Phytoestrogens	Disruption of endogenous hormone levels and the ovulatory cycle, changes in behaviour
Phytostanols	Lowered absorption of liposoluble vitamins antioxidants
Phytosterols	Diarrhea, constipation, skin problems
Relaxation	Worsening of psychological problems
Yoga	Bone fractures, ligament tears
Vitamin B6	Arrhythmia, acne, allergic reaction, drowsiness or sedation, headache, heartburn, loss of appetite, nausea, rash, recurrences of ulcerative colitis, vomiting
Vitamin D	Nausea, vomiting, weakness, kidney problems
Vitamin K	Difficulties in breathing or swallowing, enlarged liver, skin rashes, dizziness, irritability, muscle stiffness

for routine use. For this and other reasons, much of AT practised today is arguably unethical.[2]

Methodological Problems in Evaluating the Effectiveness of Alternative Therapies

Advocates of ATs often argue that it is unfair to insist on rigorous evidence for their treatments; not only are there no funds to carry out such necessary research, but there are also significant methodological problems in testing ATs for effectiveness. These arguments are, however, only partly correct.

---

[2] www.amazon.co.uk/More-Harm-than-Good-Complementary-ebook/dp/B078ZQXQNP/

As to the methodological problems, they mostly exist in some areas of ATs. Oral dietary supplements, including herbal remedies, for instance, can and should be tested much like conventional medicines, i.e. by conducting placebo-controlled RCTs. When it comes to other treatments, such as yoga, hypnotherapy or acupuncture, things can get more complex. What, for example, might be a reasonable placebo control for a trial of hypnotherapy? In some instances, this might mean that placebo controls and patient-blinding are simply impossible. However, this does not mean that RCTs comparing such ATs with standard care cannot be done.

In our experience, the biggest problem lies in the mindset of alternative therapists who often are reluctant to conduct rigorous tests of their interventions. Whether this sentiment originates from the fear that such tests might be negative or from a wider anti-scientific attitude seems irrelevant; the fact is that it represents an important obstacle to progress in this area.

Common Misunderstandings about Alternative Therapies

Because of the current popularity of ATs, it is tempting to assume that thousands of people cannot be mistaken in assuming that these treatments are effective. However, the appeal to belief, practice or popularity is a classic fallacy. Belief can be wrong, practice can be misguided and popularity is certainly not a reliable indicator for effectiveness. The history of medicine is littered with examples which demonstrate how misleading these fallacies can be.

If a menopausal woman enjoys an AT and subsequently feels better, what could be more logical than to assume that the treatment was the cause of her improvement? This conclusion seems obvious to patients and therapists alike – yet it is fallacious. Apart from the treatment per se, a whole range of factors can cause or at least contribute to a clinical improvement in that patient: the placebo effect, the natural history of menopause, the regression towards the mean, to mention just three. In other words, the patient can get better after administering ineffective or even mildly harmful remedies; and the word 'subsequently' has not the same meaning as 'consequently'. Causal inferences based on anecdotes are highly problematic and rarely a sound basis for robust conclusions about the effectiveness of ATs.

Enthusiasts of ATs claim that their treatments have stood the 'test of time' and that this test is more relevant than that of a clinical trial. A long tradition of use can, of course, be an *indicator* for the safety and efficacy of a treatment, but it can never be a *proof*. On the contrary, a long history might also mean that the origins of that therapy reach back to a time when our understanding of anatomy, physiology etc. was in its infancy. This, in turn, might lessen the chances for any such intervention to be plausible or effective.

An entire industry has developed around the notion that ATs are natural and therefore safe. The implication is that conventional treatments are unnatural, heavily based on chemicals which are potentially harmful. Nature, by contrast, is seen as benign and 'natural remedies' are therefore to be preferred. This argument is as effective for marketing purposes as it is wrong. Firstly, by no means are all ATs natural. For instance, there is nothing natural in sticking needles into a patient's body (as in acupuncture) or endlessly diluting and shaking a remedy (as in homeopathy). Secondly, nature is not necessarily benign. Even 'natural' herbal extracts are not necessarily safe – just think of hemlock!

Conclusions

Many women suffering from menopausal symptoms use ATs regularly. These women deserve reliable information about the effectiveness and the risks of ATs. Despite much advertising to the contrary, very few ATs have been shown to be effective and none are entirely free of risks. Researchers need to re-double their efforts in critically evaluating ATs for a whole range of climacteric symptoms with the aim of improving health and quality of life in this population.

References

1. Posadzki P, Lee MS, Moon TW, et al. Prevalence of complementary andalternative medicine (CAM) use by menopausal women: a systematic review of surveys. *Maturitas* 2013;75:34–43.

2. Ernst E, Hung SK. Great expectations: what do patients using complementary and alternative medicine hope for? *Patient* 2011;4:89–101.

3. Ernst E, Pittler MH, Wider B. *The Desktop Guide to Complementary and Alternative Medicine: An Evidence-Based Approach.* 2006. Mosby Elsevier.

4. Borrelli F, Ernst E. Alternative and complementary therapies for the menopause. *Maturitas* 2010;66:333–43.

5. Clement YN, Onakpoya I, Hung SK, Ernst E. Effects of herbal and dietary supplements on cognition in menopause: a systematic review. *Maturitas* 2011;68:256–63.

6. Whelan AM, Jurgens TM, Bowles SK. Natural health products in the prevention and treatment of osteoporosis: systematic review of randomized controlled trials. *Ann Pharmacother* 2006;40:836–49.

7. Zehnacker CH, Bemis-Dougherty A. Effect of weighted exercises on bone mineral density in post menopausal women: a systematic review. *Journal of Geriatric Physical Therapy* 2007;30 (2):79–88.

8. Williams AL, Cotter A, Sabina A, et al. The role for vitamin B-6 as treatment for depression: a systematic review. *Family Pract* 2005;22:532–7.

9. Kim MS, Lim HJ, Yang HJ, et al. Ginseng for managing menopause symptoms: a systematic review of randomized clinical trials. *J Ginseng Res* 2013;37:30–6.

10. Posadzki P, Alotaibi A, Ernst E. Adverse effects of homeopathy: a systematic review of published case reports and case series. *Int J Clin Pract* 2012;66:1178–88.

Menopause in Primary Care

Sarah Gray

The other chapters of this book cover the diagnosis and management of menopause-related problems, the science behind them and the risks and benefits of the various interventions available. 'Doing nothing' will result in the physiological and psychological sequelae of the loss of ovarian function.

How 'doing something' happens will vary according to the prevalent health system.

When a woman has recognized what is happening to her mind and body and decides that she wishes to discuss this further, she may then make an appointment with a recognized expert in the field of menopause. In most countries this will require personal resources or insurance.

If a recognized expert or the funding to see them is not available, general gynecology tends to be next line of approach. Dependent upon the training, updating, experience and approach of the individual clinician this may be entirely appropriate.

However, the holistic approach of primary care provides a very credible alternative. Menopause is often emotive and the emphasis on consultation skills within primary care in conjunction with experience of multisystem medical problems and risk assessment means that menopause sits well within this setting. The argument of this chapter is that managing the menopause should be an extended primary care role particularly in health systems where gynecology is primarily seen as surgical.

Primary care is the point of access for women with undifferentiated symptoms and to a variable degree according to the health system will assess, make a diagnosis and manage the problem presented. The cessation of reproductive function is universal and there is a strong case to be made that training should be available such that menopause is recognized, and initial support provided within the primary care sector wherever in the world that may be.

Role

The role of primary care within the field of menopause can be broken down as follows

1. To act as the first point of contact for a woman with symptoms that are affecting her and provide a diagnosis.
2. Once menopause has been recognized by the woman and her health care professional to provide
   a. Discussion, risk assessment and first-line management options.
   b. Onward referral to a clinician with greater expertise if necessary.

Diagnosis

Primary care sifts undifferentiated symptoms. Its strength is an ability to manage uncertainty but generally there is an attempt to understand what is happening. This may take several visits and often a symptom diary. A clear presentation may enable diagnosis at first consultation. As this book illustrates there are many symptoms that can arise as a result of the decline in ovarian function. Historically, trials of menopause treatments have been required to look at individual symptoms – usually numbers of flushes as their primary end point. There is more to menopause than flushing and this simple message needs to be promulgated both to clinicians and women.

When I teach menopause at is most basic to primary care clinicians, I talk about

1. Brain-mediated symptoms – such as temperature regulation, sleep regulation, mood, memory and ability to cope
2. 'Below the waist' symptoms – vaginal dryness, bladder irritability, sexual difficulty
3. Structural symptoms – joints, muscle, skin and energy

I emphasize that any one woman may have none, some or all, but if she has a variety of these and is in the 45–55 age group and there has been a change to her bleeding pattern, then menopause should be at the top of the list of differential diagnoses.

This may be simplistic, but a simplistic approach may be needed to move some colleagues on from the attitude of 'What do you expect at your age? Put up with it . . .' Recognition of menopause and an understanding of its impact may provide the answer the patient was looking for and may satisfy her.

Investigation

Menopause was stated by NICE [1] to be a clinical diagnosis. Holistic assessment is required, and this is the strength of primary care. The various symptoms and observations across a variety of body systems will build a picture rather like a jigsaw. It would be unlikely that a diagnosis made on the grounds of bleeding pattern, symptom profile and impact would be overturned by either blood tests or imaging and can be proposed at a first consultation. We should aim for the primary care clinician to have enough knowledge, along with an ability to listen and to integrate information, to be able to do this.

Investigation may have a role in evaluating risk. There are a variety of validated risk assessment tools and primary care will be particularly familiar with those looking at cardiovascular disease, fracture risk and may have experience in memory assessment, breast risk and others. Haematological and biochemical tests taken for other conditions may well be available and interpretation of these is an everyday activity. Access to imaging and more specialized investigation will vary with the health system but they are often available and can be appropriately selected either to enable the management decision in primary care or to assist the assessment of a more specialist clinician.

Communication

Communication skills are further strengths of the primary care clinician who has of necessity to understand what is being told to him/her and explain to the patient in language that they will comprehend. An explanation may be all that is needed.

Awareness of trustworthy information sources is important. Signposting can enable and empower the woman to research for herself. She may then come back to make decisions with a greater understanding of how the science and opinion applies to her.

Once decisions are made, a clear explanation of what to do, what to expect, what to worry about and how to seek help are all important both in the general context and for menopause. At least in the UK these are key elements of primary care training and when it occurs, clinical record assessment will look for evidence that this has taken place.

The overriding principle is that a different clinician seeing the patient should understand not just what has been decided but how and why this decision was made. This facilitates longitudinal care and that is essential for menopause, which may result in consultations over 20 years.

Training

To facilitate both diagnosis and communication the issue of knowledge should be focused on. Misinformation and misperception regrettably are still common. The fallout of the 'HRT scare' has been that menopause has been portrayed as natural and to be endured and that intervention is risky: 'hormones are dangerous'. Arguably, this has affected health care professionals to a greater extent than women. Textbooks have referenced the original papers and not the unravelling. Specific product characteristic (spc) licensing documents for registered pharmaceutical products are required to quote risks derived from these same original papers and not the subsequent evidence. Patient information leaflets are even more alarming. The non-specialist who is not up to date will perpetuate the myths and yet this is precisely the person who most needs to be informed as they will be asked by the patients for advice.

Somehow, there needs to be a grass-roots-up education program for clinicians at the point of first contact. This should start with recognition and diagnosis. An important feature of a good clinician is insight. This enables them to be able to recognize the limits of their own competence and seek help from others when they don't know. For many, their lack of knowledge strangles the application of insight, depriving their patients of information and opportunity.

If it is realized that menopause is an issue and it is impacting significantly on the patient's quality of life, but the primary care clinician is not sure what to do next, then onward referral to another with greater expertise should occur. If this stage fails, then there is a potential for misdiagnosis and even the risk of mistreatment. We can only guess at the number of women treated with antidepressants who are not truly depressed but present with sleep disturbance and mood change.

Risk Assessment

If a primary care clinician is prepared to discuss management options, then first a risk analysis is needed. This may itself lead on to referral if the patient is deemed too high a risk for the clinician to manage themselves. The following categories should be addressed looking for current problems and risk factors.

- Gynecology: menstrual history, contraceptive use both now and in the past, pregnancies, gynaecological intervention, family history

- Cardiovascular: current problems, previous events, family history (concentrating on first-degree family members affected below the age of 45 for venous events and 60 for arterial)
- Lifestyle profile: body mass index (BMI), tobacco and alcohol use, exercise, diet
- Metabolism: looking for issues which may affect cardiovascular risk, absorption and pharmacokinetics
- Breast: current problems, previous events, family history (concentrating on first- and second-degree family members affected below the age of 50)
- Bone: fracture risk assessment, e.g. FRAX (the World Health Organization Fracture Risk Assessment tool [2])
- Mental health: history including previous tolerance to hormone therapy plus impact of symptoms

An efficient clinical software system with summary, problem, medication and lifestyle sections can make this much simpler than it appears.

Consider the following scenario presented within primary care

---

Age 49

- Severe flushing – daytime and at night
- Sleep disturbance – getting to sleep but waking four to five times, then sweating
- Tired all the time – irritable, angry, readily tearful, anxious, lacking motivation and confidence
- Forgetful, struggling to concentrate
- Some urinary urgency and frequency
- Vaginal dryness such that sex is uncomfortable
- Sexual interest disappeared
- Aching all over but no joint changes
- Bled (minimally) three months ago, previous bleed six months before that, no true period for over a year

Desperate for help

This illustrates a typical perimenopausal bleeding pattern, a raft of very typical symptoms, and enables a clinical diagnosis to be made with confidence by anyone with a basic understanding of menopause – well within the skills of primary care.

The symptoms are impacting on the woman's ability to function and she is asking for help.

Risk profile review then comes into play. Here are three examples

---

Scenario 1

- BMI 24.3 BP 118/72
- Never smoked, minimal alcohol, exercises regularly
- No other medication
- No significant previous medical history
- No significant family history
- Contraception – vasectomy but has taken an ethinylestradiol/levonorgestrel combined contraceptive without problems in the past

Scenario 2

- BMI 32 BP controlled with medication at 132/80
- Smokes 10 per day, alcohol 32 units a week, walks but no vigorous exercise
- Type I diabetes – long- and short-acting insulin
- Hypothyroid – levothyroxine – 125 mcg/day
- Fatty liver – monitored
- Family – mother menopause at 42 and T1DM
- Two vaginal deliveries in twenties and no bleeding problems since
- Condoms for contraception

Scenario 3

- BMI 18.3 BP 118/72
- Never smoked, minimal alcohol, exercises regularly
- Mother diagnosed with breast cancer age 51 – still alive at 82 but very troubled with thoracic kyphosis and back pain attributed to vertebral collapse
- Always had very lumpy breasts, one screening mammogram reported as dense with negative fine needle aspirate
- Has a copper bearing-intra uterine device in situ

Scenario 1 is clearly the low-risk uncomplicated patient who could be offered a first-line cyclical HRT preparation by any clinician with very basic knowledge. Scenario 2 is medically complex but could be offered a cyclical HRT combination by an informed primary care clinician. The complexity is medical rather than endocrine and would fall more logically into a primary care rather than gynecology remit due to the experience with multisystem medical conditions. The proviso here is that the estrogen component should be delivered by a non-oral route and the choice of progestin for endometrial opposition should be carefully considered. Scenario 3 is that of a patient at higher risk of both breast disease and osteoporosis and it would be entirely reasonable for the risk assessment, counselling and negotiated management plan be performed in the more specialist setting due to the higher level of knowledge required.

Management

If the primary care clinician is prepared to offer management options then, firstly, they need to know what is available to them. Their choice of products may be restricted by licence in the country, reimbursement restrictions, formulary requirements, costs as well as production issues. They should have a basic understanding of the components of these products and how they are absorbed and delivered to the tissues.

From what is available, a clinician should pick a selection of suitable products to become familiar with. They should understand their similarities and differences to enable trouble-shooting and regime modification. National menopause societies and/or primary care organizations may be able to help with this.

An individualized management plan needs to be negotiated, agreed and then documented so that at any follow-up consultation it can be understood what has been done and why. Safety net advice should allow women to recognize significant problems and report appropriately but also to note unexpected but not worrying symptoms for discussion at review. Generally, review is recommended at 3 months after initiation or significant regimen change and annually once stable.

Annual review of all medication is recommended, and HRT can be integrated within this system.

Conclusion

The diagnosis of menopause should be viewed as a key function of primary care. Education and training should be integral to the medical curriculum for general practitioners (as is the case in the UK for the membership of the Royal College of General Practitioners [RCGP]). Emphasis and importance should be applied with effort made to ensure that this is put into practice and competency assessed. In health systems where office gynecology provides a first point of contact for matters relating to women's health, the same applies. With knowledge the clinician should be able to recognize their own limits of competence and be aware of who or where to refer patients for further risk assessment and management advice.

Primary care is a broad term, and non-medical professionals such as physician's assistants, pharmacists, nurses, physiotherapists, paramedics and others will increasingly be seeing women as the point of first contact and they too need appropriate education. Consider, in addition, support and administrative staff – receptionists, phlebotomists, call handlers – a system-wide sympathetic response to any initial enquiry is needed. Greater dissemination of information should enable them to respond appropriately.

The effort to disseminate knowledge is worth making. If you are reading this as an interested clinician, you will have been greeted by patients who say 'thank you so much, you have given me my life back'. This response provides professional satisfaction as well as indicating the degree of help for the patient. There are not many areas in medicine where so much can be achieved for so many with such minimal resource implications. We should aim for this to be a common experience in primary care where diagnosis and management of menopause sit well.

References

1. NICE NG23. Menopause: diagnosis and management. www.nice.org.uk/guidance/ng23

2. FRAX. www.sheffield.ac.uk/FRAX/

Index

.

Printed in the United States
by Baker & Taylor Publisher Services